Human Sexuality Across the Life Span

Implications for Nursing Practice

Human Sexuality Across the Life Span
Implications for Nursing Practice

Loretta P. Higgins, R.N., M.S.
Ph.D. candidate, Boston College
Associate Professor, Boston College

Joellen W. Hawkins, R.N.C., Ph.D., F.A.A.N.
Professor, Boston College

with

Ronna E. Krozy, R.N., M.S.
Ph.D. candidate, Health Education, Boston University
Associate Professor, Boston College

Roberta M. Orne, R.N., M.S.
Assistant Professor, University of Connecticut

Barbara Tuttle, A.C.S.W.
Director of Social Work, Rockville General Hospital
  Rockville, Connecticut
Sex Therapist in Private Practice

Queen E. Utley, R.N.C., M.S.
Family Nurse Practitioner, Nursing Wellness Center
  Mansfield, Connecticut

 Wadsworth Health Sciences Division
Monterey, California

Wadsworth Health Sciences Division
A Division of Wadsworth, Inc.

Printed in the United States of America
10 9 8 7 6 5 4 3 2 1

Library of Congress Cataloging in Publication Data

Higgins, Loretta Pierfedeici.
  Human sexuality across the life span.

  Bibliography: p.
  Includes index.
  1. Sex (Psychology) 2. Sex (Biology) 3. Life cycle,
Human. 4. Human reproduction. 5. Psychosexual disorders.
6. Sick — Psychology. 7. Nursing. I. Hawkins, Joellen
Watson. II. Title. [DNLM: 1. Sex behavior — Nurses'
instruction. 2. Sex disorders — Nursing. 3. Nursing
process. WY 150 H636h]
BF692.H54 1984   612'.6'024613   84-2379

ISBN 0-534-03225-7

Sponsoring Editor: James Keating
Production Services Coordinator: Marlene Thom
Production: Ron Newcomer & Associates,
          San Francisco, California
Manuscript Editor: Libby Pischel
Interior and Cover Design: Nancy Warner
Illustrations: Brown & Sullivan
Typesetting: Progressive Typographers, Inc.,
          Emigsville, Pennsylvania
Printing and Binding: R. R. Donnelley & Sons Co.,
          Crawfordsville, Indiana

To Lillian Beck Fuller, R.N.,
a pioneer in sex education.

Preface

Sexuality is as much a part of our lives as human beings as breathing, eating, and communicating. Our sexuality begins with birth, or even before, and ends with death. Acknowledging this, we have written this book using a developmental framework addressing sexuality across the life span.

Over the past few decades, nurses have been involved in the development of conceptual models for clinical practice. These models draw on numerous theories from the social and biological sciences. They reflect a holistic concept of the client, whereas the medical perspective is disease-oriented. Thus, the crisis model was chosen for the organizing framework for this book.

The Crisis Model for Nursing Practice

Crisis theory evolved out of the work of Erich Lindemann and Gerald Caplan. Their observations of individuals experiencing crisis as the result of either developmental and/or situational events and the coping patterns exhibited by those individuals led to the development of the constructs that constitute crisis theory. Erik Erikson, James S. Tyhurst, John and Elaine Cumming, and Karl Menninger also contributed to the crisis theory development. In 1970, Aquilera and Messick published the first edition of their book describing the application of crisis theory to nursing practice.

The crisis model emphasizes the potential for growth that crisis represents. It incorporates developmental-task theories, role theories, biological and social-systems theories (including family), body-image theories, psychoanalytic theories, stress theories, and the principle of rites of passage.

In the course of a human life, there occur events of a predictable (developmental) or unpredictable (situational) nature. *Developmental hazardous events* are normative, developmental milestones such as pregnancy, giving birth, or menopause. *Situational hazardous events* are most often unexpected, sudden, or accidental. Examples of the latter would be contracting a sexually transmitted disease, loss of a relationship, or discovery of a breast lump.

Whether predictable or unexpected, a hazardous event may be perceived as a threat, loss, or challenge to equilibrium and sexual integrity; the effect can be real or potential. The effects of hazardous events and the impact of the insults (resulting from the hazardous event) are influenced by a number of biopsycho-social factors. Among them are client perceptions and knowledge, health and developmental status and potential for growth, age, cultural values, anticipatory planning, biophysical protective mechanisms, previous problem-solving mechanisms, and resource repertoire.

While hazardous events and somatic insults may or may not produce disequilibrium, they will most likely require new problem-solving abilities and adaptation. Thus, in clients experiencing these changes, there is potentially increased vulnerability to crisis.

Nursing's overall goal in pre-crisis intervention is to help individuals and/or families to avoid crisis through disease prevention and health promotion. Utilizing the conceptual framework of the crisis theory model for professional practice, the nurse is well equipped to:

- assess perceptions of real or potential hazardous events, effects of body insult, and developmental stage.
- identify client/family problems, strengths, and needs.
- solve problems with clients/families and plan strategies to counter the negative effects of the insult and gain new knowledge, insight, and/or skills.
- intervene by assisting clients/families to maximize existing internal and external resources, mobilize those needed to reach realistic solutions, and reduce the hazard or restore equilibrium.
- evaluate the process, outcomes, and need for revision in assessment, planning, or intervention.

This approach to professional practice has a client-centered, rather than the more traditional problem-centered, focus. The nurse assumes the role of client health advocate and encourages active client/family participation. There are several problems the nurse commonly encounters in this role. Clients whose value system or cultural background differs from that of the nurse may choose solutions that conflict with those viewed as "more appropriate" by the provider. Other clients may choose to abdicate an active role in problem-solving altogether and prefer to be passive recipients of the nurse's plans.

When crisis occurs, nursing interventions are directed toward mobilization of additional internal and external resources and reduction of the stimulus (if possible). When the individual/family reaches post-crisis, nursing interventions focus on support measures aimed at healthy resolution or convalescence, enhancement of generativity, and promotion of the growth potential of the crisis. Measures to reverse or lessen breakdown, maladaptation, and chronicity and to promote rehabilitation are emphasized. If the process triggered by the developmental and/or situational event is not reversible, nursing interventions are aimed toward attainment of maximum possible level of wellness or support for a dignified end to life (see Crisis Theory Model on page x).

Organization and Features of This Book

This book is organized to view sexual development across the life span. The chapters are designed to look at groups of developmental and/or situational events. Whereas it may be argued that all events have the potential for crisis, the topics in the last three chapters are chosen for their importance to sexuality for the individual.

The book begins with a perspective of sexuality and sexual development from conception to old age. The focus then narrows to examine specific risks and issues for sexuality related to developmental and situational life events such as pregnancy, menopause, chronic disease, sexual assault, and exploitation. Included is a lengthy discussion of the role of the nurse in performing a sexual assessment as part of giving care. Ethical and moral issues in sexuality are also examined as they relate to the nurse's role as a health-care professional. Illustrations, charts, and tables are included to enhance the text and make it useful for immediate clinical application. It has many practical features: a communication aid, a guide for conducting a sexual health history as part of health assessment, a self-assessment tool to be used by clients, and guides for prevention of assault, teaching breast self-exam, and testicular self-exam. The appendices provide information about sexually transmitted diseases, contraceptive methods, abortion, and audiovisual aids.

The book is designed as a guide for nurses in their roles as providers of health care. It is intended to be informative, provocative, consciousness-raising, and perhaps even controversial. All of the authors are engaged in clinical practice with clients who are dealing in some way with issues of sexuality. This book is an attempt to share some feelings and experiences as health-care professionals and as sexual human beings. If it succeeds in touching you on at least one of those levels, it has achieved its purpose.

Acknowledgments

We are grateful to our clients for all they have taught us and to our students, colleagues, and friends for what they have added to this book.

To our families and those close to us, we are grateful for the unwavering support and tolerance of our need for time to write.

A special thank you to our typist, Janice Bittner, who is capable, patient, and supportive in a special way.

Mary Pat Fisher deserves our special and warmest praise for a marvelous job of developmental editing.

To Ed Murphy and Jim Keating, thank you for supporting this project and for patience in seeing it through.

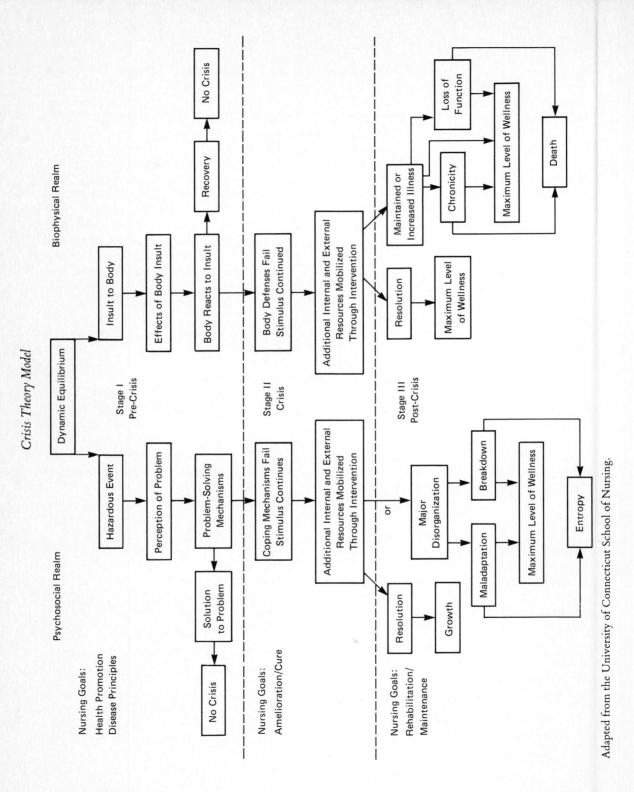

Crisis Theory Model

Biophysical Realm

Psychosocial Realm

Nursing Goals:
Health Promotion
Disease Principles

Nursing Goals:
Amelioration/Cure

Nursing Goals:
Rehabilitation/
Maintenance

Stage I
Pre-Crisis

Stage II
Crisis

Stage III
Post-Crisis

Dynamic Equilibrium

Insult to Body — Effects of Body Insult — Body Reacts to Insult — Recovery — No Crisis

Body Defenses Fail Stimulus Continued — Additional Internal and External Resources Mobilized Through Intervention

Resolution — Maximum Level of Wellness

Maintained or Increased Illness — Loss of Function — Maximum Level of Wellness — Death

Chronicity — Maximum Level of Wellness

Hazardous Event — Perception of Problem — Problem-Solving Mechanisms — Solution to Problem — No Crisis

Coping Mechanisms Fail Stimulus Continues — Additional Internal and External Resources Mobilized Through Intervention

Resolution — Growth

or

Major Disorganization — Breakdown — Maximum Level of Wellness

Maladaptation — Maximum Level of Wellness — Entropy

Adapted from the University of Connecticut School of Nursing.

Contents

8.

Human Sexuality and Nursing
Interventions: Post-Crisis   231

Joellen W. Hawkins

Appendices

Introduction

Understanding Sexuality
    Social Shaping of Sexuality
    Early Psychological Theories
    Recent Sex Research

Sexual Differentiation of the Embryo and Fetus

Development of Sexual Identity in the Child
    Biological Sex
    Gender Identity
    Social Sex-Role
    Sexual Orientation

Sexuality in Infancy

Sexuality in Early Childhood

Later Childhood Years

Sex Education

Adolescence
    Becoming a Physically Mature Female
        Adult female sexual anatomy
        Menstruation
        The process of pubertal development
    Becoming a Physically Mature Male
        Adult male sexual anatomy
        Hormonal patterns
        The process of pubertal development
    Adolescent Sexuality
        Motives for sex
        Decision-making
    Pregnancy
        The absence of contraception
        Risks of teenage pregnancy
        Teenagers as parents
        Assistance in teenage pregnancies

Summary of Implications for Nursing Practice

CHAPTER 1

Development of a Sexual Being: Growing Up Female; Growing Up Male

Loretta P. Higgins with Barbara Tuttle

Introduction

Human sexuality is a maze of biological, social, and psychological factors. To begin to unravel this maze, this chapter will present a brief overview of general aspects of sexuality and then look in greater detail at the course of its early development, from the sex cell through adolescence. Included are concepts of anatomy and physiology, sexual curiosity, the development of persons as sexual beings, the metamorphosis of puberty, and taking responsibility for one's sexuality. The role of the nurse is interwoven with this discussion, emphasizing teaching, counseling, and support, primarily in a community setting. The focus of the chapter is normal growth and development, but aberrations are included as appropriate.

Understanding Sexuality

Widespread attempts to understand sexuality have focused on how it is variously shaped by the society in which one lives, on psychological theories of what our sexuality means to us as individuals, or on measurable sexual behaviors and physiological responses.

Social Shaping of Sexuality

Throughout history, few areas of life have been as surrounded with secrecy, mythology, prohibitions, and misinformation as human sexual functioning. Rituals to ensure fertility have been a common part of many ancient and modern religions or ceremonial customs; even today, we throw rice at weddings as a blessing for a fruitful union. Tribal ceremonies introducing young adolescents to the customs and expectations of adult sexual roles have frequently been cloaked in secrecy and myth. In many societies, choosing a permanent sexual partner has been considered too important a decision for the individuals involved, and such choices have been relegated to the mandates of age-old customs.

The reasons for so much emphasis on controlling sexual functioning are mainly fourfold: the human race depends on sexual drives and reproduction for its continuity; second, sexual responses may involve strong emotions involving self and others in an intimate relationship; third, sexual interactions affect the establishment and preservation of a family unit that involves property rights as well as security and psychological growth for its members; and, fourth, the area of human sexuality has maintained its ability to induce fear, largely due to a lack of knowledge about reproduction and sexual functioning. Such powerful and mysterious forces as sexual attraction and the resulting sexual behaviors have been considered in need of authoritative controls. These controls have been communal (church, state, and family) and personal, and, until recently, the resultant taboos prevented a scientific approach to the study of sexuality.

On closer examination of social dictates of sexual behavior, one may find a vast range of "correct" attitudes and behaviors that have been considered absolute. For example, in the comparison of four tribal societies, Mead (1949) found that differences in sexual roles and behaviors were sometimes greater between societies than between males and females in the same society. Among the Arapesh, a tribe found in New Guinea, both sexes were taught to use their whole bodies in order to procreate. Both mothers and fathers played an overall protective role with their children. In fact, the father did not work after the birth of a child but slept beside the mother (Mead

1949, 86–87). Among the Manus of the Admiralty Islands, women's and men's roles were very similar: both were active participants in religious and economic activities (Mead 1949, 92).

From the earliest lessons of childhood through the behaviors of old age, these societies shaped the expectations and feelings of their members about their own bodies, sexual pleasure, tenderness toward sexual partners, and the ages and conditions under which sexual contact was allowed (see Figures 1-1 and 1-2).

In both tribal and Western societies, beliefs

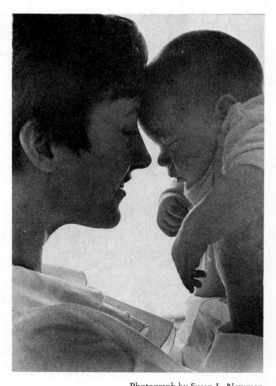

Photograph by Susan L. Newman.

FIGURE 1-1
Sexual roles and customs pervade all of our lives from birth . . .

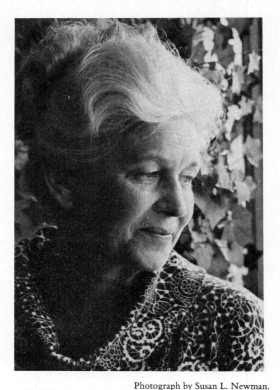

FIGURE 1-2
. . . to our later years.

Photograph by Susan L. Newman.

about male-female sexual differences help shape the roles expected of men and women. However, in the more complex societies, such as North American culture, communications of "proper" attitudes toward sexual behaviors and feelings are not as standardized as in tribal societies. Hence, it may be more difficult in a complex industrialized society for males or females to feel the reassurance of cultural approval for their own sexual behaviors, feelings, and roles. The rapidly changing demands of family, workplace, and economy also exert pressure from society on traditional sexual roles; the resulting role changes affect

sexual behaviors and feelings. As Mead (1949) pointed out, in North American culture it is possible for a person to choose a partner from millions of possibilities, each with a different set of expectations. A generation after this observation, there are few social mechanisms to help a person choose a sexual partner or to reinforce a choice once made, and even fewer guidelines to indicate "normalcy" in sexual matters.

The legal system in the United States has tried to enforce certain views of normalcy in both sexual behavior and sex roles. However, different standards for males and females have been legally enforced. For example, there have been different penalties for prostitutes and their clients, separate definitions of and punishment for adultery by women and fornication by men, and an absence of laws protecting men from rape by women. Ideas about normalcy have also been apparent in the prevalence, until recently, of laws forbidding certain sexual behaviors or the choice of a same-sex partner, and in the reluctance of lawmakers and the judicial system to deal with sexual abuse in and out of the family (including marital rape) in the same fashion as any other physical assault.

Laws regarding sexual behavior generally fall into three major categories: those dealing with sexual offenders and deviates; rights to life, property, and privacy; and access to materials considered erotic or pornographic. Sadoff (1975) defines sexual offenders as those having committed crimes involving sexual behaviors, such as rape or child molestation. He defines sexual deviates as persons engaging in illegal but noncriminal behaviors, such as homosexuality. (It seems incredible that in 1975, when Sadoff was writing, homosexuality — an issue of personal choice — was still illegal in 49 states, and that in 1983, individuals who identify themselves as homosexuals are still struggling with both legal and cultural discrimination.)

Sex-related laws regulating the rights to life, to property, and to privacy control issues such as abortion, contraception, sterilization, illegitimacy, marriage, and divorce. In addition, there are now debates about regulating artificial insemination, surrogate childbearing, and test-tube conception. Recent court cases involving "palimony" demonstrate how attitudes have changed in the face of traditional societal values that still espouse premarital virginity and different expectations about male and female sexual needs, desires, feelings, and behaviors.

Society has also struggled with the issue of defining pornography and obscenity and with regulating access to materials designed to be erotically stimulating. Lipton (1975) notes that rapidly changing social standards are making these issues even more difficult; nevertheless, the Presidential Commission on Obscenity and Pornography, which was appointed in the late 1960s, recommended repealing laws forbidding the sale, exhibition, or distribution of explicit materials to consenting adults. Recent debates have focused on separating violent behaviors from sexual behaviors in considering what is really obscene.

Religious institutions have also endorsed particular views of "normalcy" and therefore of morality in sexual behavior and sex roles. Franzblau (1975) notes that the Judeo-Christian religions stress that the sanctity of marriage and the family are essential if a moral universe is to be created. However, differing views on such issues as marital sex roles, abortion, birth control, and homosexuality indicate wide diversity in the ways in which religious groups try to determine their own value systems.

The electronic, film, and printed media have attempted to fill the needs people have for reassurance and information in modern western cultures, which lack the strict proscriptions and requirements of smaller, closed societies. But rather than clarifying sexuality for the public, much of what is presented in our society only adds to the confusion. Although primitive cultures accepted mythical explanations for sexual functioning, their members were afforded a security based on the knowledge that certain attitudes and approaches to sexuality were proper and had no acceptable alternatives. In our culture today, we need widely disseminated, accurate information about both sexual functioning and behavior if we are to exorcise harmful myths and encourage healthier attitudes and confidence about these important areas of human life. Indeed, as we cross the barriers to knowledge about human sexual physiology and behavior, we can make more information available that, as in every other area of our human functioning, will enable us to fulfill our own potential as healthy human beings.

Early Psychological Theories

Until recently, although much of the reproductive anatomy was understood, sexual physiology was essentially unexplored territory to scientists. The field of psychology, however, was already testing the frontiers of the unconscious mind, including motivation and psychopathology. The lack of knowledge about physiology allowed the development of psychological theories in the area of sexual behavior that are very controversial today.

For example, Brecher (1969, 1975) focused on three different yet influential views of sexual behaviors held by three theorists born in the mid-1800s: Krafft-Ebing, Freud, and Ellis. Krafft-Ebing (1840–1902) was a forensic psychiatrist whose exposure to violent crimes involving pathological sexual behaviors led him to define sexual behavior as a "collection of loathsome diseases." His book, *Psychopathia Sexualis*, which became popular in many countries, declared his view that sex was normal only during marriage for procreation and that only men should have orgasms; any deviations from the pattern were perversions.

Thus, he grouped rapists, torturers, and murderers with homosexuals and implied that even foreplay could be a prelude to lust murders. He showed masturbation to be a factor in the development of all deviations (see Figure 1-3), saying that it would cause one to "sink into dementia, or become subject to severe degenerative neuroses and psychoses." Brecher (1975) noted that two new editions of Krafft-Ebing's work were published as re-

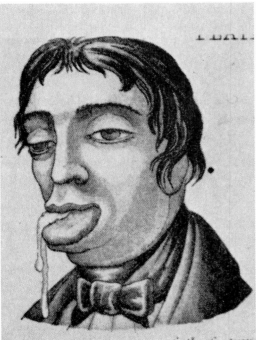

FIGURE 1-3
Association between sex (masturbation) and dementia is graphically depicted in an 1853 drawing.

SOURCE: From *Sexual Choices,* 2nd ed., by G. D. Nass, R. W. Libby, and M. P. Fisher. Copyright © 1984, 1981 by Wadsworth, Inc. Reprinted by permission of the publisher, Wadsworth Health Sciences, Monterey, California.

cently as 1965 and are still used as references by some physicians.

Freud (1856–1939), in comparison, felt that variation from what he considered normal sexual behavior was an indication of pathology or arrested development. For example, in *Three Essays of Sexuality* (1905), Freud declared that the shifting of the locus of excitement and orgasmic release in females from the clitoris to the vagina was a sign of emotional maturity and health. He considered libido to be masculine in nature, whether the source or object was male or female. Thus, females were supposed to repress their libido at puberty, while males were experiencing an increase in sexual drive. The females' repression supposedly converted their childish masculine focus on the clitoris to femininity via focus on the vagina; however, Freud stated that the necessary repression made females more prone to neurosis and hysteria. One wonders how many women suffered the label of "neurotic" and underwent years of psychoanalysis to change from "clitoral" to "vaginal" orgasms.

Freud also posited a "castration complex" in boys, "penis envy" in girls, and a competition with the same-sex parent that was repressed due to either fear of castration or presumption of previous castration in boys and girls from 3 to 5 years of age. He proposed that the "latency" period that followed (from ages 6 to 11) was characterized by a lack of interest in sexual matters due to the repression brought on during the earlier "Oedipus/Electra" period. Recent research raises doubts about these theories. Goldman and Goldman (1982) surveyed children in Australia, Sweden, North America, and England to assess their understanding of sexual differences between boys and girls, conception and childbirth, and genetic determination of sex. They found that children from ages 5 to 15 were not uninterested in sex but rather had an interest that increased with age during those years. They also found that English-speaking children of ages 7 to 9 were still unaware of genital differences indicating gender differences; this lack of opposite sex genital knowledge contrasts with Freud's theories of castration fears resulting in adult hostility between the sexes.

According to Brecher (1975), a third opinion of the meaning of sexual behavior was apparent in the works of Havelock Ellis (1859–1939). Ellis was tolerant of both masturbation and homosexuality, and felt that sexual behaviors were only the business of consenting adults in private.

Recent Sex Research

Another approach to understanding sex is to study it scientifically, through the quantifications of behaviors and measurements of physiological responses.

Alfred Kinsey and his colleagues are usually considered the pioneers of sex research in modern times. Beginning in the 1930s, these researchers collected case histories on 5300 white males and 5940 white females. The investigation grew out of Kinsey's experiences as a college professor and the questions his students had concerning aspects of human sexuality. Unlike the work of Freud and Ellis, the sample for the work of Kinsey and his co-workers came from groups of healthy individuals in the general population.

Earlier research on samples of the general population included the Russian survey from the early part of the 20th century and case histories by Katherine Davis, Hamilton, Dickinson, Terman, and Landis, all done in the 1920s and 1930s. Each of these studies employed case history and interviewing techniques (Kinsey, Pomeroy, and Martin 1953, 6).

Masters and Johnson conducted their initial research on a population of adult men and women willing to serve as subjects. The researchers made observations of anatomic and physiologic response to effective sexual stimulation and recorded these responses (Masters and Johnson 1966, 9). Masters and Johnson began their investigation by taking sexual, occupational, and medical histories of a group of subjects and then selected a smaller group for the anatomic and physiologic study (1966, 10).

Several large-scale surveys of sexual behaviors, practices, and attitudes have been conducted in recent years. These include Hite's questionnaire based on studies of female (1976) and male (1982) sexuality, and the study by Tavris and Sadd of women's sexuality from a questionnaire published in *Redbook* magazine (1977). Friday has published reports of the sexual fantasies of men and women collected through interviews and personal accounts sent to her (1973, 1975, 1980). The most recent of the survey studies is that of *Playboy* (The Playboy Readers 1983).

Instead of concentrating on general theories or specific measurements of sexuality or the hypothesized effects of societies' attempts to control sexual behavior, many sex researchers now study sex from a more detailed developmental perspective: what happens when in a person's life, and what factors contribute to the observed patterns? What has been learned to date begins with the period before birth, when the biological distinctions and similarities between males and females first appear.

Sexual Differentiation of the Embryo and Fetus

An individual's genetic sex is determined at the moment of conception. The fact that the sperm determines the sex of the child is a relatively recent discovery. The fundamentals of conception had previously been explained in various ways. Some societies believed that the female contained the whole human being and needed no help from the male. Others believed that the sperm contained the whole person and the female was merely the incubator. After it was generally understood that both the male and the female played equal roles in the genesis of life, there was still a misunderstanding about how the child's sex was determined. Fortunately, our knowledge of the process of fertilization is "light-years" beyond the early mystical beliefs, and many facts are finally known.

The sex cells (*sperm* and *ova*), or *gametes,* of human beings contain 23 chromosomes each, half the number found in other body cells. When fertilization occurs, the *zygote* resulting from the fusion of the egg and sperm contains 46 chromosomes. In addition to the 22 chromosomes called *autosomes,* the sex cells contain a *sex chromosome.* The ovum contains an X chromosome; the sperm contains either an X or Y. If an X sperm (or *gynosperm*) fertilizes the egg, a female is conceived. If a Y sperm (or *androsperm*) fertilizes the egg, a male is conceived. A female has 22 pairs of autosomes and two sex chromosomes, XX. A male also has 22 pairs of autosomes, but his sex chromosomes are XY.

Researchers have observed some differences between the sex chromosomes. The androsperm is smaller and faster than the gynosperm and prefers a mildly alkaline environment. The larger and slower gynosperm has a longer life span and prefers an acidic environment. This knowledge has prompted much speculation about the ability of couples to determine the sex of their child by following some rules for intercourse, such as precise timing around ovulation or using an acidic douche before intercourse if a baby girl is preferred (Prenatal Sex Determination 1975). The effectiveness of these precedures is highly questionable at the present time ("Waiting for a Male" 1979).

During the first six weeks of embryological life, there is no anatomical distinction between the male and female. The first gender differentiation occurs at about six weeks when, in an embryo with a Y chromosome, the testes develop. By the eighth week, it is possible to distinguish gender visually. By the ninth week the testicles begin to function. If these embryonic gonads are removed before other male sex structures begin to develop, the embryo will become a biological female even in the presence of the Y chromosome.

The presence of circulating *androgens* (male hormones) influences the development of the external genital structures, which are the structures leading to sex assignment at birth. See Figure 1-4 for an illustration of this process. *Testosterone* is the major androgen in the male fetus. The testosterone secreted by the developing testes is believed to be responsible for the division of the mesonephric (Wolffian) ducts into the ducts of the epididymis, the vas deferens, the seminal vesicle, and the common ejaculatory duct. The paramesonephric (Müllerian) duct degenerates in the male due to a secretion of the testicles. The skin folds become the urethra and foreskin and the outer swellings become the scrotum after fusing in the middle.

If any one of the many steps in the synthesis of testosterone is omitted, the external genitals may be ambiguous. For example, if enough testosterone is produced for the development of the external genitals but then such secretion ceases, for whatever reason, a child would be born with normal male external genitalia but no testicles (Lippe 1979, 96).

Normally, the testicles begin their migration from inside the body to the scrotum during the seventh month of gestation. Each testis takes along its vas deferens, vessels, and nerves (Allan 1969, 179). The condition resulting from failure of the testicles to descend is called *cryptorchidism.*

If the chromosomal structure of the embryo is XX (female), the ovaries begin to

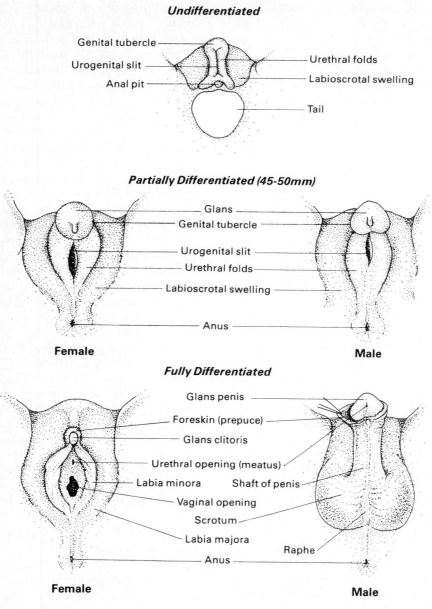

Undifferentiated

Genital tubercle
Urogenital slit
Anal pit

Urethral folds
Labioscrotal swelling
Tail

Partially Differentiated (45-50mm)

Glans
Genital tubercle
Urogenital slit
Urethral folds
Labioscrotal swelling
Anus

Female   **Male**

Fully Differentiated

Glans penis
Foreskin (prepuce)
Glans clitoris
Urethral opening (meatus)
Labia minora   Shaft of penis
Vaginal opening
Scrotum
Labia majora
Raphe
Anus

Female   **Male**

FIGURE 1-4
Development and differentiation of male and female external genitals.

SOURCE: From *Sexual Choices,* 2nd ed., by G. D. Nass, R. W. Libby, and M. P. Fisher. Copyright © 1984, 1981 by Wadsworth, Inc. Reprinted by permission of the publisher, Wadsworth Health Sciences, Monterey, California.

develop at about the 12th week (Money and Ehrhardt 1972, 5). The mesonephric ducts degenerate, while the paramesonephric ducts develop into the female genital tract. The structure homologous to the penis in the male becomes the clitoris in the female. The labia majora and vestibule in the female are homologous to the scrotum in the male.

Development of Sexual Identity in the Child

Sexual identity is a complicated term that is best understood broken down into four components: biological sex, gender identity, social sex-role, and sexual orientation. All are different aspects of female-male distinctions.

Common use of the term *opposite sex* in our culture implies that there is a polarity between the two sexes. The obvious difference between the sexes lies in the differing reproductive capacity of each. The less distinct difference involves the influence of the female hormones (estrogens and progestins) and the male hormones (androgens) on behavior. Even though our knowledge has many gaps, it seems clear that there are probably more behavioral and physical differences between individual members of the same sex than there are between the two sexes in general. The argument of "nurture versus nature" has given way to an almost universal understanding that there is an interaction between genetics and environment. The argument regarding sexual differences and their origin, however, is in full swing, with studies and opinions found in increasing numbers in professional and lay books and magazines.

Biological Sex

The first component of sexual identity is *biological sex,* which includes genetic determina-

tion and sexual organs. These aspects of sexual identity are determined at conception. As described earlier, female and male sexual organs are physically differentiated during fetal life under the influence of differing chromosomal patterns and hormonal secretions.

Occasionally, however, chromosomal and hormonal influences create a combination of male and female characteristics, or *hermaphroditism.* A "true" hermaphrodite possesses both testes and ovaries, or at least gonadal tissue of both sexes. For example, deprivation of androgen in a genetically male fetus results in regression of the Müllerian system and lack of development of the Wolffian system, resulting in male hermaphroditism (the gonads are testes but the external genitalia are either ambiguous or female in appearance). A female embryo exposed in utero to excess androgen develops masculinized external genitalia. Usually this is the result of a malfunctioning adrenal cortex or a side effect of synthetic progestin given to the mother to prevent miscarriage. The individual whose gonads are ovaries but external genitalia are ambiguous or male is called a female hermaphrodite. *Androgenital syndrome* is the term used for masculinization of the female due to the presence of excess androgens in the embryonic environment (McCary and McCary 1982, 45).

Gender Identity

The second component of sexual identity, *gender identity,* is the child's conviction or understanding of her or his sex. It is generally agreed that the important period of time for the development of gender identity is from 18 months (onset of language acquisition) to 3 or 4 years (Money and Ehrhardt 1972, 16). The development of this identity occurs as the child identifies with members of the same sex. The essence of a positive gender identity is a feeling of pride in one's own genitals and a knowledge that sex differences are primarily defined by the reproductive capacity of the sex organs (Money and Ehrhardt 1972, 14). Thus, it matters little if mother is a truck driver and father stays home and paints if each parent is a secure and proud member of her or his own sex.

Although gender identity usually develops by age 4, Money and Ehrhardt (1972) stress that this is not due to any single cause but rather is a result of the interaction between many factors and conditions that continue throughout life. Some of these are chromosomal makeup, the effect of hormones on the genitals and on the brain, cues from one's own body and from others' behavior (sex assignment), and one's own experiences and feelings. These all combine to produce the concept each person has of his or her own "maleness" or "femaleness" and to create the feelings and beliefs each person holds about having that particular gender identity.

On occasion a child is born whose genital anatomy does not clearly identify its sex. For example, an enlarged clitoris is at first thought to be a penis or a small penis may be mistaken for a clitoris. When an error is made in the announcement of sex and it is discovered and corrected in the neonatal period, a *sexual reannouncement* has occurred. If a child is older when the decision is made, it is called a *sex reassignment.* Since the sense of gender identity begins at about 18 months of age, this age is considered to be the latest that sex reassignment should occur. One of the most dramatic cases reported in the literature is that of a male twin who was the victim of a circumcision accident that destroyed his penis. He was reassigned as a girl. Even though her genotype is XY, her gender identity is female (Money 1977, 32). Despite the potential psychological trauma of sex reassignment for both the child and its parents, Money (1977, 27 and 33) points out that because our society "maximizes sex differences, it is easier for a sex reassignment to be accepted than for a person

to develop a personal identity without being male or female."

Social Sex-Role

The third aspect of sexual identity is *social sex-role* (the way one is expected to behave because of one's sex). This is largely determined by the culture in which one lives and is initially assimilated by the individual during the ages of 3 to 7 years (DeCecco and Shively 1977, 83).

Differing expectations of each sex begin even earlier. For nine months of pregnancy (unless an amniocentesis is done), there is much speculation about the sex of the child. In the delivery room interest in the sex of the newborn ranks almost equally with concern about the infant's well-being. A name for the baby is chosen on the basis of sex, as are the colors he or she will wear. This attitude is accurately described by Money and Ehrhardt (1972, 12):

> Dimorphism [the occurrence of two distinct forms—male and female] of response or the basis of the shape of the sex organ is one of the most universal and pervasive aspects of human social interaction. It is so engrained and habitual in most people that they lose awareness of themselves as shapers of a child's gender-dimorphic behavior, and take for granted their own behavior as a no-option reaction to the signals of their child's behavior which they assume to have been preordained by some eternal verity to be gender-dimorphic.

Rodgers (1975) describes a girl's early childhood years as a "honeymoon" period. Because girls have greater skills in the verbal, perceptual, and cognitive areas than boys, they please adults more than boys do. Therefore, at an early age girls become dependent on adult approval, whereas boys, who are more likely to be scolded, learn independence earlier. "The childish ways that a little boy is pressured to give up are precisely those behaviors usually identified as feminine" (Rodgers 1975, 1657).

At the same time that girls are awarded for being pleasing as children, Horney believed that girls develop a sense of inferiority due to society's expectations. As examples, she cites ". . . preference for boys in many families, the restriction of woman's activity, male monopoly of the professions, and the like" (Moulton 1975, 213).

Whether such behaviors stereotypically associated with "femaleness" and "maleness" are innate, learned, or both is difficult to determine. Fagot (1982) discusses the many problems in the study of sex-role development: the variables are numerous, rating scales that work with one age group may not work with another age group, and social class influences test-taking abilities. However, research has revealed that both behavioral and cognitive explanations should be sought for the development of sex role. It is also generally understood that one's life is constrained by the boundaries of society. In addition, the work of developmental psychologists is beginning to influence the work of sex-role researchers.

Another important avenue to understanding the basis and nature of sex roles is anthropology. In the societies that have been studied there has always been assignment of roles on the basis of sex. Upon closer perusal, one notices that the role divisions are not universal. In some societies women are considered too weak to work outdoors; in others women are considered the appropriate ones to bear heavy burdens. Mead (1950) also observed that regardless of the type of work men do in any given society, that work is considered to be important. Work that women perform, regardless of the type, is seen as less important.

Our knowledge of sex role development is still in its infancy. It is an issue of considerable emotional import and great controversy. The story of X, a work of fiction which describes nonsexist child-rearing, stands in contrast to those who believe that sex roles are biologically determined (Gould 1980).

Given the plethora of conflicting opinions of experts, it is no wonder that parents and caregivers alike become confused about child-rearing. However, as gender stereotypes blur, there is increasing interest in the concept of *androgyny*. The word originates from a uniting of male (andro) and female (gyno). Although the 1960s and 1970s were characterized by expressions of androgyny in the sense that some hairstyles and clothing were indistinguishable by sex, a wider meaning is more appropriate. Androgyny can mean a blending of traditional sex roles to free individuals from the limitations imposed by stereotypes (Nass, Libby, and Fisher 1981, 13–14).

Sexual Orientation

The fourth aspect of sexual identity — *sexual orientation* — is one's physical and emotional preference for other individuals (DeCecco and Shively 1977, 83). There is some controversy concerning when sexual orientation becomes established. It is possible for a person to be physically attracted to one sex while having feelings of love for the other sex.

The subject of sexual orientation attained legitimacy as a research focus in the works of Kinsey and his fellow researchers (1948, 1953) when they conducted the first extensive surveys of male and female sexual behaviors. The Kinsey group stressed an important and constructive definition of sexual orientation; they stated that homosexuality, heterosexuality, and autoerotic sexuality were defined by the source from which one received erotic stimulation, rather than by a fixed, immutable self-identity (1953). This definition, plus their development of a behavior scale ranging from total orientation to same-sex stimulation (6), through bisexuality (3), to total orientation to the other sex for stimulation (0) marked a turning point in the consideration of same-sex behaviors (1948).

The reasons given for homosexual orientation have changed over the years (Marmor 1975). The Greeks believed in organic bisexuality due to the undifferentiated nature of the early fetus. In the 19th century, Krafft-Ebing popularized the notion that a degenerative disease of the nervous system caused homosexuality (1922). Freud (1905) thought it was due to arrested development or regression to a previous homoerotic stage; he felt that psychic bisexuality existed in all persons. Later researchers attributed the causes to chromosomal abnormalities, lower hormonal levels, or parental influences. None of these theories based on the negative assumption that homosexuality is an aberrant pattern has proved conclusive.

Mead (1950), Money and Ehrhardt (1972), Bell and Weinberg (1978), and Masters and Johnson (1979) have attempted to explain how males and females express same-sex attraction and have tried to compare the course of such relationships to heterosexual relationships. Recently, Bell (1982) stated that hormonal events in utero, combined with sex-role conformity or nonconformity in childhood, may predispose a person to a homosexual or a heterosexual orientation.

Bell has also suggested another reason for same-sex attraction. He states that it is the age at which romantic attachments first occur (an age that varies among individuals) rather than the incidence of homosexual behaviors that appears to be linked with homosexuality in adulthood. That is, if one experiences oneself as "different" from one's own sex at the age at which one first experiences romantic attachments, one's own sex will not be "finished business" but will rather be a source of fascination or attraction, while persons close to their same-sex peers will find them to be unsuitable as romantic objects and will yearn for the other sex as "different" from themselves.

Storms and Wasserman (1982) have advanced the theory that it is the age of sexual maturation that is the important variable. Onset during a stage of close peer bonding might lead to the use of same-sex cues in developing an erotic fantasy system. These markedly differing viewpoints, themselves so very different from earlier theories, indicate the difficulties sexologists face in trying to understand the complexities of sexual orientation.

Sexuality in Infancy

The infant is a sensual human being whose gratifications come from feeding, warmth, closeness, and caressing. The infant whose needs are met tends to develop a high level of self-esteem and a feeling of security. During the first year of life babies find pleasure in sucking, touching soft blankets, twirling their hair, or favoring a certain soft toy. By the end of the first year, as part of learning about their bodies, infants discover their genitals (Kneeman 1965, 249). Random genital play may occur just as babies play with their hands and feet. The randomness of genital play is characteristic of infancy (Martinson 1977, 75) (see Figure 1-5).

Some parents, even at this early stage of their child's development, may feel uncomfortable with their infant's genital manipulation. Alert and sensitive caregivers will realize that the education of parents about this aspect of their child's development may start the family on a healthier psychosexual course. Children are very adept at picking up nonverbal cues from their parents. If parents are

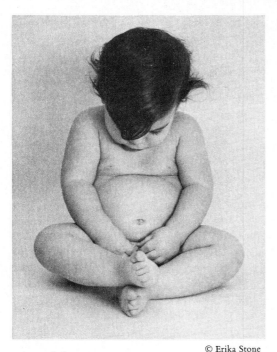

FIGURE 1-5
Genital exploration.

uncomfortable, or even if they use distraction as a technique, the connection that genitals are undesirable and should not be touched may be made. One study showed that in order for genital play to occur the first year, there had to be a "close *and* balanced" mother-child relationship (Spitz 1949, 99).

As infants acquire language skills they should be taught the names for their genitals just as they are taught the names for their other body parts. In 1920 Sanger wrote that mothers should begin teaching their children about sexuality and abandon the approach that the body is neuter (p. 2). That excellent advice applies no less at the present time.

Freud also asked why parents felt constrained to withhold from their children in-

formation about sexuality. He theorized that parents reacted in that manner out of "habitual prudery and a guilty conscience in themselves about sexual matters," or perhaps out of "theoretical ignorance on their part to be counteracted only by fresh information" (Freud 1978, 19).

Parents' lack of knowledge about sexual matters is an important concept for the nurse to keep in mind. The growing family often has contact with nurses—the nurse in the clinic, pediatrician's office, community center, school, or hospital. Parents will probably not bring up concerns about genital play or the education of their children in aspects of sexuality, including reproduction. Often, it is the nurse who must open the topic for discussion. She or he can clarify any present concerns the family may have and also provide some anticipatory guidance by including sexuality when growth and development are discussed.

Sexuality in Early Childhood

As children grow out of the infant stage into early childhood, genital play becomes less random and more purposeful. By the end of the second year the child is entering a new phase. The genitals come into a sharper focus, often because of toilet training. This is a phase of primary genital arousal. This arousal is often initiated by voluntary control of the urinary and anal sphincters (Peltz 1977, 41). The word *masturbation* may then apply to this activity. Masturbation is a word that for many people is charged with negative implications (see Chapter 4 for additional discussion). A thorough definition of masturbation was written by Tausk (1951, 63): Masturbation is ". . . that kind of sexual manipulation of the genitals or of an erogenous zone which has no partner as an indispensible prerequisite, and the aim of which consists in the direct discharge of sexual excitation."

Gibney (1972, 128) sees masturbation as the response of individuals to sexual needs that are not met in another way. Kinsey's findings dispute this "substitution" theory, however. He and his colleagues found that masturbation accounted for some of the sexual outlet for persons with sexual partners, as well as for those without partners (Kinsey et al. 1953, 132–190). In fact, Kinsey's statistics show that people who masturbate early in life and continue to masturbate throughout adulthood generally have the most well-adjusted sex lives (Kinsey et al. 1953, 172–190). Masturbation becomes pathological when it interferes with

a person's relationships or when it causes personality conflicts because of fear or guilt (Gibney 1972, 132), but such developments are uncommon.

During the early childhood years, masturbation seems to be a part of the normal developmental process. Without showing aversion to the activity, parents may set limits on where the masturbation activity may take place. For example, parents may not allow masturbation in a public place.

Parents' attitudes toward early childhood behaviors with sexual undertones typically mirror social attitudes toward sex in general. Notwithstanding the sexual bombardment from media advertisements, explicit art forms, and sexually suggestive clothing, American society is a repressive one regarding its outlook on sexuality. Sex is not viewed as a healthy, open aspect of development (Martinson 1977, 77). Because of this, parents may feel bewildered about the best approach to take when they find their child indulging in sex play, either alone or with others (see Figure 1-6). Many adults remember situations from their own childhood that stand out vividly, such as being "caught" playing doctor. These episodes may be recalled in positive or negative ways depending on the reaction of the discovering parent.

Martinson (1977) does not see a dichotomy between the seemingly blatant sexuality in American culture and repression among parents. Rather, he sees the repression as being a cause of obsessive sexual interest. Permissiveness and a positive approach would foster a healthier attitude. Studies have shown that sex offenders and people who have sexual problems come from sexually repressive backgrounds and received little or no factual sexual information (Green 1977, 100).

Another concern of parents which usually begins at the preschool age is that of parental nudity. Experts disagree as to its harm or benefit. Some believe that if parents are comfort-

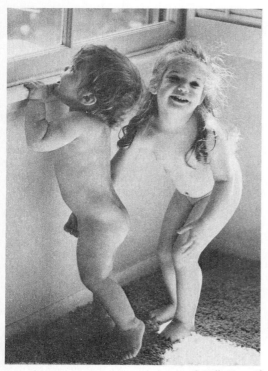

© Hella Hammid

FIGURE 1-6
Early childhood "sex play."

able with being nude in the presence of their children there is no harm (Martinson 1977). Others, through the use of clinical examples, show that some children become overstimulated and unable to handle their feelings when exposed to parental nudity (Peltz 1977, 48). Because of the dearth of evidence and the conflicting views of experts, this is an issue that parents will need to decide by themselves. Parents should consider how comfortable each family member is about this subject.

Later Childhood Years

Freud used the term *latency* in describing the childhood years between ages 5 and 10. He believed that repression of infantile genitality occurred during this period, with a cessation of sexuality and physical sexual maturation (Erikson 1963, 62 and 86). Kinsey was one of the first whose studies showed that school-aged children did, in fact, engage in sexual behavior. This behavior includes masturbation, genital manipulation with peers, manipulation with toys, blankets or other objects, same-sex and heterosexual play, and genital exhibition (comparison of anatomies) (Kinsey et al. 1965, 101–115).

As children reach kindergarten age some aspects of their behavior may change quite radically. Whereas just a short time before there may have been few or no inhibitions regarding nudity, they may suddenly become modest and insist on privacy. Boys and girls up to the age of 5 or 6 often play together, but as they enter kindergarten, play becomes more sex-segregated. In running or chasing games boys chase girls or girls chase boys. They develop relationships with members of their own sex and begin to identify with the same-sex parent. After the age of 8 a larger peer group seems to become more important than one "best friend." It is common for children of

this age to have sexual fantasies and to delight in telling "dirty" jokes (Peltz 1977, 53).

Sex Education

Sex education is usually thought of in relation to the school-age child. Like so many other topics that involve sexuality, it is often viewed in an emotional way. It has the potential for causing a community to become divided on either side of the issue. Probably few would disagree that, ideally, sex education should begin in the home. Many parents believe that it should both begin and end in the home. Unfortunately, these beliefs are not put into practice. A number of studies have been done to try to determine children's sources of sex information. They show that parents, for the most part, are not in the forefront as sources of enlightenment. Fathers have virtually no role in sex education.

Fox (1979) reviewed studies related to parental communication about sexuality with their children. This review of the literature indicated that only three studies looked at sex communication between mothers and daughters, that parents do not engage in a great deal of dialogue with their children about sexuality, and that the role of parents as sex educators is minor (pp. 21–25). Bloch (1972) studied 124 mothers of seventh grade girls. Of these women, 20% had never told their daughters anything about menstruation (giving a very liberal interpretation to *any* information given), 50% never mentioned the father's role in procreation, and 60% had not talked about birth control.

The Goldmans (1982, 57) interviewed 838 children between the ages of 5 and 15 from Australia, England, North America, and Sweden. Their purposes were to gain a deeper understanding of the children's sexual knowledge and to learn how children use their cognitive processes to explain biological phenomena. Among its many findings, the study showed that some sexual analogies used to explain conception and birth to children actually served to retard their understanding. For example, sperm were often described as tadpoles, and the word *tummy* was often used instead of uterus (Goldman and Goldman 1982, 586). The evidence from the Swedish children indicated that children are able to understand complex biological concepts at an earlier age than was previously thought (p. 391).

Besides confusing children's understanding of the biology of sex, parents often neglect such topics as intercourse or other erotic behaviors in their discussions (Nass, Libby, and Fisher 1981, 247). If parents feel embarrassed or uncomfortable when children ask questions about sexuality, children soon learn to stay away from the offending subjects. They then tend to receive their "information" (often inaccurate or actually incorrect) from peers unless their school has a sex education curriculum.

Nass, Libby, and Fisher (1981, 251) report six reasons for parental objections to school sex education programs. One concern is the qualification of the teacher. Another is presentation of topics. For example, should sexually transmissible diseases be taught as risks of sexual intercourse, or as a preventable disease? The third and perhaps most important concern is the expression of values: Should information be taught in a value-free context or with a "sex-negative" or "sex-positive" approach? A fourth concern is the teacher's age (parents seem to prefer older teachers to younger ones). A fifth concern is that some parents equate children's knowledge with performance. That is, they may worry that if a child learns about intercourse then that child will want to "try it out." The last reason is a fear that children will "grow up too fast" and lose their innocence (or ignorance). Nevertheless, the Goldmans' study recommended that

sex education be considered a complementary responsibility of both home and school (1982, 390).

No type of sex education can be successfully established in a community without parental support. Gaining parental support initially is not enough; the support must be maintained throughout the conception and implementation of the curriculum. In one community, the voters passed a referendum in favor of the development of a sex education curriculum for the elementary, middle, and high schools. It took a number of years for the teachers who had been appointed to the task to devise a curriculum. Unfortunately, the typist who was completing the final draft found the content of the work to be offensive and alerted the community. There were long, acrimonious debates in public halls and on the editorial pages of the local newspaper. The program was canceled, and, many years later, there is still no sex education in the public schools of that community.

Perhaps some preventive action might have ensured success in the community mentioned. As the curriculum was being developed the teachers might have met with interested parents, sharing ideas and audiovisual materials with them. In addition to informing parents about the process of sex education, these sessions would have provided an opportunity to share content as well. Parents who have been well informed and involved in the process may be more willing to let their children learn about sexuality.

If a school system does not have the resources to develop its own total program, it may want to use one already developed and adapt it to the needs of that community. There are other alternatives to a total sex education program. Evening programs for parents and children have proven successful in many instances. These sessions could be sponsored by the parent-teacher organization, the school nurse, teachers, or other community leaders.

Often, such an evening begins with an introductory session during which parents and children view a film together. Then the group is separated into three subgroups — girls, boys, and parents. Each group has an adult leader who is experienced in group process, teaching, and sex-education content. During the evening, books, pamphlets, and other information may be shared (Boettcher and Boettcher 1978).

Another approach to consider is the Goldmans' suggestion that courses be provided for parents to help teach children about sexuality. Children themselves perceive adults as having hang-ups in discussing sex with them. Fathers seem to need more help in this area; mothers are much more frequently sources of sex-related information (Goldman and Goldman 1982, 323 and 392). The process of sex education for people of all ages is further discussed in Chapter 5, as part of a holistic approach to promoting sexual health.

Adolescence

Adolescence is the period in life that begins with puberty and ends in adulthood. It has the potential for crisis, as each individual undergoes a kind of metamorphosis. The adolescent is in the process of becoming an adult and is gradually putting away the things of childhood. The favorite stuffed animal may be placed on a shelf and no longer taken to bed. The doll, truck, and building toys are relegated to a storage closet. There are new, more "grown-up" concerns to deal with. Some of the tasks characteristic of adolescence are feeling comfortable with a new body, feeling good about one's developing sexuality, establishing an identity of one's own, establishing relationships, defining a moral code, becoming independent of parents, and learning how to deal with increasingly adult situations

(Tanner 1962, 218; Mercer 1979, 10). The period of adolescence may be seen as the second phase of becoming an individual (Blos 1965, 145).

Adolescents often behave in ways that try the patience of their parents and teachers. Peers take on a new importance and influence. Being different from one's peer group is threatening. Adolescents feel that they must conform in dress, behavior, and attitudes in order to be accepted. Elkind (1978, 127) discusses the import of the imaginary audience to teenagers. Because the adolescent now has the cognitive ability to think about what others' perceptions may be, all the others become the imaginary audience. Because she or he is so preoccupied with self, it is assumed that everyone else is also. Teenagers therefore tend to be quite self-conscious because they feel that everyone is "watching" them. Teenagers do not seem to have the ability to sort out which aspects about themselves would be of interest to others and which aspects would not.

Puberty, the period of time marking the changes from the child body to the adult body, from being incapable of reproduction to attaining the ability to reproduce, begins the adolescent period. The age puberty commences and the length of time it takes vary with each individual. Today it is generally considered normal for a girl to begin puberty between the ages of 9 and 11 and for a boy between the ages of 13 and 15. The onset of puberty signals the beginning of marked bodily changes in hormone secretion, fat distribution, bodily hair growth, bone structure, secondary sexual characteristics, and reproductive organs.

Becoming a Physically Mature Female

The end point of puberty is the adult body, capable of reproduction. This section begins with a description of the sex organs and secondary sex characteristics of a woman, and then describes the processes that lead to that end.

Adult Female Sexual Anatomy

The organs of the female sexual/reproductive tract are both internal and external. The external organs are called the *vulva* or *pudendum.* The *mons pubis* is a fat pad that covers the symphysis bone. Hair grows in a typically female pattern over the mons; that is, in the shape of a triangle (see Figure 1-7).

The *labia majora,* or outer lips, are folds of skin covering fat pads. Hair grows in the outer surfaces; the inner surfaces are highly pigmented. The smaller, inner lips, or the *labia minora,* are thinner and contain many sebaceous glands. The *clitoris,* composed of sensitive erectile tissue, is hooded by the anterior parts of the labia minora.

The *urethral orifice* or *urinary meatus* is located between the clitoris and the introitus. *Skene's glands* are located just inside the opening on the urethral floor.

The *introitus* is the vaginal opening. The *hymen* is a fold of mucous membrane that partially covers the introitus if it has not been penetrated. In some women the hymen completely obstructs the opening and must be incised in order for menstrual fluids to be passed and intercourse to occur. On either side of the introitus are *Bartholin's glands,* which provide a small amount of the lubrication to the vagina during sexual excitement.

The *perineum* includes the structures from the mons to the coccyx. However, in commonly used terminology it refers to the area between the introitus and the anus (see Figures 1-8 and 1-9).

The internal sexual/reproductive organs are the vagina, cervix, uterus, fallopian tubes, and ovaries. The *vagina,* a musculomembranous tube-like organ with many rugae or folds, is situated between the introitus and

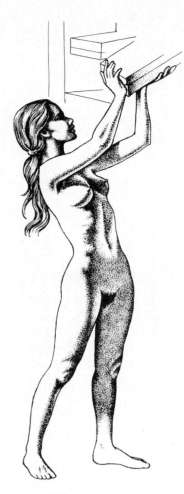

FIGURE 1-7
A sexually developed young woman.

cervix. It is about 7 to 9 cm long; the anterior segment is shorter than the posterior. At the uppermost end, the cervix protrudes into the vagina forming four spaces or fornices. The vagina is a flexible space whose walls are usually touching. It serves as a receptor for the penis and sperm, as the outlet for the menstrual flow, and the passageway for the birth of the fetus. Transudation of fluids from the vaginal walls during sexual arousal supplies lubrication for intercourse. The bladder and ure-

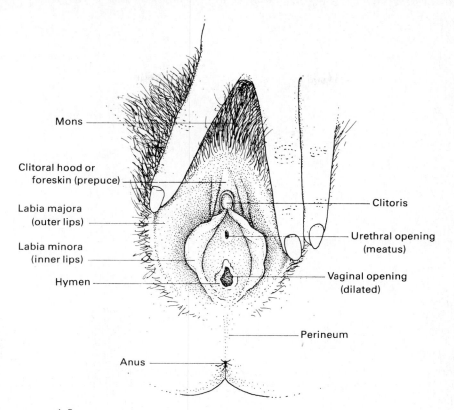

FIGURE 1-8
Female external genitals.

SOURCE: From *Sexual Choices,* 2nd ed., by G. D. Nass, R. W. Libby, and M. P. Fisher.
Copyright © 1984, 1981 by Wadsworth, Inc. Reprinted by permission of the publisher,
Wadsworth Health Sciences, Monterey, California.

thra are anterior to the vagina, the rectum posterior.

The vagina's acid environment and the presence of lacto bacilli serve to protect it against the growth of pathogenic organisms. Because vaginal cells change in response to hormonal influence, they are important diagnostic indicators.

The *cervix,* or neck of the uterus, is easily visualized during a vaginal exam. The *os* (opening) of the cervix connects the vagina and the body of the uterus. The uterine end is called the internal os; the vaginal end is called the external os.

The cervix is covered with epithelial tissue. Squamous epithelium is found in the vagina and on the outer or ectocervix, while columnar epithelium covers the inner or endocervix. The squamocolumnar junction is the point at which they meet, which is near the external os. A transformation occurs during three developmental stages of a woman's life, fetal,

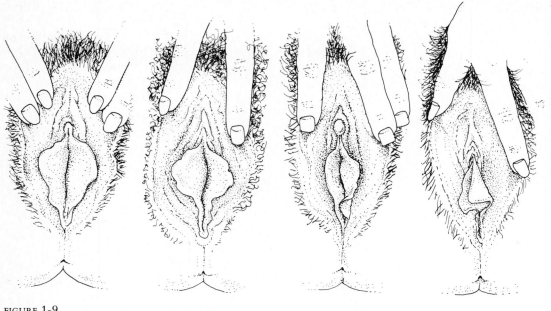

FIGURE 1-9
Variety in genitals.

SOURCE: From *Sexual Choices*, 2nd ed., by G. D. Nass, R. W. Libby, and M. P. Fisher. Copyright © 1984, 1981 by Wadsworth, Inc. Reprinted by permission of the publisher, Wadsworth Health Sciences, Monterey, California.

adolescence, and first pregnancy. The columnar epithelium may become squamous epithelium, forming a transformation zone. If the process goes awry, the new cells may be atypical. This may occur due to in utero DES (diethylstilbestrol) exposure (Reagan and Olaizola 1980, 96), or possibly due to chemical spermicide use (foams, creams, and jellies), early intercourse, or herpes Type 2. The latter two factors are associated with increased risk for cervical cancer; the precancerous warning sign is an ectropion (atypical cells from the cervical canal on the surface of the cervix) or dysplasia (hyperplasia of basal cells).

The *uterus* or womb is a thick-walled pear-shaped structure located in the pelvis, lying at right angles to the vagina. The urinary bladder is anterior and the rectum posterior. A fallopian tube opens into the uterus about two thirds of the way to the top on each side. The portion of the uterus above these insertions is called the *fundus*. The uterine walls are composed of three layers: the outer layer, which is serous and derived from the peritoneum; the muscular layer, or myometrium, which contains many blood vessels; and the inner layer, or endometrium, which is composed of epithelium, blood vessels, and glands. The endometrium is a dynamic layer, responding to hormonal influences.

The uterus has a tremendous capacity for expansion because it is the potential home of the developing embryo and fetus. The muscular layer has an important function in contracting during labor as the power in the birth process. The uterus is not in a fixed position but is suspended by ligaments, which permits its movement and growth during pregnancy.

The *fallopian tubes* extend laterally from each side of the uterus. They are the passageways for the movement of the egg from the ovary to the uterus. Fertilization also takes place in the tubes. The distal ends of the tubes are fimbriated. These fimbriae, finger-like projections extending from a funnel shape, gently propel the egg released from the ovary into the tube. The tubes are about 11 cm long and 6 mm in diameter. The inner layer is ciliated and, along with peristaltic movements of the muscular layer, helps propel the egg forward into the uterus.

The two *ovaries* lie on either side of the uterus. They are about the size and shape of an almond and are attached to the uterus by the

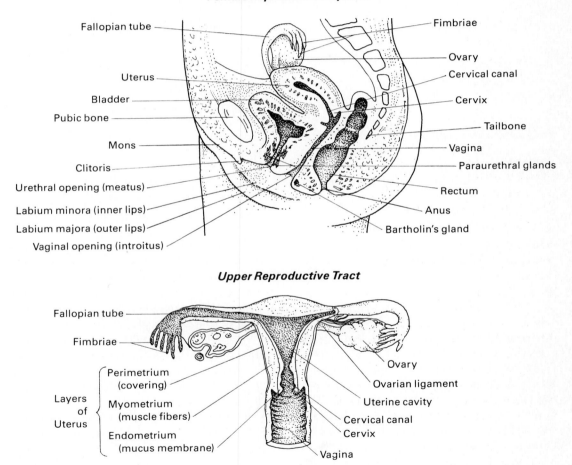

Female Reproductive System

Fallopian tube

Fimbriae

Ovary

Cervical canal

Uterus

Cervix

Bladder

Pubic bone

Tailbone

Mons

Vagina

Clitoris

Paraurethral glands

Urethral opening (meatus)

Rectum

Labium minora (inner lips)

Anus

Labium majora (outer lips)

Bartholin's gland

Vaginal opening (introitus)

Upper Reproductive Tract

Fallopian tube

Fimbriae

Perimetrium (covering)

Ovary

Ovarian ligament

Layers of Uterus

Myometrium (muscle fibers)

Uterine cavity

Cervical canal

Endometrium (mucus membrane)

Cervix

Vagina

FIGURE 1-10
Internal structure of a woman.

SOURCE: From *Sexual Choices,* 2nd ed., by G. D. Nass, R. W. Libby, and M. P. Fisher. Copyright © 1984, 1981 by Wadsworth, Inc. Reprinted by permission of the publisher, Wadsworth Health Sciences, Monterey, California.

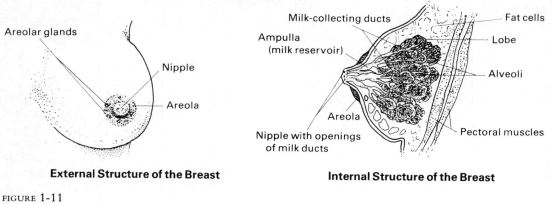

Female Breast

Areolar glands

Nipple

Areola

External Structure of the Breast

Milk-collecting ducts

Ampulla
(milk reservoir)

Fat cells

Lobe

Alveoli

Areola

Nipple with openings
of milk ducts

Pectoral muscles

Internal Structure of the Breast

FIGURE 1-11
Breast.

SOURCE: From *Sexual Choices*, 2nd ed., by G. D. Nass, R. W. Libby, and M. P. Fisher. Copyright © 1984, 1981 by Wadsworth, Inc. Reprinted by permission of the publisher, Wadsworth Health Sciences, Monterey, California.

ovarian ligament. The inner part of the ovary, the medulla, contains connective tissue, blood vessels, nerves, and lymphatic tissue. The cortex or outer portion contains thousands of minute follicles, each containing a germ cell or oocyte. The process of egg development will be discussed in detail in the section on menstruation.

The pelvic organs are richly supplied with blood vessels, nerves, and muscular tissue (see Figure 1-10).

The *breasts* or mammary glands are considered accessory organs of reproduction due to their milk-producing capabilities (see Figure 1-11). They are also important sexual organs. They are highly erogenous and may be a source of pleasure during sex play, breastfeeding, and masturbation. The breasts are the most obvious sign of a woman's maturity. The size of breasts varies dramatically among women, which may cause problems in self-esteem. Breasts are often perceived as being too small, but women with disproportionately large breasts may also have problems. Vandestienne (1982, 13) discusses some of those problems: neck and back pain, problems in

buying bras and other clothing, and unwanted attention focused on the overendowed body.

A young woman's breasts are firm and high but become softer and lower as she ages. Breast size increases during pregnancy and lactation. Small breast size does not hamper the ability to breastfeed.

The breasts are composed of glandular tissue, adipose or fat tissue, and connecting tissue. Fibrous tissue, ligaments, and underlying muscles support the breasts. The nipples are located at the center of each breast and contain about 20 openings that lead to a system of ducts and alveoli. The nipples are sensitive and become erect during breastfeeding, sexual stimulation, or exposure to cold. The areola, the pigmented skin surrounding the nipple, contains glands that secrete a substance that keeps the nipples soft and supple during lactation.

Menstruation

In addition to anatomical maturity, the adult woman's reproductive capacity also involves menstruation. The cyclical process of menstruation begins during puberty and ends during the menopause. The cycle varies in length from woman to woman, but the 28-day cycle is considered a standard and will be used here for discussion purposes. Complexity and harmony exist in the interplay of hormones, target organs, and feedback mechanisms to create the dynamics of the menstrual cycle (see Figures 1-12 and 1-13).

During the first part of the cycle the hypothalamus increases its secretion of *gonadotropin-releasing hormone* (GRH). GRH causes the pituitary to secrete *luteinizing hormone* (LH) and *follicle-stimulating hormone* (FSH). FSH stimulates the development of an ovarian follicle (an egg and its surrounding cells). This follicle, which resembles a blister on the surface of the ovary, grows rapidly and fills with fluid. Meanwhile the lining of the uterus is already in a regenerative phase that begins at the latter part of the menstrual phase. The vagina is also undergoing changes. The pH is about 4.5 during the first half of the menstrual cycle and a specimen of mucus viewed under microscope shows a fernlike pattern. The cells of the ovarian (graafian) follicle secrete estrogen. As the estrogen secretion increases, the FSH decreases but the LH increases just before ovulation at about day 12.

Ovulation occurs on about day 14. The egg is ushered into the fallopian tube by the fimbriae in the end of the tube. If the egg is not fertilized, its life span is approximately 24 hours. The cells of the ruptured follicle become the corpus luteum secreting estrogens and progesterones. Unless the ovum is fertilized, the corpus luteum has a life span of about 1.4 days, during which time the rich lining of the uterus is being maintained. The mucus secretions of the vagina thicken, the pH is more alkaline, and the fernlike pattern disappears. With the demise of the corpus luteum and the decrease in its hormonal secretions, the uterine lining sloughs away and menstruation begins. Menstrual fluid consists of mucin, blood, and epithelial cells usually ranging from 50 to 100 ml in volume. The flow normally lasts from five to seven days, but can range, in the extremes, from two to eight or nine days.

The Process of Pubertal Development

Even before any physical signs of puberty appear, hormonal changes are occurring in a girl's body. About two years before these signs, the hypothalamus increases its release of gonadotropins, thereby increasing the secretion of follicle-stimulating and luteinizing hormones. These initial hormonal releases occur primarily at night (Fordney 1981, 385). Finkelstein calls this time very early puberty (1980, 58).

One of the first signs of puberty in females is budding of the breasts. Pubic hair appearance usually follows within the year, although in some individuals pubic hair may be noticed first (Tanner 1962, 37). Hormones continue to increase. These include gonadotropins, the growth hormone, and sex steroids. Internal reproductive organs are growing, as are the external ones. The labia minora become larger and protrude through the labia majora. A clear vaginal discharge appears as the vaginal epithelium becomes thicker. The pH of the vagina changes from 6 to 7 to 4 to 5. A subcutaneous fat layer develops all over, especially in the areas of hips, buttocks, thighs, and breasts, giving the body an adult appearance (Tichy and Malasanos 1976, 388). Sebaceous glands on the face and back become more active and acne may ensue. An increase in the growth hormone may cause a spurt in growth during this midpubertal time (Finkelstein 1980, 58).

Menarche (onset of menstruation) occurs in the majority of girls between the ages of 11 and 14. The mean age has been decreasing by almost one-half year per decade (Fordney 1981, 386). There is much speculation about what specifically triggers menarche. Some hy-

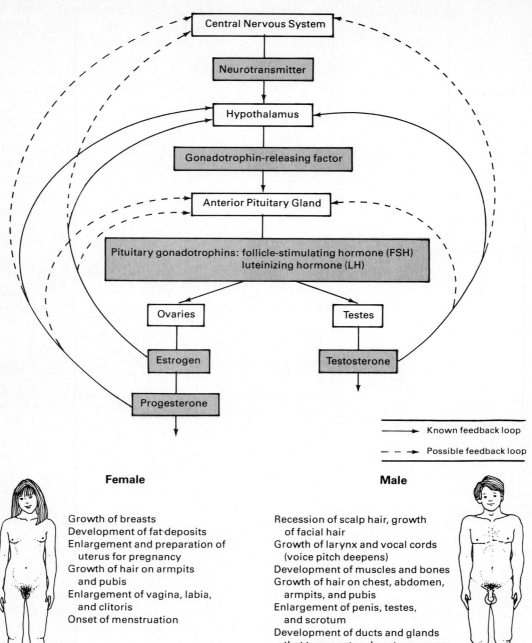

Female

Growth of breasts
Development of fat deposits
Enlargement and preparation of
  uterus for pregnancy
Growth of hair on armpits
  and pubis
Enlargement of vagina, labia,
  and clitoris
Onset of menstruation

Male

Recession of scalp hair, growth
  of facial hair
Growth of larynx and vocal cords
  (voice pitch deepens)
Development of muscles and bones
Growth of hair on chest, abdomen,
  armpits, and pubis
Enlargement of penis, testes,
  and scrotum
Development of ducts and glands
  that transport and nurture sperm
Beginning of ejaculation

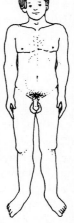

FIGURE 1-12
Puberty.

SOURCE: From *Sexual Choices,* 2nd ed., by G. D. Nass, R. W. Libby, and M. P. Fisher. Copyright © 1984, 1981 by Wadsworth, Inc. Reprinted by permission of the publisher, Wadsworth Health Sciences, Monterey, California.

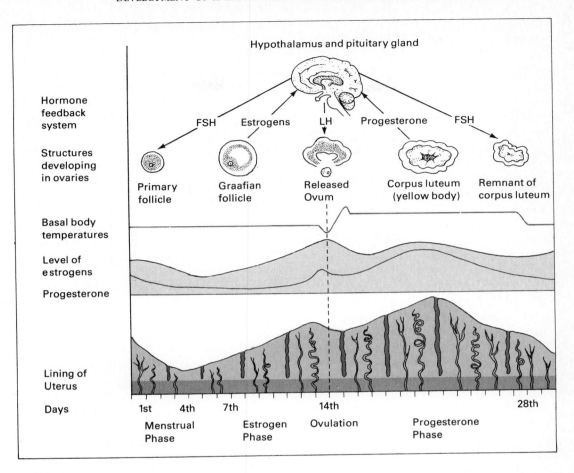

FIGURE 1-13
Hormone-regulated changes during the menstrual cycle.

SOURCE: From *Sexual Choices,* 2nd ed., by G. D. Nass, R. W. Libby, and M. P. Fisher. Copyright © 1984, 1981 by Wadsworth, Inc. Reprinted by permission of the publisher, Wadsworth Health Sciences, Monterey, California.

potheses are attainment of a critical body weight, nutrition, a genetic factor, and diet. The first few cycles or even half of the cycles during the first year of menstruation may be anovulatory. The cycles of the first year may also be quite irregular in both length and volume.

Primary dysmenorrhea, or painful menstruation which occurs near menarche with no

pathology present, is beginning to be more clearly understood. Some of the symptoms are lower abdominal pain, cramps in the legs, lower back pain, and gastrointestinal upsets. At one time in the recent past these problems were thought to be of psychological origin, and many gym teachers and perhaps a goodly number of school nurses as well encouraged girls to exercise during their discomfort.

At present, the best indications are that these unpleasant manifestations are due to the actions of certain prostaglandins. *Prostaglandins* are manufactured by a variety of body cells and exert different effects. The prostaglandins found in menstrual fluids have the capability of causing uterine contractions with resultant pain due to uterine ischemia. For those women who are disabled by dysmenorrhea, prostaglandin inhibitors offer relief. Acetylsalicylic acid (aspirin) is a known prostaglandin synthetase inhibitor and has been used successfully to prevent cramps in young women when taken three days prior to menstruation. Oral contraceptives were once widely used to eliminate dysmenorrhea in adolescents since they suppress ovulatory cycles and cause an atypical "withdrawal bleed" cycle. It is recommended that the choice be one with a low estrogen dose, however; in addition, other health considerations must be kept in mind before an oral contraceptive is prescribed (see Chapter 6). Other prostaglandin inhibitors now used are ibuprofen and mefenamic acid (Drugs for Dysmenorrhea 1979, 81; Budoff 1979). For those whose symptoms are mild, supportive therapy and recommendations such as hot baths and rest may suffice (Fordney 1980, 398). Even though endometriosis (the presence of endometrial tissue in the pelvic area outside the uterus) is not a common problem among teenagers, it must still be considered as a possible cause for primary dysmenorrhea that requires special treatment (Klein 1980, 142).

Becoming a Physically Mature Male

The process by which males mature sexually is similar to that of females, but the end results are visibly different. The sections that follow describe adult male sexual anatomy and hormonal patterns, and the pubertal changes involved in their development.

Adult Male Sexual Anatomy

Unlike the female sex organs, which for the most part are inside the body, the male sex organs are visible. They consist of the *penis* (the organ of copulation) and the *scrotum,* which contains the testicles or testes (singular: testis). The penis consists of highly distensible erectile tissue. The tip of the penis is called the *glans.* If a male is circumcised, the glans is readily apparent. If circumcision was not done, the glans is covered by the foreskin. The skin of the penis is continuous with the skin of the scrotum and is highly pigmented. The urethra, about 20 cm long, extends from the urinary bladder to the meatus at the tip of the penis (see Figures 1-14 and 1-15).

The size of the penis probably concerns boys and men as much as the size of their breasts concerns women. Penises in their unerect or flaccid state vary a great deal in size from man to man; erect penises vary less in size. The size of the penis has little effect on attaining sexual pleasure.

The *testicles,* analogous to the ovaries in the female, produce sperm in thousands of complex *seminiferous tubules.* Sperm remain in these tubules for sixty days, then they go to the *epididymis* where they remain while they mature (see Figure 1-16). The *vas deferens* continues from the epididymis and joins the seminal vesicle ducts. They become the ejaculatory ducts, pass through the prostate gland, and join the urethra. The *urethra* is the passageway for urine and ejaculate.

The ejaculate, or *semen,* is composed of sperm, water, and secretions from the prostate and bulbourethral glands. The volume varies but is usually about 3 to 5 ml per ejaculation. The alkaline pH and the content of the semen ensure the health of the sperm. Another factor ensuring the health of sperm is the temperature in the testicles. It is maintained at 1° to 2°C below body temperature for optimum sperm production. The muscles in the scrotum

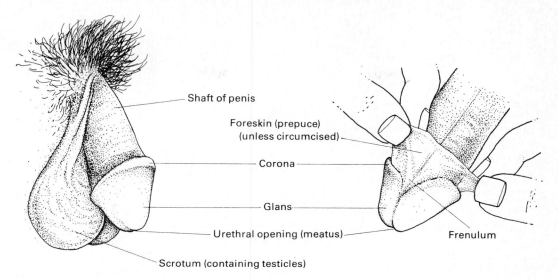

Shaft of penis

Foreskin (prepuce)
(unless circumcised)

Corona

Glans

Urethral opening (meatus)

Frenulum

Scrotum (containing testicles)

FIGURE 1-14
Male external genitals.

SOURCE: From *Sexual Choices,* 2nd ed., by G. D. Nass, R. W. Libby, and M. P. Fisher. Copyright © 1984, 1981 by Wadsworth, Inc. Reprinted by permission of the publisher, Wadsworth Health Sciences, Monterey, California.

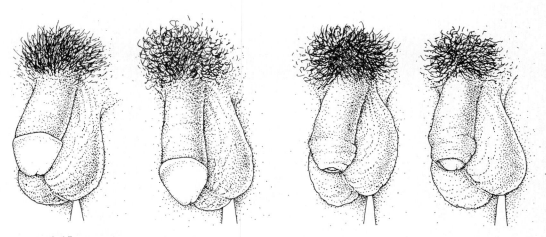

FIGURE 1-15
Variety in genitals.

SOURCE: From *Sexual Choices,* 2nd ed., by G. D. Nass, R. W. Libby, and M. P. Fisher. Copyright © 1984, 1981 by Wadsworth, Inc. Reprinted by permission of the publisher, Wadsworth Health Sciences, Monterey, California.

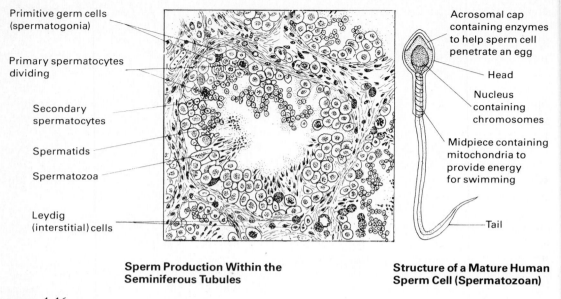

Primitive germ cells
(spermatogonia)

Primary spermatocytes
dividing

Secondary
spermatocytes

Spermatids

Spermatozoa

Leydig
(interstitial) cells

Acrosomal cap
containing enzymes
to help sperm cell
penetrate an egg

Head

Nucleus
containing
chromosomes

Midpiece containing
mitochondria to
provide energy
for swimming

Tail

**Sperm Production Within the
Seminiferous Tubules**

**Structure of a Mature Human
Sperm Cell (Spermatozoan)**

FIGURE 1-16
Production and structure of sperm.

SOURCE: From *Sexual Choices,* 2nd ed., by G. D. Nass, R. W. Libby, and M. P. Fisher. Copyright © 1984, 1981 by
Wadsworth, Inc. Reprinted by permission of the publisher, Wadsworth Health Sciences, Monterey, California.

contract in the cold, pulling the testicles closer to the body, and relax in warmth, allowing the testicles to move away from the body.

An analysis of semen can determine a man's capability for fathering a child. The specimen should be deposited in a clear, dry, wide-mouthed jar and should be analyzed within an hour. There should be over 60 million and as many as 100 to 200 million sperm per mL of semen, with fewer than 25% of the sperm having abnormal forms. At least 60% of the sperm should be motile. However, these are merely guidelines. Excellent motility, for example, may compensate for a lower number of sperm.

Hormonal Patterns

There are similarities in the functioning of the hormones that govern the female and male reproductive organs. In both genders, gonadotropin secretion from the hypothalamus stimulates the anterior pituitary to secrete follicle-stimulating hormone and luteinizing hormone. In the male, the FSH has an effect on the seminiferous tubules and is important in the development of sperm (spermatogenesis). Luteinizing hormone stimulates the testicles to produce testosterone, the principal male hormone. Testosterone is responsible for male secondary sex characteristics, for the promotion of growth, and for maintaining spermatogenesis.

The Process of Pubertal Development

The adolescent male begins puberty in much the same way the female does. In early puberty, before any physical changes become apparent, the hypothalamus increases its secretion of gonadotropins during sleep. The average age of onset of puberty in boys and girls is also similar. The development of the male genitalia may begin merely a few months after breast development begins in the female. One major and noticeable difference in development is the two-year growth spurt lead that girls have. Even so, both sexes complete the physical maturation process at about the same time (Finkelstein 1980, 65).

The sequence of changes in the male begins with a speeding of growth of the testes and scrotum and a darkening of the scrotal skin. Pubic hair appears and the penis grows. About two years after the appearance of pubic hair, axillary and circumanal hair appears (see Figure 1-17). Body hair continues to appear even

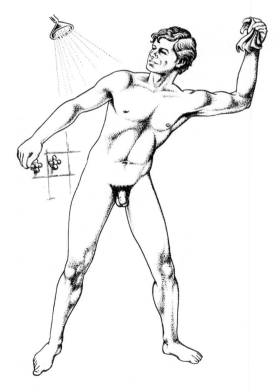

FIGURE 1-17
A sexually developed young man.

after the end of puberty. The growth of the larynx will eventually result in a deeper voice. The apocrine sweat glands enlarge and the scent of perspiration changes from the typical child odor to that of the adult. The breasts may temporarily enlarge and the areolae darken and increase in diameter. This may very disconcerting to the self-conscious adolescent male. The internal organs, the prostate and bulbourethral glands also become larger. The first ejaculation occurs about one year after penile growth begins (Tanner 1962, 29–35) (see Figure 1-18).

Adolescent Sexuality

As sexologist Herbert Katchadourian (1980, 17) has observed, "The blossoming of sexuality in each generation of adolescents is as fascinating a sight as the unfolding of spring each year: predictable and repetitive, yet nonetheless enchanting." The sexual drive observed in adolescents probably has a great deal to do with the increase in secretion of hormones, although that is not the entire explanation. Children who experience a precocious puberty do not usually exhibit an increase in sexual activity at the time. In addition to hormones, the psychosocial context is influential in the development of the sexual behavior of adolescents. Statistics show that more adolescents are becoming sexually active at an earlier age than just a decade ago. Much of this sexual activity now takes place in the home rather than the automobile (Katchadourian 1980).

Motives for Sex

Mitchell (1976, 275), who defines intimacy as "sharing, taking into confidence, and trusting," says that teenagers are not only searching for intimacy; they are "impelled toward it." Adults must help adolescents understand that achieving true intimacy is difficult. Even

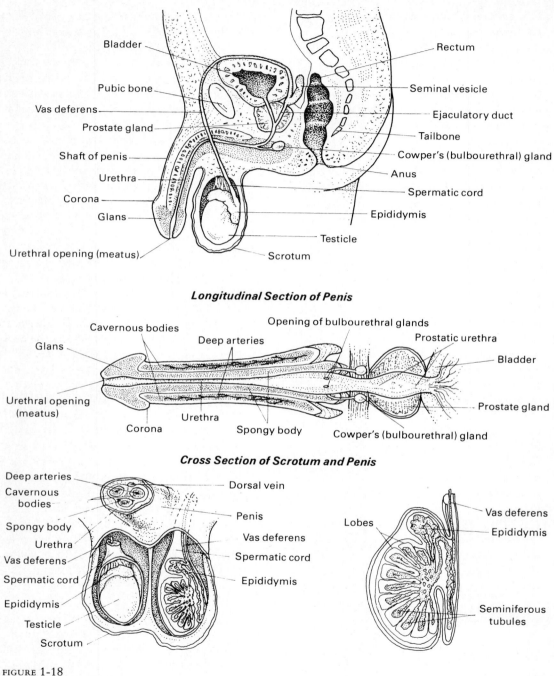

Male Reproductive Organs

Bladder
Rectum
Pubic bone
Seminal vesicle
Vas deferens
Ejaculatory duct
Prostate gland
Tailbone
Shaft of penis
Cowper's (bulbourethral) gland
Urethra
Anus
Corona
Spermatic cord
Glans
Epididymis
Testicle
Urethral opening (meatus)
Scrotum

Longitudinal Section of Penis

Cavernous bodies
Opening of bulbourethral glands
Prostatic urethra
Glans
Deep arteries
Bladder
Urethral opening (meatus)
Prostate gland
Corona
Urethra
Spongy body
Cowper's (bulbourethral) gland

Cross Section of Scrotum and Penis

Deep arteries
Dorsal vein
Cavernous bodies
Vas deferens
Spongy body
Penis
Epididymis
Urethra
Vas deferens
Vas deferens
Spermatic cord
Lobes
Epididymis
Spermatic cord
Epididymis
Testicle
Seminiferous tubules
Scrotum

FIGURE 1-18
Male reproductive system.

SOURCE: From *Sexual Choices,* 2nd ed., by G. D. Nass, R. W. Libby, and M. P. Fisher. Copyright © 1984, 1981 by Wadsworth, Inc. Reprinted by permission of the publisher, Wadsworth Health Sciences, Monterey, California.

though identity must precede intimacy, many teenagers use sexual relationships to help them establish an identity. Because parents are often fearful of the budding sexuality of their children, they attempt to control their activities by imposing curfews and dress and hair codes. Adolescents who are trying to separate from their parents may use sexual activity as a means of rebellion (Katchadourian 1980).

Sex fulfills many additional needs for the adolescent. These are the needs for dominance and submission, the need to belong, and the need to explore and acquire competence. Sex may also be a way of relieving tensions. For some, it is merely a diversion (Leppink 1979, 156 and 159).

Some teens enter sexual relationships in order to feel loved and nurtured, for peer approval, and to prove they are normal. Another "nonsexual" motivation is the desire to express anger against parents or the other sex. In some, sexual activity becomes part of a destructive pattern that may include drug abuse, dangerous behavior, or even suicide. Meanwhile, the underlying conflicts are not resolved (Heisler 1980, 384).

When caring for the sexually active adolescent, the health-care giver needs to be aware of her/his own values and evaluate the teen using objective criteria. These criteria apply to adult relationships as well. Heisler (1980, 384) defines satisfying sex as pleasurable, including interest in the partner with some stability in the relationship. Healthy sex also increases self-esteem, does not exploit anyone, is not always associated with drug abuse, and can help adolescents become mature adults. Sex that is unhealthy or destructive causes guilt, decreases self-concept, exploits the partner, or is promiscuous.

Decision-making

It seems that many adolescents wish to escape the decision-making process that must be a part of becoming responsible for one's own sexuality. Making a decision allows a measure of control in one's life, and also adds dignity to one's actions. The teenager who is not taught or supported in decision-making may enter the threshold of adulthood with negative feelings of having no control over his or her destiny. Decision-making is a growth-producing process that, although difficult, has long-term benefits.

Juhasz (1975) has described a model for sexual decision-making. This model, if used by parents and health-care providers to counsel teenagers, could help them define their own beliefs, lessen the chances of their being caught up in a moment of passion, and move them toward achieving adulthood by taking responsibility for their actions.

The first question that needs to be considered is whether to have sexual intercourse. Some related questions involve the choice of the partner and the circumstances. If the decision is to have intercourse, another question to be faced is whether to have children. The answer to this question has ramifications for society, family, teenager, and infant. If teenagers choose not to have children, they will need to make a third decision: what method of birth control will be used. This issue can become quite complex and generates other questions: How can it be obtained? Who should be responsible?

Even though the decision-making process has proceeded rationally to this point, pregnancy may still occur. If it does, teens must decide whether or not to have an abortion. This decision will be based on certain considerations such as values, religious beliefs, and economic factors.

If the decision is made to continue the pregnancy, the teens must decide if they want to keep the child. In addition, the couple must decide if they want to marry.

Another possible outcome of teenage sexual activity is the spread of sexually transmissible diseases (STD). Considered the most serious though generally nonlethal health problem facing young people today, these diseases are particularly prevalent among 16- to 24-year-olds. Education, communication between partners, and the conscious decision to practice preventive measures could cut the incidence of STD dramatically (Nass, Libby, and Fisher 1981, 474–507). Nursing interventions for STD are discussed in Chapter 6 of this book.

There are many teenagers who choose not to be sexually active. One study queried 514 high school and college women. Of these, 249 had not experienced intercourse. About 20% of these high school and college virgins cited moral reasons for not engaging in intercourse. About 28% said fear of pregnancy was the reason for abstention. One-third of the high school and one-fourth of the college virgins had not met the "right" person. This last group is most likely to engage in premarital intercourse (Herold and Goodwin 1981).

It is not unusual for teenagers to worry that they may be homosexual. About 25% of adolescents do have some homosexual experiences. If an individual eventually has a "predominant and consistent attraction and sexual arousal to the same sex rather than the opposite sex" he or she can be considered homosexual (Jensen 1981, 48). Sometimes parents worry about boys who have effeminate mannerisms and need to be reassured that these characteristics do not necessarily imply a homosexual orientation (Katchadourian 1980, 27).

Anorexia nervosa, a rare but increasing disease in young women, is a disease that prompts its victims to starve themselves. It is mentioned here because there is some thought that a link exists between conflicted adolescent premarital intercourse and the onset of anorexia. It would behoove every health-care professional to be aware of the need for a complete sexual history (see Chapter 5) on every patient who presents with anorexia nervosa (McAnarney and Hackelman 1979).

Pregnancy

Of the 29 million young people aged 13 to 19, some 12 million have had intercourse. One of the most obvious results of teenage sexual activity that has a great impact on society as a whole is teenage pregnancy. There are over 1 million pregnancies among adolescents each year in the United States (*Teenage Pregnancy* 1981, 17). This figure is further broken down by the Urban Institute to reveal that 22% of the pregnancies end with a child born to a single mother, 10% of the young women get married, 17% of the pregnancies occur to already-married teens, 13% are spontaneously aborted, and 38% end in voluntary abortion ("Births to the Unwed" 1981, B11).

The Absence of Contraception

Consistent use of effective contraceptives would prevent teenage pregnancies. Although contraception should be a concern of both male and female adolescents, it is not, simply because most methods are used by the female and she is the one who will bear the consequences.

Some teenagers do try to practice contraception. In a 1979 survey, only 27% of sexually active teens reported they had never used any contraception, 34% reported consistent use, and 39% reported sporadic use. Forty-nine percent used a method for first intercourse. Between 1976 and 1979, an increase in consistent use, use at first intercourse, and a decline in never use occurred (*Teenage Pregnancy* 1981, 11).

Many studies have been done to try to determine why many teenagers do not use contraceptives. The results indicate that lack of knowledge about where to get contraceptives did not seem to be the issue, since 82% of the 13- to 18-year-olds queried said they were aware of resources for obtaining birth control. However, the young men and women had little or no knowledge about the menstrual cycle and its relation to conception. Most of these adolescents stated that they did not want to get pregnant and expressed surprise when they did (Smith, Weinman, and Mumford 1982, 90). As Elkind (1978) says, teenagers believe in a "personal fable." That is a belief that they are special and things that happen to others — such as pregnancy — won't happen to them. In another study, teenage girls cited a variety of reasons for not visiting a birth control clinic. Two important ones were fear of having a pelvic examination and fear that their parents would find out. Only 14% of the 1200 adolescents studied went to a clinic for birth control advice before their first sexual experience. Many others reported using nonprescription methods intermittently ("Teen-Age Girls" 1981, C3).

Risks of Teenage Pregnancy

If teenage pregnancies terminated with healthy mothers and babies whose economic status enabled them to survive, there would be no need for concern. The unpleasant fact is that adolescent mothers are at high risk. There are physiological risks as well as psychological risks. Teenage girls are notorious junk-food eaters whose nutritional status may not be good. Their bodies are still developing. Some pregnancies occur in girls of 12 years of age or even younger. Cephalo-pelvic disproportion is not uncommon in these young women, whose pelvises and other structures have not yet reached maturity. Smoking, street drugs, and alcohol used by the adolescent all may be detrimental to her pregnancy (Hawkins and Higgins 1981, 263).

The negative psychological factors are legion. Unlike the planned pregnancy, the teenage pregnancy is not greeted with joy. Often it is denied by the adolescent and her parents for many months or right up to the time of delivery. One young woman and her family denied so strongly that she delivered her baby, alone, in her bathroom at home. The partner, too, may deny or simply terminate the relationship. The psychological stressors vary depending on the culture. Some cultures are more tolerant of single pregnancies than others. The pregnancy may cause a rift between parents and daughter, who may disagree on the solution to the problem. For this reason some pregnant teenagers leave home.

One study showed that high levels of support were likely to relieve the emotional stress felt by the pregnant adolescent. This study also showed the importance of dealing with adolescents as individuals, rather than viewing them as a homogeneous group (Colletta and Gregg 1981). When given support, young mothers are better able to nurture their infants (Colletta et al. 1980).

About 80% of pregnant teenagers leave school during their pregnancies, never to return. They are likely to have low levels of self-esteem, believe that external forces control them, and feel lonely, uncertain, unhappy, and depressed. Because these young women have so many unmet needs themselves, they have difficulty in giving to their infants. These young families need a great deal of support before and *after* the birth of the baby (Colletta et al. 1980).

Teenagers as Parents

There are few parents of any age who are not at least a little surprised at the total commitment and high energy level required to care for an infant. It is beyond the scope of this book to include a comprehensive discussion of teenagers as parents. However, in order to understand the extent of the problem of teenage pregnancy, the health-care provider needs to have a familiarity with some of the problems often experienced by teenage parents. These problems may place the children of teenage parents at risk.

During the first year of infancy, the child requires much physical care. After the excitement of the first week or two postpartum, reality strikes. The new mother (or father) may, in addition to having parental responsibilities, be responsible for a job and school. These adolescents often lose touch with their peers and feel left out of activities.

Young parents sometimes have difficulty empathizing with their babies. One mother dressed her baby in a frilly dress like a doll leaving her arms and legs exposed even though it was a cool day (Kuhn 1982). On a positive note, Mercer (1977, chap. 7) describes the joys young people receive from being parents and the unique questions they ask in an effort to understand their babies.

Even if the first year passes with no major problems, the second year poses new challenges. As the child is striving for its first measure of independence, the parent begins to teach her or him about values and attitudes. Teens are still in the process of working these things out for themselves. Because the child may be making demands that the parent cannot deal with, child abuse or accidents due to negligence may occur (Cram-Elsberry and Malley-Corrinett 1979, 208).

Assistance in Teenage Pregnancies

Even though the teenage pregnancy rate is rising and it is generally agreed that education is an important variable in helping the young mother become a productive member of society, school systems have not responded to these needs. Most school systems do not actively initiate programs for pregnant teenagers. Their attitudes tend to be more passive. They do comply with Title IX of the 1972 Education Amendments, by allowing preg-

nant teenagers to remain in school. Even when special programs do exist, their quality is uneven and they often do not change as new needs develop. Few evaluate their effectiveness because follow-up studies are so expensive (Zellman 1982).

Community programs that are geared toward helping the pregnant adolescent often neglect her mother. Mothers' expectations for their daughters usually do not include early, single pregnancy. Acceptance follows an initial period of denial (Bryan-Logan and Dancy 1974). Depending on how far the pregnancy has progressed and the values of the family, discussion may focus on options such as abortion, marriage, keeping the baby, or releasing it for adoption. If the new baby and the teenage mother live with her mother, role conflict may occur. The two women may have difficulty sharing the mothering role and find themselves arguing about related issues while never coming to terms with the one role issue that is causing the problem (Bryan-Logan and Dancy 1974). The community health nurse can be especially helpful in assisting mothers and daughters in both preventing and resolving these conflicts.

Teenage pregnancy can cause serious problems. Many families become stressed emotionally and economically. Health-care providers need to become involved to help ensure good health care before and after the birth of the baby.

Summary of Implications for Nursing Practice

The saga of a person's development as a sexual being begins with conception and does not end until death. Childhood and adolescence are times when important developmental tasks, both biophysical and psychosocial, are accomplished in order to prepare the individual for his or her role as a sexually mature adult. The path is not always smooth, nor is it straight. There are risks along the way with the potential for crisis. In partnership with health-care professionals the individual and his or her parents can be assisted to prevent crises. If crisis occurs, resources can be identified and used to deal with the event and promote growth to the highest possible level. Risks inherent in psychosexual development will be discussed in Chapters 6, 7, and 8. The next two chapters will focus on human development as it progresses through young and middle adulthood and maturity.

REFERENCES

Allan, F. D. 1969. *Essentials of human embryology.* 2d ed. New York: Oxford University Press.

Bell, A. P. 1982. Sexual preference: A postscript. *SIECUS Report* 11:1–3.

Bell, A. P., and M. S. Weinberg. 1978. *Homosexualities: A study of diversity among men and women.* New York: Simon & Schuster.

Births to the unwed found to have risen by 50% in 10 years. 1981. *New York Times,* 26 October B11.

Bloch, D. 1972. Sex education practices of mothers. *Journal of Sex Education and Therapy* 7(1).

Blos, P. 1965. The initial stage of male adolescence. *The psychoanalytic study of the child* 20:145–164.

Boettcher, J., and K. Boettcher. 1978. Sex education for fifth and sixth graders and their parents. *The American Journal of Maternal Child Nursing* 3:218–220.

Brecher, E. M. 1975. History of Human Sexual Research and Study. In *Comprehensive textbook of psychiatry II,* ed. A. M. Freedman, H. I. Kaplan, and V. Sadock, vol. 2. Baltimore: Williams & Wilkins.

Brecher, E. M. 1969. *The sex researchers.* Boston: Little, Brown.

Bryan-Logan, B. N., and B. L. Dancy. 1974. Unwed pregnant adolescents: Their mothers' dilemma. *Nursing Clinics of North America* 9:57–68.

Budoff, P. W. 1979. Use of mefenamic acid in the treatment of primary dysmenorrhea. *Journal of the American Medical Association* 241:2713–2716.

Colletta, N. D., and C. H. Gregg. 1981. Adolescent mothers' vulnerability to stress. *The Journal of Nervous and Mental Disease* 169:50–54.

Colletta, N. D., C. H. Gregg, S. Hadler, D. Lee, and D. Mekelburg. 1980. When adolescent mothers return to school. *The Journal of School Health* 50:534–538.

Cram-Elsberry, C., and A. Malley-Corrinet. 1979. The adolescent parent. *High-risk parenting: Nursing assessment and strategies for the family at risk,* ed. S. H. Johnson. Philadelphia: Lippincott.

De Cecco, J. P., and M. G. Shively. 1977. Children's development: Social sex-role and the hetero-homosexual orientation. In *The sexual and gender development of young children,* ed. E. K. Oremland and J. D. Oremland. Cambridge, Mass.: Ballinger.

Drugs for dysmenorrhea. 1979. *Medical Letters Drugs Therapy* 21:81.

Elkind, D. 1978. Understanding the young adolescent. *Adolescence* 13:126–134.

Erikson, E. H. 1963. *Childhood and society.* 2d ed. New York: Norton.

Fagot, B. I. 1982. Sex role development. In *Strategies and techniques of child study,* ed. R. Vasta. New York: Academic Press.

Finkelstein, J. W. 1980. Endocrinology of adolescence. *Pediatric Clinics of North America* 27:53–69.

Fordney, D. S. 1981. Adolescence. In *Gynecology and obstetrics: The health care of women,* ed. S. L. Romney, M. J. Gray, A. B. Little, J. A. Merrill, E. J. Zwilligan, and R. W. Stander. New York: McGraw-Hill.

Fox, G. L. 1979. The family's influence on adolescent sexual behavior. *Children Today* 8(3):21–36.

Franzblau, A. N. 1975. Religion and sexuality. In *Comprehensive textbook of psychiatry II,* ed. A. M. Freedman, H. I. Kaplan, and V. Sadock, vol. 2. Baltimore: Williams & Wilkins.

Freud, S. [1905] 1962. *Three essays on the theory of sexuality,* ed. J. Strachey. New York: Basic Books.

Freud, S. 1978. *The sexual enlightenment of children.* New York: Collier.

Friday, N. 1975. *Forbidden flowers: More women's sexual fantasies.* New York: Pocket Books.

Friday, N. 1980. *Men in love: Men's sexual fantasies: The triumph of love over rage.* New York: Dell.

Friday, N. 1973. *My secret garden: Women's sexual fantasies.* New York: Pocket Books.

Frye, B. A., and B. Barham. 1975. Reaching out to pregnant adolescents. *American Journal of Nursing.* 75:1502–1504.

Gibney, H. A. 1972. Masturbation: An invitation for an interpersonal relationship. *Perspectives in Psychiatric Care* 10(3):128–134.

Goldman, R., and J. Goldman. 1982. Children's sexual thinking: Report of a cross-national study. *SIECUS Report* 10(3):1, 2, 7.

Goldman, R., and J. Goldman. 1982. *Children's Sexual Thinking.* London: Routledge & Kegan Paul.

Gould, L. 1980. X. *Ms.,* May, 61–64.

Green, R. 1977. Atypical sexual identity: The "feminine" boy and the "masculine" girl. In *The sexual and gender development of young children,* ed. E. K. Oremland and J. D. Oremland. Cambridge, Mass.: Ballinger.

Hawkins, J., and L. Higgins. 1981. *Maternity and gynecological nursing: Women's health care.* Philadelphia: Lippincott.

Heisler, A. B., and S. B. Friedman. 1980. Adolescence: Psychological and social development. *The Journal of School Health* 50:381–385.

Herold, E. S., and M. S. Goodwin. 1981. Reasons given by female virgins for not having premarital intercourse. *The Journal of School Health* 51:496–500.

Hite, S. 1976. *The Hite report: A nationwide study of female sexuality.* New York: Dell.

Hite, S. 1982. *The Hite report on male sexuality.* New York: Ballantine.

Jensen, G. D. 1981. Teenagers' fears that they are homosexual. *Medical Aspects of Human Sexuality* 15(5):47–48.

Juhasz, A. M. 1975. Sexual decision-making: The crux of the adolescent problem. In *Studies in adolescence: A book of readings in adolescent development.* 3rd ed., ed. R. E. Grinder. New York: Macmillan.

Katchadourian, H. 1980. Adolescent sexuality. *Pediatric Clinics of North America* 27:17–28.

Kinsey, A. C., W. B. Pomeroy, and C. E. Martin. 1948. *Sexual behavior in the human male.* Philadelphia: Saunders.

Kinsey, A. C., W. B. Pomeroy, C. E. Martin, and P. H. Gebhard. [1953] 1965. *Sexual behavior in the human female.* New York: Pocket Books.

Kleeman, J. A. 1965. A boy discovers his penis. *Psychoanalytic Study of the Child* 20:239–265.

Klein, J. R. 1980. Update: Adolescent gynecology. *The Pediatric Clinics of North America* 27:141–152.

Krafft-Ebing, R. V. 1922. *Psychopathia sexualis: A medico forensic study.* Brooklyn, N.Y.: Physicians and Surgeons Book Co.

Kuhn, J. 1982. Stress factors preceding postpartum psychosis: A case study of an unwed adolescent. *Maternal-Child Nursing Journal* 11.

Leppink, M. A. 1979. Adolescent sexuality. *Maternal-Child Nursing Journal* 8:153–161.

Lippe, B. M. 1979. Ambiguous genitalia and pseudohermaphroditism. *Pediatric Clinics of North America* 26:91–106.

Lipton, M. A. 1975. Pornography. In *Comprehensive textbook of psychiatry II,* ed. A. M. Freedman, H. I. Kaplan, and V. Sadock, vol. 2. Baltimore: Williams & Wilkins.

Marmor, J. 1975. Homosexuality and sexual orientation disturbances. In *Comprehensive textbook of psychiatry II,* ed. A. M. Freedman, H. I. Kaplan, and V. Sadock, vol. 2. Baltimore: Williams & Wilkins.

Martinson, F. M. 1977. Eroticism in childhood: A sociological perspective. In *The sexual and gender development of young children,* ed. E. K. Oremland and J. D. Oremland. Cambridge, Mass.: Ballinger.

Masters, W. H., and V. E. Johnson. 1979. *Homosexuality in perspective.* Boston: Little, Brown.

Masters, W. H., and V. E. Johnson. 1966. *Human sexual response.* Boston: Little, Brown.

May, R. 1980. *Sex and fantasy: Patterns of male and female development.* New York: Norton.

McAnarney, E. R., and R. A. Hockelman. 1979.

Conflicted adolescent premarital intercourse. An antecedent of mild anorexia nervosa. *Clinical Pediatrics* 18:340–342.

McCary, J. L., and S. P. McCary. 1982. *McCary's human sexuality.* 4th ed. Monterey, Calif.: Wadsworth.

Mead, M. 1949. *Male and female: A study of the sexes in a changing world.* New York: Dell.

Mead, M. [1935] 1950. Sex and temperament in three primitive societies. New York: Mentor Books.

Mercer, R. T. 1977. *Nursing care for parents at risk.* Thorofare, N. J.: Charles B. Slack.

Mercer, R. T. 1979. *Perspective on adolescent health care.* Philadelphia: Lippincott.

Mitchell, J. J. 1976. Adolescent intimacy. *Adolescence* 11:275–280.

Money, J. 1977. The "givens" from a different point of view: Lessons from intersexuality for a theory of gender identity. In *The sexual and gender development of young children,* ed. E. K. Oremland and J. D. Oremland. Cambridge, Mass.: Ballinger.

Money, J., and A. A. Ehrhardt. 1972. *Man and woman: Boy and girl.* Baltimore: Johns Hopkins University Press.

Moulton, R. 1975. Early papers on women: Horney to Thompson. *The American Journal of Psychoanalysis* 35:207–223.

Nass, G. D., R. W. Libby, and M. P. Fisher. 1981. *Sexual choices.* Monterey, Calif.: Wadsworth.

Peltz, M. 1977. Sexual and gender development in the latency years. In *The sexual and gender development of young children,* ed. E. K. Oremland and J. D. Oremland. Cambridge, Mass.: Ballinger.

Peltz, M. 1977. Sexual and gender development in the nursery school years. In *The sexual and gender development of young children,* ed. E. K. Oremland and J. D. Oremland. Cambridge, Mass.: Ballinger.

The Playboy Readers' Sex Survey, Part I. 1983. *Playboy,* Jan.

Prenatal sex determination implementation and implications. 1975. Evansville, Ind.: Mead Johnson.

Reagen, J. W., and M. Y. Olaizola. 1980. Using cytology to study DES daughters. *Contemporary OB/GYN* 15:95–103.

Rodgers, J. A. 1975. Struggling out of the feminine pluperfect. *American Journal of Nursing* 75:1655–1659.

Sadoff, R. L. Sex and the law. In *Comprehensive textbook of psychiatry II,* ed. A. M. Freedman, H. I. Kaplan, and V. Sadock, vol. 2. Baltimore: Williams & Wilkins.

Sanger, M. H. [1920] 1980. *What every girl should know.* New York: Belvedere.

Smith, P. B., M. L. Weinman, and D. M. Mumford. 1982. Social and affective factors associated with adolescent pregnancy. *The Journal of School Health* 52:90–93.

Spitz, R. A. 1949. Autoerotism. *Psychoanalytic Study of the Child* 3/4:85–120.

Storms, M. D., and E. Wasserman. 1982. Quoted in New theory of the causes of sexual orientation, ed. S. Prescod. *Sexuality Today* 6(5).

Tanner, J. M. 1978. *Education and physical growth.* New York: International Universities Press.

Tanner, J. M. 1962. *Growth at adolescence.* Oxford: Blackwell Scientific Publications.

Tausk, V. 1951. On masturbation. *The Psychoanalytic Study of the Child* 6:61–79.

Tavris, C., and S. Sadd. 1977. *The Redbook Report on Female Sexuality,* New York: Delacorte.

Teen-age girls found reluctant to get sex advice. 1981. *New York Times,* 27 October C3.

Teenage Pregnancy: The problem that hasn't gone away. 1981. New York: The Alan Guttmacher Institute.

Tichy, A. M., and L. J. Malasanos. 1976. The physiologic role of hormones in puberty. *The American Journal of Maternal Child Nursing* 1:384–388.

Vandestienne, G. 1982. Breast reduction—when less is more. *Ms.,* 10(8):13–15.

Waiting for a male: It's conceivable. 1979. *Science News* 116(2):24.

Zellman, G. L. 1982. Public school programs for adolescent pregnancy and parenthood: An assessment. *Family Planning Perspectives* 14:15–21.

Adult Sexual Response

Barbara Tuttle

Introduction

Adolescence, characterized in physical terms by the changes that occur during puberty, is a time of preparation for adult sexual roles. The surge of hormones that assures the normal secondary sex characteristics of both males and females creates a new dimension of human sexuality: that of taking pleasure in and desiring others.

In later chapters, the wide variety of sexual behaviors and sexual problems will be discussed more fully. First, however, it will be helpful to understand the physiology of the natural, automatic sexual response potential available to every healthy adult regardless of sexual orientation or interpersonal status. Sexual responses cannot be willed; neither, given sufficient physical stimulation under circumstances ranging from neutral to erotic and in the absence of physical aberrations, will they be blocked, except by psychological interference. We will first examine the vascular and muscular changes of the sexual response cycle and then look at the hormonal, neuro-chemical, psychological, and interpersonal factors influencing the course of these responses. These factors pertain to all normal adult sexual response; Chapter 3 examines special considerations in older people's sexuality, and Chapters 6, 7, and 8 discuss pre-crisis, crisis, and post-crisis medical situations involving patients' sexuality.

Vascular and Muscular Changes in Sexual Response

Masters and Johnson published the findings of their landmark research in 1966 in *Human Sexual Response,* a difficult text which enumerates physiological changes leading to, during, and following orgasm. In the course of their research in the 1960s, they measured thousands of male and female responses. They categorized these under the "stages" of excitement, plateau, orgasm, and resolution. Building on their work, Kaplan (1979) states that although these stages are useful as descriptions of observable events, to understand the underlying physiological systems, it is more helpful to focus on desire, excitement, and orgasm.

In addition to Kaplan's "desire" stage, other theorists also mention a preexcitement "transitional" stage of psychological receptivity to erotic stimuli. Knoepfler (1981) explained a great number of cases of dysfunction during the desire stage as inability or unwillingness to receive erotic stimuli.

Although all these categories are useful when examining theories about the psychological, neurological, hormonal, vascular, and muscular determinants of sexual response, we will use a progression of measurable physical changes in males and females (see Figures 2-1 and 2-2) as a framework for examining what happens during sexual arousal. Masters and Johnson found that the primary physiological changes in sexual response are caused by vascular congestion, while the secondary changes are due to muscle tension (see Tables 2-1 and 2-2 for a list of physiological changes based on Masters and Johnson's research).

The Excitement Phase

There are both similarities and differences in males' and females' sexual response patterns. The first sign of the excitement phase for

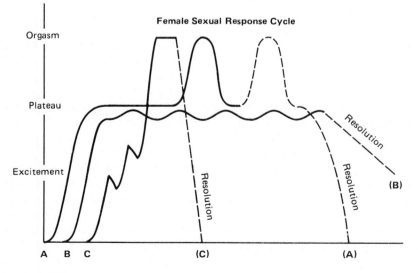

FIGURE 2-1
Female sexual response cycle.

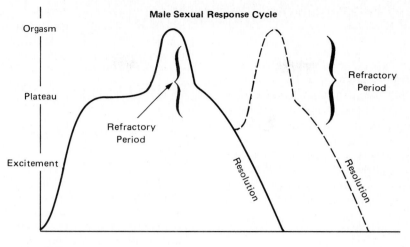

FIGURE 2-2
Male sexual response cycle.

males is erection; for females it is lubrication within the vagina (less easily noticed). These rapid changes are caused by the dilation of genital blood vessels. Both males and females may also experience other vascular and muscle changes: nipple erection, swelling and increased sensitivity of the external genitals, swelling of the breasts (females), and elevation of the testicles and thickening of the scrotum (males). To analyze these responses in greater detail, we will examine each sex separately.

Female

Vaginal lubrication is the first response a female exhibits when she experiences psychological or physical stimulus she deems erotic. Within the first 10 to 30 seconds of such stimuli, vasocongestion within the estrogen-rich mucosal lining causes a transudation of fluid — a "sweating" response within the vagina. There are no secretory glands in the vaginal walls that produce lubrication (Kolodny, Masters, and Johnson 1979). Another early genital change caused by the increasing vascular congestion is swelling of the labia

minora. Extragenital body changes include nipple erection (not always both simultaneously) and an increased definition and extension of the breast venous pattern, especially in nulliparous women. The heart rate starts to increase due to this parasympathetic activation and blood pressure elevation begins and will continue until orgasm; the amount of increase correlates to the rising tension.

The excitement phase may be quite brief or of long duration (see Figure 2-3). As this phase progresses, the vascular congestion causes flattening of the rugal pattern of the vaginal walls, they deepen in color, and the vagina lengthens and distends. The uterus, which has developed some excitability, partially elevates into the false pelvis. It should be remembered that the vagina contains a potential, rather than actual, space. These changes cause an enlargement in vaginal size which, along with the production of increased lubrication, prepare the vagina for intercourse and allow it to accommodate any size penis.

The clitoral glans becomes tumescent; the reaction is more rapid and extensive with direct stimulation. There is usually a distinct

TABLE 2-1   *Female Sexual Response**

	Vascular Congestion	Muscle Tension
Excitement	Nipples become erect; breasts increase in size; areolar engorgement; sex flush. Increase in heart rate and blood pressure. Engorgement of labia majora and minora, with movement away from vaginal outlet. Increase in clitoral diameter. Beginning of lubrication; lengthening and distending of vagina.	Some voluntary tension as stimulative attempts. Uterus partially elevates; uterine excitability develops.
Plateau	Vasocongestion maintained, with some increases (except for slowed lubrication). Sex flush spreads. Secretions from Bartholin's glands. Increase in uterine size. Mucosa at lower third of vagina engorges as part of orgasmic platform.	Hyperventilation. Increase in general and specific tension; carpopedal spasm. Contraction/contortion of arms, legs, neck, and face. Retraction of clitoris. Full elevation of uterus. Pubococcygeus muscle increases in tension as part of orgasmic platform.†
Orgasm	Blood pressure and heart rate at maximum, for that episode.	Hyperventilation at maximum. Loss of voluntary control: contractions/spasms of muscle groups including rectum, orgasmic platform, and uterus. An initial contraction of the outer third of the vagina and possibly further contractions at 0.8 second intervals may follow; number of contractions depends on intensity of the orgasm. Involuntary distention of urethral meatus.
Resolution	Widespread moisture film appears; not related to exertion. Sex flush, sex skin disappear. Decrease in breast size; involution of nipple erection. Return of labia majora to midline position. Clitoral detumescence (slower). Descent of anterior vaginal wall. Orgasmic platform rapidly disperses. Loss of uterine congestion.	Voluntary muscle tension release. Involuntary muscle tension release (slower). Clitoris returns to pudendal overhang position. Rapid descent of uterus; gaping of cervical os. Orgasmic platform disperses.

* The above data are derived from Masters and Johnson (1966) and have been separated into categories of primary (vasocongestive) and secondary (myotonic) system changes, based on Kaplan's (1974) biphasic emphasis. Her third phase, desire, is not included here, as there appears to be little vascular or muscle involvement before the excitement state.
† See Perry and Whipple (1981).

TABLE 2-2 *Male Sexual Response**

	Vascular Congestion	Muscle Tension
Excitement	Heart rate and blood pressure increase. Penile erection. Constriction and thickening of scrotal sac.	Some voluntary tension for stimulative attempts. Distention of urethral meatus. Partial elevation and rotation of testes.
Plateau	Sex flush (25% incidence). Erection may be partly lost/regained. Increase in coronal tumescence and testicular size. Secretions from Cowper's gland.	Hyperventilation. Carpopedal spasm. Muscles of legs, arms, abdomen, neck, and face contort/contract. Complete elevation of testes.
Orgasm	Heart rate and blood pressure at maximum, for that episode.	Hyperventilation at maximum. Contractions of vas deferens, seminal vesicles, prostate. Increase in size of urethral bulb. Urinary sphincter closes. External bladder sphincter relaxes; fluid propelled from urethral bulb and penile urethra. Contractions of perineal bulbospongiosus and ischiocavernosus muscles and urethral sphincter. Penile contractions occur at approximately 0.8 second intervals to expel semen.
Resolution	Sex flush disappears. Involuntary perspiratory reaction, not related to exertion. Loss of some of penile tumescence (another ejaculation not possible) with slower return to unstimulated size. Scrotal detumescence.	Voluntary muscle tension release. Involuntary muscle tension release (slower). Descent of testes.

* The above data are derived from Masters and Johnson (1966) and have been separated into categories of primary (vasocongestive) and secondary (myotonic) system changes, based on Kaplan's (1974) biphasic emphasis. Her third phase, desire, is not included here, as there appears to be little vascular or muscle involvement before the excitement state.

increase in the diameter of the clitoral shaft, and, in some cases, it also elongates.

As the labia minora swell to cause an actual extension of the vaginal barrel, the labia majora also become congested, flattening and elevating away from the vaginal opening. This is more marked in multiparous females (Masters and Johnson 1966, 146).

Throughout her body, the female exhibits further changes due to increases in vascular congestion. The nulliparous female experiences an increase in breast size, and most females experience some areolar engorgement.

Indeed, this can be so pronounced as to partially or completely obscure the nipple erection. A "sex flush" also appears on most females. This is a maculopapular rash which starts on the epigastrium, spreads to the breasts, neck, and face, and later may extend further.

Male

Within the first 30 seconds after a male experiences either psychological or physiological stimuli he deems erotic, he begins to experi-

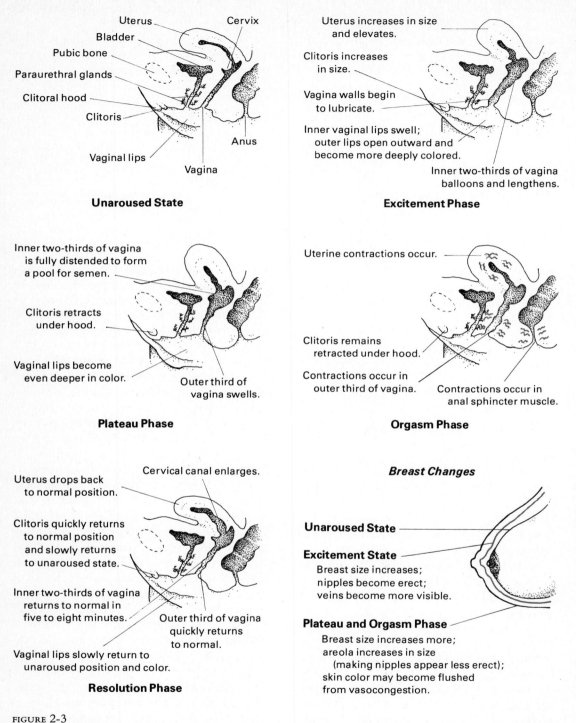

Unaroused State

Uterus
Cervix
Bladder
Pubic bone
Paraurethral glands
Clitoral hood
Clitoris
Anus
Vaginal lips
Vagina

Excitement Phase

Uterus increases in size and elevates.

Clitoris increases in size.

Vagina walls begin to lubricate.

Inner vaginal lips swell; outer lips open outward and become more deeply colored.

Inner two-thirds of vagina balloons and lengthens.

Plateau Phase

Inner two-thirds of vagina is fully distended to form a pool for semen.

Clitoris retracts under hood.

Vaginal lips become even deeper in color.

Outer third of vagina swells.

Orgasm Phase

Uterine contractions occur.

Clitoris remains retracted under hood.

Contractions occur in outer third of vagina.

Contractions occur in anal sphincter muscle.

Resolution Phase

Cervical canal enlarges.

Uterus drops back to normal position.

Clitoris quickly returns to normal position and slowly returns to unaroused state.

Inner two-thirds of vagina returns to normal in five to eight minutes.

Outer third of vagina quickly returns to normal.

Vaginal lips slowly return to unaroused position and color.

Breast Changes

Unaroused State

Excitement State
Breast size increases; nipples become erect; veins become more visible.

Plateau and Orgasm Phase
Breast size increases more; areola increases in size (making nipples appear less erect); skin color may become flushed from vasocongestion.

FIGURE 2-3
Female sexual response.

SOURCE: From *Sexual Choices,* 2nd ed., by G. D. Nass, R. W. Libby, and M. P. Fisher. Copyright © 1984, 1981 by Wadsworth, Inc. Reprinted by permission of the publisher, Wadsworth Health Sciences, Monterey, California.

ence his first vasocongestive change: the beginning of an erection. The penis is comprised of two corpora cavernosa, the corpus spongiosum (which contains the urethra) and the glans, all contained in a dense fascial covering. When parasympathetic activation causes arterial dilation, the inflow of blood into the vascular spaces in the erective corpora causes erection of the penis. This erection is maintained if outflow and inflow maintain a state of equilibrium. Vasocongestion in the scrotal sac skin causes a reduction of the ridges (rugae) and some flattening due to thickening of the integument. The male also starts experiencing increases in heart rate and blood pressure, caused by the rising tension.

In a sense, erection is a great equilizer. Masters and Johnson found that smaller penises underwent a greater increase in size than did large penises, and thus they became much more similar in size. The appearance of the erection does not mean the male is immediately desirous of intercourse, but only that intercourse becomes possible.

As in the female, the male's excitement phase may be very brief, or may be a long period of rising tension. During the latter, a male's erection may partially or completely be lost and regained several times. This can be worrisome for the male who doesn't understand that even during growing excitement, the degree of fullness still depends on the inflow and outflow of blood to the penis; sometimes this relationship may be out of balance. Loss of part of the erection is especially likely if asexual, distracting stimuli are perceived; however, refocus on erotic stimuli will aid in regaining a firm erection.

During this period of maximum vasocongestive change, there is some distension of the urethral meatus, as the penis lengthens and increases in diameter. The testes, in the constricting scrotal sac, partially elevate toward the perineum and rotate anteriorly and the spermatic cords shorten (see Figure 2-4). Some

males may experience erection of their nipples at this time, although no breast engorgement was reported by Masters and Johnson.

For both males and females, there is little involuntary muscle tension during the excitement phase. However, there may be voluntary contractions of muscle groups in the perineal area in an attempt to increase stimulation. General body tension can build slowly or quickly during the excitement phase (for typical patterns, see Figures 2-1 and 2-2).

The Plateau Phase

Plateau is the prolongation of excitement at a continuously high level, just below the threshold for orgasm. In either sex, it may be brief or may be of longer duration, if sufficient stimulation continues. Again, erection may come and go during this phase and lubrication in the female may vary or even subside at times. This stage is marked not only by continued vasocongestion but also by increased muscle tension, which is the second important physiological concomitant of sexual response. Indeed, the increase in general and specific myotonia as a high level of excitement is reached is what distinguishes this stage. Excitement continues at this high plateau until the threshold of tension precipitating orgasm is attained, if sufficient stimulation continues, or until the changes slowly reverse, if stimulation ceases. Not only do high levels of general body tension distinguish this plateau phase for both males and females, but so do contractions of specific muscle groups. A gripping reflex of the hands (and feet) called "carpopedal spasm" may occur, particularly when in a supine position. Late in the plateau phase, hyperventilation (respiratory rates up to 40 per minute), tachycardia (rates from 110 to 180), and blood pressure elevation (increases in systolic of 30 to 100 mm Hg and diastolic of 20 to 50 mm Hg) may occur or become much more

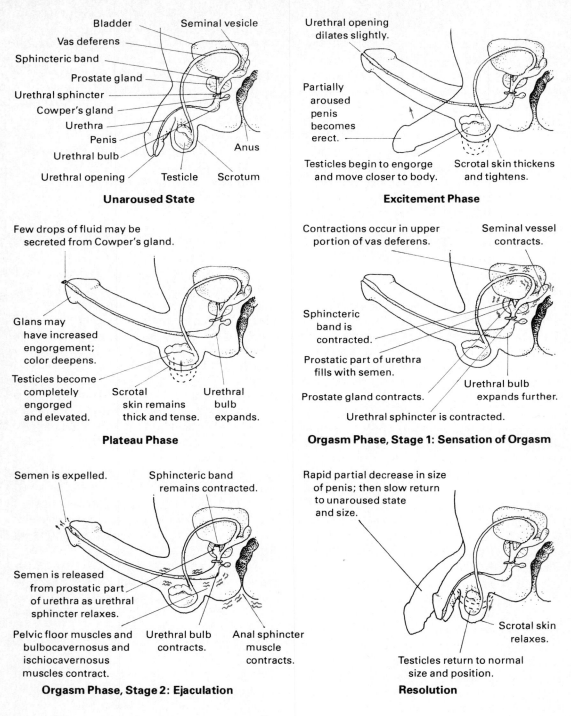

Unaroused State

- Bladder
- Seminal vesicle
- Vas deferens
- Sphincteric band
- Prostate gland
- Urethral sphincter
- Cowper's gland
- Urethra
- Penis
- Urethral bulb
- Urethral opening
- Testicle
- Scrotum
- Anus

Excitement Phase

Urethral opening dilates slightly.

Partially aroused penis becomes erect.

Testicles begin to engorge and move closer to body.

Scrotal skin thickens and tightens.

Plateau Phase

Few drops of fluid may be secreted from Cowper's gland.

Glans may have increased engorgement; color deepens.

Testicles become completely engorged and elevated.

Scrotal skin remains thick and tense.

Urethral bulb expands.

Orgasm Phase, Stage 1: Sensation of Orgasm

Contractions occur in upper portion of vas deferens.

Seminal vessel contracts.

Sphincteric band is contracted.

Prostatic part of urethra fills with semen.

Prostate gland contracts.

Urethral bulb expands further.

Urethral sphincter is contracted.

Orgasm Phase, Stage 2: Ejaculation

Semen is expelled.

Sphincteric band remains contracted.

Semen is released from prostatic part of urethra as urethral sphincter relaxes.

Pelvic floor muscles and bulbocavernosus and ischiocavernosus muscles contract.

Urethral bulb contracts.

Anal sphincter muscle contracts.

Resolution

Rapid partial decrease in size of penis; then slow return to unaroused state and size.

Scrotal skin relaxes.

Testicles return to normal size and position.

FIGURE 2-4
Male sexual response.

SOURCE: From *Sexual Choices,* 2nd ed., by G. D. Nass, R. W. Libby, and M. P. Fisher. Copyright © 1984, 1981 by Wadsworth, Inc. Reprinted by permission of the publisher, Wadsworth Health Sciences, Monterey, California.

pronounced (Masters and Johnson 1966, 277–278). Muscle conractions of the extremities may occur and contortion of the facial muscles may cause a grimacing effect.

Female

During this stage the vagina continues to have minor increases in width and depth in a "ballooning" of its inner two-thirds. Further elevation of the uterus causes a "tenting" effect of the inner anterior wall over the potential "seminal pool" in midvagina (see Figure 2-3).

The outer one-third of the vagina narrows due to increasing vasocongestive swelling to form what Masters and Johnson (1966) labeled the "orgasmic platform." This swelling creates a gripping action on the penis during intercourse, another example of how the vagina accommodates itself to any size penis.

The Bartholin's glands may secrete one to two drops of mucoid fluid near the vaginal opening at this time, especially during intercourse. The labia minora undergoes a decided color change, which is referred to as the "sex skin," increasing to bright red (nulliparous) or a deep wine color (multiparous). The labia majora may continue to increase in size.

The clitoris retracts under the clitoral hood until it is completely hidden. Although the new position against the pubic symphysis may hide it from sight or direct touch by self or partner, stimulation to the mons area and labia or continued stimulation of the attached labia minora-clitoral hood structures through penile thrusting can bring continued stimulation of the clitoris. Although many positions used during intercourse do not allow enough clitoral stimulation, a change in position or manual manipulation of the mons area can bring sufficient stimulation to proceed to orgasm. As will be discussed more fully later, stimulation of an especially sensitive area of the vagina may also lead to orgasm.

During the plateau stage, the sex flush may spread to the abdomen, shoulders, buttocks, thighs, and back; females may experience a further increase in breast size, particularly if they have never nursed a child.

Male

As the plateau phase continues in the male, there is a slight increase in tumescence of the coronal (ridge) of the glans penis, sometimes accompanied by a darkening in color (see Figure 2-4). The testes complete their anterior rotation and elevation to a point where they rest firmly against the perineum. Cowper's glands secretion also frequently occurs, with the release of a few drops of fluid from the urethral meatus. Kolodny, Masters, and Johnson (1979) observed that this secretion sometimes contains live spermatozoa, which is important to note since many couples use withdrawal of the penis as a form of birth control.

When a male exhibits a sex flush, it usually occurs on the epigastrium during the late plateau phase. This maculopapular rash sometimes spreads to the chest, neck, and face.

Orgasm

When sufficient physical and psychological stimulation continues past the critical threshold levels of tension, orgasm occurs. Both males and females experience a series of genital contractions during orgasm, and the male ejaculates during this phase. Since most validated research has focused on males, we will examine male orgasm first.

Male

The male, it may be recalled, is at the near maximum (for that sexual episode) of heart rate (110 to 180 beats per minute), blood pressure (an increase of 40 to 100 mm Hg systolic and 20 to 50 mm Hg diastolic), and muscular tension just before orgasm. Sex flush and nipple tumescence may have occurred, along with a darkening of the coronal area of the penis. The testes are completely elevated and the male may be hyperventilating, with respiratory rates up to 40 per minute (Masters and Johnson 1966, 277–278).

The male next experiences the *emission stage* — a sensation Masters and Johnson called "the moment of ejaculatory inevitability." As the urethral bulb increases in size, contraction of the internal (secondary) organs causes seminal fluid to be deposited in the prostatic urethra, whereupon the internal urinary sphincter closes (preventing retroflex ejaculation to the bladder). This causes the sensation of imminent ejaculation. Indeed, the sequence of physiological events is now usually inevitable and cannot be halted, except by those men who have learned to consciously withhold ejaculation (Robbins and Jensen 1978).

In the usual course of events, *ejaculation* follows emission. Immediately after emission of fluid to the prostatic urethra, the external bladder sphincter relaxes and the fluid flows into the urethral bulb and urethra. Strong contractions of the muscles at the base of the penis (perineal, bulbospongiosus, and ischiocavernosus) propel and expel the ejaculate. The contractions start at 0.8 second intervals and continue with decreasing force and frequency for several seconds. Similar involuntary contractions of the rectal sphincter occur simultaneously. About two-thirds to three-quarters of a teaspoon (3 to 5 ml) of ejaculate is the average amount expelled (extra fluid observed after intercourse actually results from the more copious female lubrication). The ejaculation phase is accompanied by very pleasurable subjective sensations (see Figure 2-4).

Female

Female orgasm is still less well-understood than male orgasm, but it is known that the physiology corresponds more closely with male functioning than was previously thought. Like the male, the female at high levels of excitement is near maximum (for that episode) levels of muscular tension, blood pressure, and heart rate, and is also straining for release of this tension. Masters and Johnson (1966) found that sufficient clitoral stimulation, whether accompanied by vaginal stimulation or not, resulted in involuntary contractions of the orgasmic platform and rectal sphincter (depending on intensity of the experience) at the same 0.8 second intervals experienced by males during ejaculation, accompanied by pleasurable sensations. Female contractions were found to occur three to 15 times, with diminishing strength and frequency.

Graber and Kline-Graber (1979) note that the orgasmic platform contractions of the female orgasm are due to the pubococcygeus muscle, which underlies the engorged mucosa. Kegel (1952) had studied this muscle intensively and had recommended specific exercises to strengthen the muscle in order to improve muscle tone and sexual feeling (see Figure 2-5). Similarities between the pelvic floor muscles of the male and female are shown in Figure 2-6.

In addition to contractions of the orgasmic platform and rectal sphincter, there also is involuntary distension of the urethral meatus and contraction of the uterus (Masters and Johnson 1966). These uterine contractions start at the fundus, continue through the midline, and end at the lower segment, in a way similar to uterine contractions during labor (see Figure 2-3).

Theorists such as Kaplan (1979) have stressed the similarities of male and female responses. Kaplan postulated that the two parts of male orgasm were mediated by different neurological mechanisms — emission by the sympathetic nervous system and the smooth muscles of the reproductive organs, and ejaculation by an unrelated unknown re-

Kegel Exercises for Females

1. Insert one finger into the opening of your vagina. Contract the vaginal muscles so that you can feel them squeeze your finger. Remove your finger, contract the same muscles, and hold the contraction for 3 seconds. Relax. Repeat this sequence 10 times.
2. Quickly contract and release the same muscles 10 to 25 times. Relax and repeat.
3. While imagining what it would feel like to draw something into your vagina, contract the muscles that would be involved. Hold the contraction for 3 seconds. Relax. Repeat this sequence 10 times.

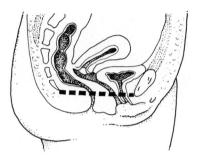
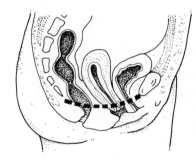

Female with Good Tone in Pelvic Floor Muscles   **Female with Poor Tone in Pelvic Floor Muscles**

FIGURE 2-5
Kegel (pelvic floor) exercises for females.

SOURCE: From *Sexual Choices,* 2nd ed., by G. D. Nass, R. W. Libby, and M. P. Fisher. Copyright © 1984, 1981 by Wadsworth, Inc. Reprinted by permission of the publisher, Wadsworth Health Sciences, Monterey, California.

flex stimulation of the striated muscles. She claimed the latter mechanisms also controlled the female orgasm. Other researchers have been looking for female physiological changes corresponding to both the emission and ejaculation phases occurring in males, as well as other parallels between males and females during the orgasm stage, for the following reasons:

1. During the fetal development, the same types of tissue differentiate into different genital/reproductive structures; however, the underlying vascular and muscular components remain remarkably similar.
2. Many of the extragenital changes during sex response are almost identical.

3. As the neurological components of response have become better understood, innervation of vascular and muscle changes during excitement and plateau stages have shown definite parallels.
4. During resolution (the release of tension following orgasm, to be discussed in the next section), reversal of changes also occurs in similar fashion, with the main differences due to the male's refractory period.

Although results of the many new findings have not been compiled into a more comprehensive explanation of female orgasm, some of the research has produced interesting, even startling, results. Freud's (1905) distinction

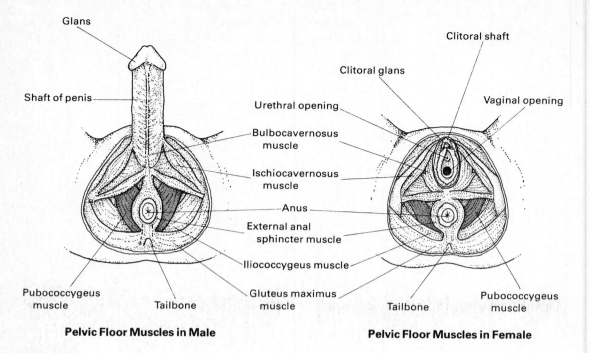

Pelvic Floor Muscles in Male

Pelvic Floor Muscles in Female

FIGURE 2-6
Pelvic floor muscles in male and female.

SOURCE: From *Sexual Choices*, 2nd ed., by G. D. Nass, R. W. Libby, and M. P. Fisher. Copyright © 1984, 1981 by Wadsworth, Inc. Reprinted by permission of the publisher, Wadsworth Health Sciences, Monterey, California.

between "clitoral" and "vaginal" orgasms has been one area of controversy. Grafenberg (1950) and Hoch (1980) found an area of increased sensitivity to stimulation along the anterior wall of the otherwise fairly insensitive vagina. Stimulation of this "G" spot (named for Grafenberg) was found to produce an excitement "of a different quality" but similar intensity to that of clitoral stimulation (Hoch 1980). Hoch also found some women for whom this "G spot" stimulation was more effective than direct clitoral stimulation. He reminds us that Kinsey (1953) also had mentioned this area of increased sensitivity. Although Kegel (1952) had mentioned vaginal sensitivity at the "4 and 8 o'clock" locations, recent research has not corroborated his findings (Hoch 1980; Perry and Whipple 1981). Hoch theorizes that his findings provide a link between "clitoral" and "vaginal" orgasms, stating that both clitoral and vaginal areas are part of the same sensory component of the orgasmic reflex (the muscular contractions being the motor component) (see Figure 2-3).

Gillian and Brindley (1979), during studies measuring vaginal vascular responses to clitoral vibratory stimulation, found sustained reflex contraction of the pelvic floor. They questioned whether this could be a counterpart to the contraction of the bulbocavernosus muscle in males.

Perry and Whipple (1981) suggest that two separate reflexive pathways mediate orgasm in both males (Kaplan 1974) and females. They hypothesize that the uterine contractions in females are a result of impulses via the pelvic nerve which activate the "G" spot, bladder, urethra, and the proximal portions of the pubococcygeus muscle. They suggest that the pudendal nerve discharge is activated by clitoral stimulation and affects the bulk of the pubococcygeus muscle.

More startling still have been the recent findings in the area of female "ejaculation." Sexologists have long known that many females experience loss of fluid through the urethral meatus during orgasm. It had long been thought that this fluid was urine, a concept that frequently led to much distress for the female, particularly when amounts were copious. Perry and Whipple (1981) are two of the latest researchers to note that this fluid does not appear to be urine; Grafenberg had mentioned this in 1950 when he attributed female ejaculation to secretions of the "intraurethral glands" in the anterior vaginal wall. He stated that stimulation of the Grafenberg spot was connected somehow with these urethral expulsions. Perry and Whipple have attempted to link this female "ejaculation" to the "uterine orgasm" (contractions of the uterus that are part of a woman's orgasmic response). Further research in this area is highly likely and should be helpful in increasing understanding of female orgasm. Whether two types of female orgasm really exist, are separable, and include (on occasion) ejaculation remains to be verified.

Sexual Response After Orgasm

Females and males differ in the amount of further sexual response possible after orgasm. Many females, on some occasions, are capable of successive orgasms if they remain at a plateau level and stimulation continues. Males, however, usually enter a "refractory" period, when a full erection may be regained but

ejaculation is impossible (Kolodny, Masters, and Johnson 1979). The refractory period usually increases in duration with age; it may be short or almost nonexistent in the young male. However, there is great variability between men and even between occasions with individual men.

Resolution

Right after orgasm, return to the former tensionless state happens quickly, with one additional change: both males and females may experience an immediate sweating. This film spreads over the body and is not related to exertion but is more like the appearance of transudate within the vagina early in the excitement. Some females also experience a slight continuation of lubrication at this time. Both of these responses may be related to existing vasocongestion during a time of rapid decrease in voluntary muscular tension. Deep congestive changes are slower to reverse than the more superficial vascular changes and the reduction of muscle tension (see Figures 2-3 and 2-4). If no orgasm occurs and stimulation ceases, the female's genitals take much longer to return to homeostasis than the male's. Without the tension release of orgasm, some vasocongestion may persist, sometimes for several hours. Although there may be some minor discomfort for both males and females if orgasm does not occur, there is nothing physically harmful about continued high levels of sexual arousal that are not followed by the orgasmic discharges of tension.

Cycle Variations

It is important to note that any time during excitement or plateau, decrease in the fullness of an erection may occur due to distractions or change in type of stimulation or of body position. These are not physical signs of lessening arousal. In the same manner, a decrease in lubrication can also occur in spite of the fact that the female may be attaining or maintaining high levels of arousal.

Any person is capable of many different patterns of response on different occasions. As Figures 2-1 and 2-2 show, the same person might experience a rapid build-up of excitement, a brief plateau stage, and a rapid resolution following orgasm on one occasion, and experience a more leisurely build-up of excitement, a high tension plateau phase of different duration, and might or might not have an orgasm before returning to homeostasis on another occasion. In addition, the underlying physiological levels of vasocongestion or myotonia may not correspond at all with the person's subjective experience. A female may be approaching plateau levels of excitement but, due to lack of awareness of her internal lubrication and of other genital changes, may be unaware of her arousal. Similarly, the ebb and flow of an erection may give false cues to a male or his partner about his level of excite-

ment. Situational factors—such as choice of partner, expectations, and distractions—also affect the subjective experience.

Age also has an effect on sexual responses. For example, a young adult male may have quicker responses, the possibility of a shorter refractory period, or firmer erections than he might experience in later life, but he can expect to remain sexually responsive throughout his life. Similarly, although a female may go through a reproductive cycle that has a profound effect on many aspects of her life, she, too, may expect to be sexually responsive for the rest of her life.

Hormonal Factors and Desire

One of the factors underlying sexual responsiveness is hormones. Although the effects of hormones upon sexual development and upon reproduction are well understood, ongoing research is needed to understand more clearly the role of the endocrine system on sexual

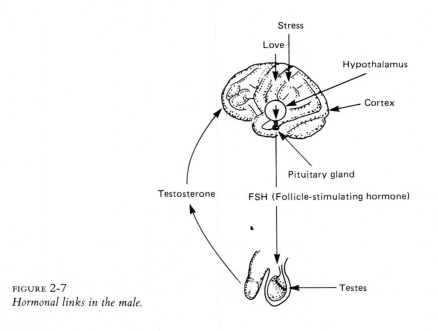

FIGURE 2-7
Hormonal links in the male.

behavior. Indeed, Masters and Johnson discussed postmenopausal hormonal changes in their landmark book (1966), but not the role hormones play in sexual functioning.

Kaplan (1979) stresses the role androgen plays, for both males and females, during the preexcitement "desire" phase. She states that in the absence of testosterone, there is little sexual desire, for either males or females. She also cites (1979) research indicating that luteinizing hormone releasing factor (LH-RF) may enhance sexual desire in the absence of testosterone. The mechanisms by which these hormones interact with neurotransmitters in the sex centers of the brain to increase desire are not yet clear, nor are the complex biological interactions that physically inhibit desire (see Figure 2-7).

Kolodny, Masters, and Johnson, in their excellent *Textbook of Sexual Medicine* (1979), stress that changes in sexual functioning may be the first symptoms indicating an underlying medical problem. Masters (1981) noted that low libido and impotence in several of his patients were symptoms of pituitary tumors or other pituitary abnormalities. The diagnoses were made based on low levels of testosterone with exceedingly high levels of prolactin.

Neuro-chemical Factors

Kaplan (1979) has also stressed the underlying neurological systems in her "triphasic" explanation of sexual response. She claims the sexual response cycle may be best understood when divided into desire, excitement, and orgasm phases based on different neural wiring circuits. She claims that the desire (receptive/initiating) phase is mediated by brain centers that have excitatory and inhibitory neurotransmitters which are interconnected with other parts of the brain similar to those mediating other drives. Thus, a person's total experiences, thoughts, and feelings can affect sexual desire and erotic feelings, and vice versa. Heiman's (1980) research with females in the areas of physiological arousal and subjective awareness of arousal led her to the hypotheses that these two entities fluctuate somewhat separately, and that if internal cues are ambiguous or weak, situational cues may be relied on to help the female interpret the presence of arousal. Therefore, she, too, indicates that cognitions may influence or be influenced by physiological responses (see Figure 2-8).

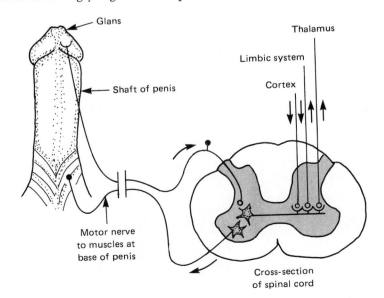

FIGURE 2-8
Sexual response reflexes for the male.

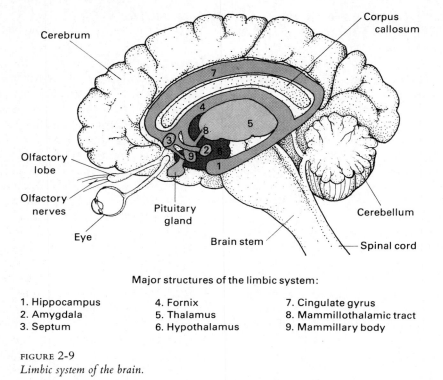

Major structures of the limbic system:

1. Hippocampus   4. Fornix   7. Cingulate gyrus
2. Amygdala   5. Thalamus   8. Mammillothalamic tract
3. Septum   6. Hypothalamus   9. Mammillary body

FIGURE 2-9
Limbic system of the brain.

SOURCE: From *Sexual Choices,* 2nd ed., by G. D. Nass, R. W. Libby, and M. P. Fisher.
Copyright © 1984, 1981 by Wadsworth, Inc. Reprinted by permission of the
publisher, Wadsworth Health Sciences, Monterey, California.

In contrast to the preexcitement phase mediation by brain centers, Kaplan claims the excitement and orgasm phases are produced by reflex vasocongestion and by reflex muscular contractions, mainly in the genital area. She states that arousal and orgasm are mediated by parasympathetic impulses involving two spinal cord centers ($s_2 s_3 s_4$ for arousal and T_{11}, T_{12}, $L_1 L_2$ for orgasm), which cause genital blood vessel dilation. She claims that orgasm has a separable reflex pattern, with efferent messages entering the sacral portion of the spinal cord (pudendal nerve) and efferent impulses arising from T_{11}-L_2. However, she also claims orgasm in the male is governed by sympathetic reflex systems and by the higher brain centers (see Figure 2-9). Kaplan's state-

ment that arousal is controlled by the parasympathetic system and orgasm by the sympathetic system is very important. Her work contributes to the ability of professionals to differentiate problems of desire, arousal, and orgasm in clients experiencing difficulties. It is possible for one phase to be experienced normally and another to be problematic.

Wiedeking, Ziegler, and Lake (1979) support the theory of sympathetic activity at the later stage of arousal, and Krosnick and Podolsky (1981) stress both parasympathetic and limbic (psychic) origins for excitement. Several parts of the nervous system are thus thought to be involved in sexual response. As Krosnick and Podolsky note, erection may occur due to psychic stimuli originating in the limbic area, while reflex erection occurs when stimulation of the penis activates impulses that travel to the spinal cord via the pudendal nerves. The ability of these systems to operate separately also makes it possible for a person to have inhibited response in just one of the phases: desire, excitement, or orgasm (Kaplan 1979).

While having different loci of control make the response cycle somewhat vulnerable, this also means that persons with lesions at one part of the spinal cord may still experience other parts of the response cycles, and persons psychologically inhibited from excitement may still experience erection and lubrication due to the parasympathetic reflex. Knowledge of the existence of varying control centers for sexual response is important from both a diagnostic and a treatment standpoint. For example, a change in sexual functioning may be the first indication of a major disease such as diabetes or multiple sclerosis (Lundburg 1981). In addition, health-care professionals should be aware that the sexual response cycle is vulnerable to a number of medications that affect sexual neurophysiology (Seagraves 1977).

Psychological and Interpersonal Factors

In addition to their biological aspects, adult sexual responses are influenced by psychological factors and the characteristics of past and present sexual interaction with others. The infant or young child may easily experience pleasure by touching all parts of his or her body, especially the genitals. Before such behavior is socially discouraged, pleasure is easily obtained and is a natural part of early experience. The adult, however, may have accumulated layers of prohibitions, myths, memories of discomfort, or interpersonal sexual conflicts, all of which affect the way he or she thinks about his or her own identity as a sexual being. These thoughts, feelings, and experiences comprise the personal sex value system which determine one's receptivity to opportunities for sexual stimulation (Sarrel and Sarrel 1979).

Other factors such as depression, illness, fatigue, and environmental changes or pressures may affect a person's interest in sexual activity. An example could be the numerous effects of a recent pregnancy on the parents' sexual interest: the mother's absorption in her new child; the possibility of painful intercourse due to birth trauma to the vagina and her lower level of estrogen, resulting in vaginal dryness; the ongoing physical demands of nursing her baby and the fatigue associated with round-the-clock feedings; her husband's pressure to return to a more active sexual life; his adjustments to a sexual partner who is now a mother and his own concerns about being a good father; the disappearance of uninterrupted privacy; the increased financial responsibility; and fear of another pregnancy too soon. These potential influences are examples of how a major life event can affect the willingness of one or both partners to engage in sexual behavior, even in a "happy" marriage in which both partners are in good health.

Under ordinary circumstances, the first factors necessary for a complete sexual response cycle are unimpaired physical capability to respond, a psychological willingness to engage in sexual activity, receptivity to stimuli considered erotic, and (except for autoerotic behavior) the presence of a willing partner in an environment conducive to intimacy.

Some physiological responses may be caused by high stress even though the above factors are absent. For instance, erections may accompany fear during battle in much the same way urination or defecation can occur. Increases in vascular activity and muscle tension at such times make such a response possible and may bewilder the male who confuses the reflexive nature of such an erection with a response to erotic stimuli.

On the other hand, sexual response may not occur even when it is ostensibly desired by both partners. In such situations, sometimes sexual responsiveness is blocked by subtle interpersonal fears, resentments, or hostilities between the sexes. The Goldmans (1982) found a surprisingly high degree of hostility between young boys and girls which they thought might be a reflection of sexual hostility in the adult world. One might wonder whether that hostility may be due less to childhood psychological development than to social factors such as control and sex role competition.

Women may have learned to assume a rather passive role in sexual activities, and they have frequently felt lack of ownership of their own anatomy. This sense of lack of control over their bodies may be due partly to the fact that their genitals are hard for them to observe, and partly to the paternalism of male doctors. Along with male scientists and theorists, male doctors have often decided how women feel, or ought to feel, during sex.

Men, too, have suffered from stereotypical views of their sexual physiology. Historically, much pressure has been placed on the male's ability to respond with an erection at any time, and proceed to orgasm. Unlike females, males have frequently not been allowed to show vulnerability — physical or psychological — and so have often been more cautious in showing their emotions in intimate relationships. Both sexes have suffered from the unfortunate existence of competition and goal orientation in their sexual behaviors.

The clinical significance of present interpersonal behavior has only been a major focus of psychology and therapy since the 1950s. Previously, theorists and researchers concentrated on individuals almost as if their sexual responses occurred in a vacuum; for example, the only influence noted about the effects of significant others was from childhood. Now, the interactions with significant others throughout a lifetime are seen to have primary importance for individuals in terms of psychological validation, social identity, and physical and mental health. New fields of interpersonal treatment have arisen, such as family therapy, marital counseling, and sex therapy. Good interpersonal transactions are very important for a healthy self-image, which, in turn, affect one's ability to cope with life events. Good interpersonal functioning and a good self-image cannot be overstressed because they are of prime importance in determining one's quality of living; a person's sex value system is of prime importance to both. The "sex value system" is based on an individual's sexual thoughts, feelings, experiences, and activities. It is the basis for each person's beliefs about his or her own sexuality and expectations about sexual activities with others (Sarrel and Sarrel 1979).

Historically, sexual activity has frequently been fraught with anxiety, frustration, and disappointment because of the lack of information people have had about what is "normal" sexual behavior. Kinsey and his associates (1948, 1953) made the first major contributions to this area of knowledge in their reports detailing who did what with whom and when. Hite's reports (1976, 1982) went further, and focused on what males and females think, feel, and like about sex. Still, all individuals continue to have different sex value systems and may experience great distress when differing expectations collide. As Friday points out in her books about male and female fantasies (1973, 1975, 1980), the longing men and women feel for each other is marked by ambivalence that started in earliest childhood and continues throughout adulthood, as each sex tries to understand the other while meeting needs of its own.

Holistic Understanding of Sexual Response

Theorists and researchers from many different philosophical vantage points have been involved in attempts to understand and explain sexual functioning. Freud considered it in a psychoanalytic framework and found sexual drives to be genetically determined and adult sexual behavior to be based on the psychological development of early childhood. The Goldmans, focusing on psychosocial development within an Eriksonian mode, have found social learning to be of primary importance. Bell, in attempts to understand homosexual behavior, has focused on both biological determinism (hormonal effects on the fetus) and on later childhood interpersonal attachments. Barbach (1980) and Kegel have shown that cognitive learning also influences sexual functioning for adults; Barbach has shown clinically that females can learn orgasmic response, while Kegel has indicated that females can increase orgasmic pleasure by strengthening the pubococcygeus muscle.

Describing sexual behaviors and roles has been the province of other theorists and researchers. Mead has shown the effects of cultural determinants. Kinsey, Hite, and others have indicated the wide range and incidence of specific behaviors and have given us more knowledge about the affective components of sexual response. Heiman has stressed the interplay of physiology, emotions, and context.

Masters and Johnson established a whole new field of scientific inquiry when they undertook their landmark research on the physiology of sexual functioning. Many researchers are following in their footsteps, studying both normal functioning (Perry and Whipple, Hoch) and dysfunction (Seagraves, Lundberg).

Kaplan, the Sarrels, and the LoPiccolos (1978) have joined Masters and Johnson in publishing books relating their theories and experiences in applying psychotherapy to the treatment of sexual dysfunction. Kolodny, Masters, and Johnson have attempted to show the effects of illness and disease on sexual functioning.

From all of these sources we may see that sexuality is physical, cognitive, affective, and behavioral; it is multidetermined, possibly influenced by unconscious drives, genetic factors and hormonal events, social context, and expectation. As Sarrel (1975) notes, being sexual is a life-long process; each human has the potential for natural sexual response including orgasm (ejaculation requires physical maturity) from early childhood through old age. Sexual response occurs in the same manner whether it is a result of heterosexual or homosexual contact or automanipulation (which usually results in more intense responses). Sexual response also happens during sleep, as well as when we are awake.

Males and females have equal potential to be sexually responsive. Evolution has provided humans with advances and trade-offs: we, alone, are capable of continuous arousability, but we are also subject to psychological interference, including fear of intimacy. With this increase in desire and the ability to choose or abstain from sex, we have also developed guilt, shame, and socially enforced proscriptions. As we have developed countless variations in arousability and behavior, we have also developed psychologically caused dysfunctions.

Throughout life, sexual functioning and behaviors will be influenced by myriad factors: money, religion, law, age, trauma, developmental experiences, interpersonal relations, role, body image and self-esteem, family behavior patterns, peer pressures, exposure to erotic imagery, life cycle events, and disuse. It is important to remember that these may be just as influential in determining sexual functioning as injuries, fatigue, general nutrition, chemical use (medications, alcohol, or drugs), clinical depression or anxiety, endocrine balance, disease, or disability. It is also important for health-care providers to be sensitive to patients' subjective experiences and responses affecting their lives as well as to their physiological functioning.

Summary of Implications for Nursing Practice

Through evolution, humans have moved from just procreational to recreational and relational aspects of sexuality. Touch is still extremely important to the quality of human life and growth. As Lief (1975) notes, the pleasures of all the senses, the experiences of being touched, and the rewards of an intimate relationship are all just as important as orgasm, and all parts of the body, not just the genitals, are important in the giving and receiving of pleasure. Nurses need to be aware of this importance, particularly when giving care to patients whose debilitation is depriving them of basic physical comforts. Sensitivity here can promote the well-being of the patient through the judicious use of touch, while avoiding either unconscious sexual stimulation or increasing feelings of isolation or rejection in the patient.

Sexual functioning is probably the most complex and varied of all human behaviors. It may be terribly important to an individual and still not mentioned to a health-care giver. In order to encourage patients to be open about their sexual problems or concerns, providers must become knowledgeable about and comfortable with all aspects of human sexual expression. Providers must also take responsibility for introducing the subject of sexuality and conveying its appropriateness as a topic of concern for the patient. Patients are often embarrassed to initiate discussion, and yet are relieved when concerns can be openly discussed. Perhaps most important, giving good care means being responsive to others, and that involves in-depth thinking about one's own sex value system and its effect on caring for others whose value systems may be different, but are equally important.

REFERENCES

Barbach, L. 1980. *Women discover orgasm.* New York: The Free Press.

Bell, A. P. 1982. Sexual preference: A postscript. *SIECUS Report* 11:1–3.

Bell, A. P., and M. S. Weinberg. 1978. *Homosexualities: A study of diversity among men and women.* New York: Simon & Schuster.

Freud, S. [1905] 1962. *Three essays on the theory of sexuality,* ed. J. Strachey. New York: Basic Books.

Friday, N. 1975. *Forbidden flowers: More women's sexual fantasies.* New York: Pocket Books.

Friday, N. 1980. *Men in love: Men's sexual fantasies: The triumph of love over rage.* New York: Dell.

Friday, N. 1983. *My secret garden: Women's sexual fantasies.* New York: Pocket Books.

Gillan, P., and G. S. Brindley. 1979. Vaginal and pelvic floor responses to sexual stimulation. *Psychophysiology* 16(5):471–481.

Goldman, R., and J. Goldman. 1982. Children's sexual thinking: Report of a cross-national study. *SIECUS Report* 10(3):1, 2, 7.

Graber, B., and G. Kline-Graber. 1979. Female orgasm: Role of pubococcygeus muscle. *Journal of Clinical Psychiatry* August:33–39.

Grafenberg, E. 1950. The role of urethra in female orgasm. *International Journal of Sexology,* vol. 3.

Heiman, J. 1980. Female sexual response patterns: Interactions of physiological, affective, and contextual cues. *Archives of General Psychiatry* 37(11):1311–1316.

Hite, S. 1976. *The Hite report: A nationwide study of female sexuality.* New York: Dell.

Hite, S. 1982. *The Hite report on male sexuality.* New York: Ballantine.

Hoch, Z. 1980. The sensory arm of the female orgasmic reflex. *Journal of Sex Education and Therapy* 6(1):4–7.

Kaplan, H. S. 1979. *Disorders of sexual desire and other new concepts and techniques in sex therapy.* New York: Simon & Schuster.

Kaplan, H. S. 1974. *The new sex therapy.* New York: Brunner/Mazel.

Kegel, A. H. 1952. Sexual functions of the pubococcygeus muscle. *Western Journal of Surgery, Obstetrics and Gynecology* 60:521–524.

Kinsey, A. C., C. E. Martin, W. B. Pomeroy, and P. H. Gebhard. 1953. *Sexual behavior in the human female.* Philadelphia and London: Saunders.

Kinsey, A. C., W. B. Pomeroy, and C. E. Martin. 1948. *Sexual behavior in the human male.* Philadelphia: Saunders.

Knoepfler, P. 1981. Transition: A prephase of the human sexual response cycle. *Journal of Sex Education and Therapy* 7(1):15–17.

Kolodny, R. C., W. H. Masters, and V. E. Johnson. 1979. *Textbook of sexual medicine.* Boston: Little, Brown.

Krosnick, A., and S. Podolsky. 1981. Diabetes and sexual dysfunction: Restoring normal ability. *Geriatrics* 36(3):92–100.

Lief, H. I. 1975. Introduction to sexuality. In *Comprehensive textbook of psychiatry II,* ed. A. M. Freedman, H. I. Kaplan, and V. Sadock, vol. 2. Baltimore: Williams & Wilkins.

LoPiccolo, J., and L. LoPiccolo. 1978. *Handbook of sex therapy.* New York and London: Plenum.

Lundberg, P. O. 1981. Sexual dysfunction in female patients with multiple sclerosis. *International Rehabilitation Medicine* 3(1):32–34.

Masters, W. 1981. Paper presented at the Seminar on Human Sexuality. Boston, 18 October.

Masters, W. H., and V. E. Johnson. 1966. *Human sexual response.* Boston: Little, Brown.

Mead, M. 1949. *Male and female: A study of the sexes in a changing world.* New York: Dell.

Perry, J. D., and B. Whipple. 1981. Pelvic muscle strength of female ejaculators: Evidence in support of a new theory of orgasm. *Journal of Sex Research* 17(1):22–39.

Robbins, M. B., and G. D. Jensen. 1978. Multiple orgasm in males. *Journal of Sex Research* 14(1):21–26.

Sarrel, L. J., and P. M. Sarrel. 1979. *Sexual unfolding.* Boston: Little, Brown.

Sarrel, P. M. 1975. Sexual physiology and sexual functioning. *Postgraduate Medicine* 58(1):67–72.

Seagraves, R. T. 1977. Pharmacological agents causing sexual dysfunction. *Journal of Sex and Marital Therapy* 3(3):157–176.

Wiedeking, C., M. G. Ziegler, and C. R. Lake. 1979. Plasma noradrenalin and dopamine-beta-hydroxylase during human sexual activity. *Journal of Psychiatric Research* 15(2):139–145.

BIBLIOGRAPHY

Barbach, L. 1975. *For yourself: The fulfillment of female sexuality.* New York: Signet.

Brecher, E. M. 1975. History of human sexual research and study. In *Comprehensive textbook of psychiatry II,* ed. A. M. Freedman, H. I. Kaplan, and V. Sadock, vol. 2. Baltimore: Williams & Wilkins.

Brecher, E. M. 1969. *The sex researchers.* Boston: Little, Brown.

Franzblau, A. N. 1975. Religion and sexuality. In *Comprehensive textbook of psychiatry II,* ed. A. M. Freedman, H. I. Kaplan, and V. Sadock, vol. 2. Baltimore: Williams & Wilkins.

Lipton, M. A. 1975. Pornography. In *Comprehensive textbook of psychiatry II,* ed. A. M. Freedman, H. I. Kaplan, and V. Sadock, vol. 2. Baltimore: Williams & Wilkins.

Marmor, J. 1975. Homosexuality and sexual orientation disturbances. In *Comprehensive textbook of psychiatry II,* ed. A. M. Freedman, H. I. Kaplan, and V. Sadock, vol. 2. Baltimore: Williams & Wilkins.

Masters, W. H., and V. E. Johnson. 1979. *Homosexuality in perspective.* Boston: Little, Brown.

Masters, W. H., and V. E. Johnson. 1970. *Human sexual inadequacy.* Boston: Little, Brown.

Money, J., and A. Ehrhardt. 1972. *Man and woman, boy and girl: The differentiation and dimorphism of gender identity from conception to maturity.* Baltimore: Johns Hopkins University Press.

Sadoff, R. L. 1975. Sex and the law. In *Comprehensive textbook of psychiatry II,* ed. A. M. Freedman, H. I. Kaplan, and V. Sadock, vol. 2. Baltimore: Williams & Wilkins.

Storms, M. D., and E. Wasserman. 1982. Quoted in New theory of the causes of sexual orientation, ed. S. Prescod. *Sexuality Today* 6(5).

Sexuality and the Older Adult

Queen E. Utley

Introduction

History reveals that sex has always played a major role in human affairs. By looking at our customs, religion, art, mores, and laws, one can see that sex holds a place of distinction. Yet today's society still lacks an understanding of the sexual needs, capacities, and expressions of older people. From birth, when the cry "It's a girl," or "It's a boy," rings out in the delivery room, an individual is considered a sexual being, but once that individual progresses to old age, suddenly he or she is considered sexless. The idea that an individual loses sexual drive or interest as he or she grows older is a very common misconception held by young and old alike. Still others believe that sexual

activity in an older person is immoral. Many of the myths that surround this subject need to be dispelled. This chapter describes the sexuality issues characteristic of older adults and ways in which caregivers can help address these issues.

Recognizing Sexuality in the Elderly

The fact is that sexual interest and activity are not rare in persons over 60 years of age. The Duke longitudinal studies conducted in the 1960s indicate that the likelihood of continued sexual expression in later life is related to a high degree of sexual activity and interest in early life (Palmore 1970). In other words, the sexual behavior patterns established during young adulthood are likely to be maintained throughout old age.

Nevertheless, the health professional's approach to sexuality in the elderly is often colored by societal myths and attitudes. It sometimes appears as though health professionals have chosen not to acknowledge the sexual concerns of older adults. In health institutions lack of privacy, segregation of sexes, and prohibition of conjugal visits are all evidence that sexuality in the elderly is essentially ignored. In primary and acute care settings, providers tend not to acknowledge the existence of sexual needs or concerns among older adults. A sexual history is not included as part of the general health history, and clients are not counseled about the effects of aging and/or disease states on their sexual selves. Ignoring the sexuality of an older individual limits the perception of that individual to less than that of a whole person. Human health or well-being depends to some degree on congruence between physical, spiritual, and psychosocial needs. Psychosocial needs include being cared about, being loved, and having an opportunity to express those needs.

A first step in changing our professional approach and attitudes about sexuality and the older adult is to evaluate our definition of sexuality. Caregivers need to think in terms of intimacy for older adults, rather than limited concepts of sex. Sexuality is typically defined too narrowly, often as specific erotic behaviors such as sexual intercourse, masturbation, and oral-genital stimulation. It is more appropriate to broaden this definition to include all aspects of life that give physical and emotional pleasure. Sexuality includes how people feel about themselves and others, and how they view sex roles. Physical contact, such as caressing, simple handholding, kissing, touching, and other kinds of stimulation to the sense organs are essential parts of the sexual drive.

Even when intercourse is no longer possible due to disease or illness, the need for other aspects of a sexual relationship still persist. The need for closeness, being cared for, touching, and sensuality is still very prevalent among the elderly (see Figure 3-1). Most individuals benefit from a close, intimate relationship. An intimate sexual relationship gives pleasure, is a means of exercise, and can offer release from tension and anxiety. Satisfying sexual activity, such as intercourse, closeness, touching, or giving of self in other ways is also a means of increasing self-concept and self-esteem. This is especially important for the older adult who has been stripped of many of the things society uses to dictate self-esteem and self-concept. In our society a youthful appearance, a job, and a spouse are some symbols which help to enhance one's self-concept and self-esteem. An elderly person may have lost one or more of these symbols.

Many theorists see intimacy and sexuality as an important part of development. Erikson (1963) views intimacy as a critical developmental stage. Intimacy is a close relationship with another person, which may or may not include intercourse. It is a desire to be with and be enjoyed by that person, to share and confide in him or her. Studies have shown that infants who are cuddled, fondled, and loved are more likely to gain weight, thrive, and develop normally (Peterson and Payne 1975). Might the same be true for older adults? Might they better thrive, maintain normal weight, and accomplish the developmental tasks of the later years if they are cared for and loved?

Situational Changes and Altered Relationships

Developmental and situational hazardous events occur during later adulthood that directly or indirectly can affect the sexuality of the older adult. Retirement, widowhood, and divorce are but a few of the hazardous events

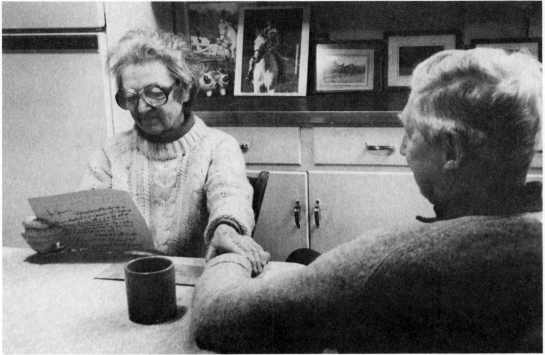

© Maureen Fennelli/Photo Researchers, Inc.

FIGURE 3-1
Definitions of love, intimacy, and caring may change over the years.

that can lead to role changes and self-esteem problems.

Widowhood and Remarriage

In widowhood, there is a loss of one's sexual partner as well as loss of a partner for most social events. Many older individuals desire to remarry or establish new relationships, but some do not know how to go about meeting new people. Because most social activities are geared toward couples, the opportunity to meet available partners and build new interpersonal relationships is limited. In addition, older women fear being taken advantage of financially in ill-fated liaisons. Still others have expressed fear of marrying another older

person who is not in good health. These women found themselves caring for husbands who were in poor health prior to their deaths and do not want to go through the same situation again.

When a widow or widower is fortunate enough to find a companion and move into a new relationship in late adulthood, the new marriage may be a source of sexual conflict. In a remarriage, the previously married spouse may have the same sexual expectations of the new partner as of the previous one. The following case illustrates this potential conflict:

Liz, an attractive 59-year-old female who had been a widow for five years, recently married John, age 65, a friend whom she had known for many years. This was

John's first marriage. They had been married two months when Liz presented for a health maintenance visit. Liz's complaint was that she had married a "pig in a sack." The interview revealed that the two had not engaged in intercourse before the marriage and thus far John had been unable to gain an erection. After further inquiry, Liz admitted that she expected John to respond sexually as had her first husband. She stated that her first husband was able to have one or two erections during intercourse without any assistance from her. Liz saw her role as being passive in the sexual relationship. She was uncomfortable with active participation and refused to give John any assistance with penile stimulation or other encouragement during the sexual act.

In exploring the relationship with Liz, it became apparent that she was unable to talk with John about her expectations. He had expressed none to her and seemed content to share her companionship. John had recently retired and, according to Liz, seemed to be unable to occupy his time. Furthermore, she knew he had not had a physical examination in a number of years.

The nurse practitioner was able to persuade John to come in for a physical. In the course of the visit, he admitted that he feared he wasn't "man enough" for Liz. After several visits, he was able to open up to Liz about his fears. Liz was able to talk about her expectations and began to appreciate John for what he could bring to the relationship instead of comparing him with her first husband. John became active in the senior center and soon was involved in the foster grandparents program. Liz and John worked together to incorporate suggestions for sexual stimulation into their lovemaking. Liz began to enjoy stroking and caressing John rather than just being a recipient of such attention. She began to look forward to long relaxed sessions of intimacy.

On their first anniversary, Liz came in to thank the nurse practitioner for the best year of her life.

Both John and Liz needed education and support to assist them in accepting a new sexual identity in their relationship. This is but one example of the problems that can arise when older adults become involved in new sexual relationships.

Retirement

Other transitions in the later years can affect sexuality. Retirement means a loss of the work role. In a society in which an individual is judged by what he or she does, such a loss can lead to a decreased self-image, which will affect one's perception of his or her sexual self and ability to attract others. Retirement can also mean retiring from the parent role as children become adults. It may also mean assuming responsibility for an older parent. In addition, a change in traditional male and female roles can occur with retirement: older men may begin to adopt household chores that have traditionally been ascribed to women. Certainly, this change has an impact on self-image and the way one's spouse views the retiree. At the same time, retirement can be an opportune time for rebuilding a caring sexual relationship with one's partner. Outside demands should be decreased, leaving more time and energy available for relationships.

Divorce

Another factor that may affect an older person's sexuality is divorce. Divorce rates now include a larger percentage of older adults who have sought divorce after being married to the same partner for 25 or 30 years. It is reported that "though most divorces occur during the first years of marriage, older people are divorcing more, too. From 1963 to 1969, divorce among women 55 years and older increased by over 34%. Six percent of all divorces in 1969 involved couples who had been married for 25 years or more" (Oaks 1976, 84). There is still little research on the effect of divorce on older adults. However, divorce does lead to an altered sexual image, as well as loss of a sexual partner. Experiences in working with older adults indicate that they divorce for a number of reasons, but not without guilt and shame for coming to such a decision.

> Nan, a 76-year-old, states, "I'm divorcing my 80-year-old husband. You must think I am really cruel to do this. I am not divorcing him so much for what he is doing now, but for the things he has done to me through the years. I asked for a divorce years ago and he threatened to take my child away from me. Well, I am not taking his cruelty any longer, regardless of how many years I have left to live."

Older divorced women are at a higher risk for lack of intimacy because it is more difficult for them to build new intimate relationships. "In 1970 the ratio was 80 men to every 100 women between the ages of 55 and 64. By the time they were 74, there were only 72 men to every 100 women" (Shomaker 1980, 313). It is somewhat less difficult for older divorced men to find new partners, because older women outnumber older men by a large ratio. In addition, society finds it more acceptable for older males to choose younger female partners than for older women to choose younger partners.

Biophysiological Sexual Changes

Some natural physiological changes occur with aging, although the desire for or interest in sexual activity does not change significantly. Research by Masters and Johnson has shown a number of physiological changes that occur in the elderly during the human sexual response cycle. It is of utmost importance that the health provider is knowledgeable about these changes and implications. The four stages of the human sexual response cycle as explained by Masters and Johnson (1966, 1970) (also described in Chapter 2) will be discussed in the following summary.

Males

In the excitement phase the older male takes longer to achieve a full penile erection. The plateau phase is longer than it is for a younger man, which means that, once gained, penile erection can be maintained for a longer period of time without ejaculation. The orgasmic phase is shortened, but there is no evidence that the erotic pleasure of the experience is decreased. However, there is decreased seminal fluid volume, fewer sperm, decreased ejaculatory pressure and force during the orgasmic phase, and a diminution of intensity in the orgasmic experience. The resolution phase occurs more rapidly and the refractory period is extended. This extended refractory period means that an older male cannot regain a second erection as quickly as he could when he was younger. On physical examination, a loss of pubic hair and a reduction in size and firmness of testicles may also be noted.

Females

For many years, menopause — the cessation of menstruation — has been proclaimed a significant factor decreasing older women's sexual drive. This is a myth. Cessation of the menstrual cycle or a hysterectomy does not affect libido. Society considers the ability to reproduce an intricate part of female sexuality. Because of this, the cessation of reproductive capability is symbolically associated with being old and asexual. In reality, postmenopausal women report that they enjoy sex more fully than at any previous time during their lives.

Although postmenopausal women may continue to enjoy sex, they will experience some changes in their sexual responses. In the older female, there is decreased vaginal lubrication and elasticity during the excitement and plateau phases, probably due to the hormonal changes that occur after menopause. The vagina becomes thin and atrophic. There is some shrinkage of the vaginal length and width, and a loss of the corrugated appearance of the vaginal wall. The vaginal mucosa becomes light pink, with a glossier tint than seen in younger females. Due to the decrease in hormones, the cervix and uterus shrink in size. This results in a less distinguishable cervix upon physical examination. Shrinkage of the clitoris is also noted in older females, but with no apparent change in its ability to give pleasure. There is also a loss of pubic hair and the breasts begin to lose firmness to varying degrees.

In the sexual response cycle, the orgasmic phase is shortened and fewer vaginal contractions occur, but there is no loss of sensation. The resolution phase subsides more rapidly than in a younger woman.

In addition to these physical changes, menopause usually occurs at a point in a woman's life when a number of developmental and situational hazardous life events are occurring. There is often the loss of the role of mother (the children have left home), physiological changes of aging begin to occur (weight gain, dry and wrinkled skin, and so on), and other events, which can lead to a high degree of stress at this time. The health practitioner has a responsibility to educate the older female client about the physiological, emotional, and developmental factors involved throughout the climacteric. These mid-life changes for both men and women and suggested nursing interventions are discussed in detail in Chapter 6.

Health Factors that Affect Sexuality: Special Concerns for the Older Adult

Although sexual needs and desires do not undergo an abrupt change as a result of the aging process, many health factors can influence the desire for sex and the amount of sexual activity engaged in. In addition to past sexual activity, physical health, medications, and emotional and mental well-being affect one's desire or ability to engage in sexual activity. Research done by Masters and Johnson (1970), Carey (1975), Yeaworth (1975), and others, reveals some of the health factors that are definite deterrents to sexual interest and responsiveness.

Mental and Emotional Problems

Mental fatigue as a result of occupational, financial, or other personal concerns can lead to decreased sexual drive for brief or extended periods of time. Three emotional conditions frequently seen in the elderly—anxiety, depression, and grief—can also alter sexual response. Treatment of these problems can lead to improved sexual interest and performance.

Overeating or Alcohol Abuse

Overindulgence in food or drink can result in repression of both sexual desire and performance. Although alcohol can lower inhibitions and increase desire, it may also interfere with performance. Secondary impotence has been seen in male clients with a history of alcohol abuse. Rossman (1975) reports that impotence occurs due to impairment of hepatic function so that endogenous estrogens are not properly conjugated and metabolized. Obesity has also been related to impotence and decreased sexual interest.

Medication

Drugs can also affect the sexual ability of both males and females. The effect of drugs on the male is more recognizable because impotence in the male is more readily identified. Adverse drug effects in the male can lead to inability to ejaculate, erectile impotence, and failure to achieve orgasm. Major tranquilizers (haldol, mellaril, thorazine), steroids, hormones, anticholinergic drugs (pro-banthine, atropine), antiadrenergic drugs (antihypertensives, ergot alkaloids), neuropathy-producing drugs (vincristine), and antimetabolic drugs (myleran) all can contribute to sexual dysfunctions. Hypertensive medication is often the culprit in the elderly, causing impotence or inhibition of ejaculation in males. Although the effect of drugs on females is less observable, decreased libido and failure to achieve orgasm are reported side effects of hypertensive medications and psychotropic drug therapy in females.

When assessing drug-induced sexual problems, the practitioner must first determine if the problem existed before treatment started. Second, it is necessary to assess for developmental and/or psychosocial influences that may be interfering with usual sexual patterns. If an individual is being treated for depression with psychotropic drugs, the practitioner should consider whether the sexual problem is a result of illness or drug therapy. Time has to be allowed for the depression to lift after initial therapy has begun. Lowered dosages, discontinuation of drug, change in medication, and specific periods without a drug can all be appropriate interventions for drug-induced sexual problems in older adults (see Chapter 8 for discussion of hypertension and heart disease).

Declining Health

A change in health status or altered physical state due to chronic illness, acute disease process, or surgical procedure can influence sexual functioning. Older individuals are at higher risk for chronic illness and disabilities than other age groups. Chronic debilitating diseases — such as stroke, arthritis, diabetes, and hypertension — are major problems for the elderly and may have a negative effect on sexual functioning. For example, diabetes has been related to impotence in males. This effect is thought to be caused by autonomic neuropathy involving nerve fibers that supply the penis and bladder. Prostatectomy is an example of a surgical procedure that can lead to sexual impairment (such as impotence or retrograde ejaculation), depending upon the kind of surgical approach. If the incision is made through sex-related nerve centers, impairment is likely to occur. An older male considering such surgery would need to be informed about the procedure so that he and his surgeon could make the best choice. If the surgery is undertaken because of a malignancy, the chances of maintaining potency are not as great.

Cardiovascular disease, respiratory disease, hormonal imbalance, and neurologic, hematologic, and psychological disorders are all conditions that can influence sexual functioning. In many cases, these health problems need not mean an end to sexual activity. For example:

> Bob, a 66-year-old male, had a mild myocardial infarction two years ago. Since that time he suffered mild angina at periodic intervals and was medicated as necessary with nitroglycerin. Bob had an inordinate fear of having another myocardial infarction or severe angina pain if he engaged in sex with his wife. Nevertheless, he stated that he frequently felt aroused sexually and desired intercourse with his wife. With assistance from the nurse practitioner, he learned about normal sexual response, total energy expenditure during intercourse, and how nitroglycerin could be used prophylactically. After gradually

beginning to experience a climax through masturbation in the privacy of his own home, Bob gained the confidence to resume active sexual relations with his wife.

Some practical recommendations for clients with such conditions are given in Chapter 8.

Chronic illness and disability in older adults will affect body image, self-worth, and sexual role identity, which can become a source of conflict for partners. The healthy partner may begin to resent the inability of the chronically ill partner to participate in sexual activity. The chronically ill partner in turn may become very sensitive or even anxiety ridden about his or her inability to meet the sexual needs of the partner. The nurse can assist through anticipatory guidance, education, and counseling. Knowledge of the emotional and sexual conflicts that might arise with chronic illness and disability helps allay fears in the older adult.

History Taking with Older Adults

In caring for an older adult, age does not eliminate the need for a holistic perspective, including sexuality. Chapter 5 presents a complete sexual history and examination; included here are considerations pertaining specifically to older adults.

A sexual history is a part of any general health history and should not be considered a separate entity. In order for a sexual history to be meaningful, it must be viewed in the context of the total person and his or her environment. For example, it would be difficult for the practitioner to understand how a person was adjusting to changing sexual needs during later years if there was no understanding of whether the individual was coping with other developmental tasks and life events (that is, death of a spouse, declining health, and physical well-being) of one's age group. Separating the sexual history from other health history taking suggests that sex is not a part of the total human experience.

The sexual history is elicited with sensitivity toward the individual and his or her own sexual attitudes (see Chapter 5). It does not involve minute details of an individual's sexual experience. Rather, its aim should be to gather information about the basic personality, preference, concept of interpersonal relationships, and any desirable changes in sexual lifestyle. Older people must be seen as individuals, understood and respected in terms of their past and present lifestyles, coping capacities, and internal and external resources. The practitioner must discern what the client's needs and desires are. In addition, throughout the health history, the practitioner needs to be alert to any misinformation and myths the client has about sexuality. This is very important in order to plan appropriate counseling and education.

Following are some examples of open-ended questions that can be used to gather a meaningful sexual history as part of the older adult's total health record: What is your sexual lifestyle like? Has your sexual lifestyle changed recently? Are you happy with your sexual lifestyle? Would you like to make any changes in your sexual lifestyle? Older clients are not as likely to be embarrassed or upset by being asked about sexuality as some practitioners anticipate them to be. A client is more likely to answer sexuality questions easily if some rapport has been established with the interviewer. This can be done by asking nonthreatening questions about general health history before asking sexuality questions. This allows the practitioner to establish a rapport with the client in a warm and sensitive atmosphere. However, it is best not to leave all the sexuality questions until the end of the interview because this distinction may be interpreted as meaning that sexuality is not a part of one's total health history.

In an interview for a sexual history, a client should not be made to feel that she or he is compelled to discuss sexual concerns. By asking about an older individual's sexual lifestyle, the interviewer, in effect, says that sexuality is an open and acceptable topic to be discussed. From clinical practice with older adults, it is evident that a number of older adults may not choose to discuss sexuality concerns during the initial interview, but very often return at a later time to share concerns.

Physical Examination of the Older Adult

Sexual concerns that are of biophysical origin are rare. Temporary sexual problems in older adults are usually the result of psychosocial concerns. However, the possibility of biophysical problems should not be excluded. As part of the nursing assessment, a complete physical examination should be given to find out if the client has the necessary physiological resources available for healthy sexual functioning (see Chapter 5 for details). The physical examination should be not only a time of discovering if the necessary sexual parts of the body are normal, but also a time to educate the client about normal functioning of body parts. Older adults grew up when sexuality was not an open topic of discussion and some still know very little about their bodies. Males and females may expect the examination to be uncomfortable because of past misconceptions and negative experiences. Older women recount experiences where they have been ridiculed and treated with insensitivity during gynecological examination. Therefore, the practitioner should be most careful to convey a sense of caring and sensitivity to the client, by his or her attitudes and skills used in the examination.

In the female, the breasts, abdomen, clitoris, external genitalia, vagina, cervix, and rectum should be examined. Particular attention should be paid to the vaginal canal of older women. Many women suffer from prolapsed pelvic structures due to decreased elasticity and thinning of tissues and stretching of ligaments. Structures such as the bladder, uterus, rectum, and urethra may relax and protrude into the vagina, interfering with sexual activity. The extent of the interference depends on the severity of prolapse and accompanying symptoms.

Some postmenopausal women think and have been told by health-care providers that they do not have to continue having Pap smears. To the contrary, some regular periodic pattern should be established for doing gynecological assessments and Pap smears for older female clients. The frequency will be determined by past and family history and previous Pap findings. Although this group is not at high risk for cervical cancer, the risk becomes greater for uterine cancer. Endometrial cancer usually afflicts women more than 50 years of age. The American Cancer Society explains the limits of Pap smears in revealing endometrial cancer: "The Pap test is highly effective in detecting early cancer of the uterine cervix and only 40% effective in detecting endometrial cancer" (1982, 16).

The examination of the male should include inspection of the scrotum, testes, and penis. A rectal examination is also to be included, with particular attention given to the prostate. Any hard irregular nodules would suggest a neoplasm, while a swollen, tender gland could be indicative of prostatitis.

With all older clients special attention should be given to the following areas: genital-urinary functioning and normalcy, neurophysiological functioning (such as sensory perception), and capacity for mobility and strength. The major emphasis of the physical examination would be determined from the presenting problem and the health history (rarely is the presenting problem sexual; more often the "real" problem is discerned as the visit progresses). A physical examination may not necessarily be a part of assessment. For example, the sexual complaint might only necessitate educating the individual, which would be evident after taking a sexual history. If the physical examination indicates further need for evaluation, the nurse practitioner can make the appropriate medical referral.

Intervention

Temporary sexual concerns are frequently seen in the elderly that can be handled by the nurse. Primary care providers are in strategic and accessible positions within the health-care system. Older adults are more apt to seek help where they feel less threatened and fewer anxieties are provoked. What more natural place, then, to first seek sexual counseling than with the primary care provider? By the very nature of the nurse's role, she or he is often considered approachable about such matters.

The nurse provider must be aware and accepting of the fact that many older people continue to desire and have an active sexual life. In addition, she or he must first come to terms with her or his own sexuality before assisting others in exploring their sexual needs. Self-awareness is important for effective and comfortable exploration and intervention with a client. The nurse practitioner's sexual value system should not be the standard for intervention and management. Intervention for the nurse practitioner consists mainly of education, guidance, and counseling.

Education and Counseling

Early education and counseling are beneficial in preparing the middle-aged and older adult for developmental/situational events that affect sexuality and in preventing some of the problems that might occur. Knowledge of sexual physiology and natural changes that occur with the aging process need to be understood to alleviate anxiety, increase confidence, and foster appropriate adjustment. For example, the older male and his partner may recognize that it takes longer for him to reach an erection and that he needs more tactile stimulation. Rather than becoming frustrated at his not being able to reach an erection as quickly as he did when younger, both partners can relax, engage in prolonged foreplay, and understand that once an erection is reached, he will be able to maintain it longer. It is also important for the male and his partner to understand the change that occurs during resolution and not try to force a second erection during an extended refractory period.

The changing sexual responses of the older female may also dictate some changes in sexual patterns. More stimulation during foreplay to enhance lubrication can occur without undue anxiety when the older female and her partner recognize that vaginal lubrication will be naturally delayed. It is necessary for the older female and her partner to be aware that attempting coitus without adequate vaginal lubrication can lead to irritation of the urethra, which results in cystitis-like symptoms of burning and an urge to urinate. If a woman does not engage in sexual activity for prolonged periods of time, she may experience some pain, tenderness, or discomfort at first as a result of decreased vaginal lubrication and possible decrease in vaginal length and width. In this case a water-soluble vaginal lubricant or saliva may be indicated. Water-soluble lubricants do tend to dry up very quickly, so clients need instruction in their use. Another alternative is the use of estrogen creams, although some studies have questioned their efficacy and safety (Schiff 1980).

In order to make realistic, rational, and informed choices about their sexual needs, older persons must be enlightened. The nurse as primary practitioner is one source of sexual information. Most older adults grew up in an era when learning about one's sexual self was not an acceptable thing to do. Information-sharing by the nurse could be an older person's first formal learning experience in sexual health. At the onset, the practitioner may have to start with very basic information. It is important to correct, in a nonjudgmental way, misinformation that may have been acquired through the years.

Sensitive listening and acceptance of any concerns require the practitioner to communicate a nonjudgmental attitude. A warm, understanding atmosphere is crucial, and can be established early in an interview or counseling session, although developing trust and confidence is a slower process. One way to establish this warm, understanding atmosphere is a process described by Rodin and Janis (1979) as gaining referent power: "(1) Make statements that identify affinities between self and client in the realm of values, attitudes, and beliefs. (2) Convey a benevolent attitude toward the client in a spirit of caring. (3) Make statements of acceptance despite any shortcomings the patient has shared" (Turner 1980, 43).

Exploring Alternatives

Sexual needs vary from one older individual to the next; not everyone needs to be encouraged to engage in sexual activity. Clients can be advised to share interpersonal warmth and enjoy the satisfaction of body contact as long as the desire and capacity to do so continue.

However, some older individuals accept the fact that they themselves have no desire for sexual activity and do not become upset by it or wish to make changes.

If a client wishes to do so, exploration of a new means of sexual expression is in order. Open discussion of alternative avenues such as masturbation, fantasy, and group social activities, become important. Combinations of alternatives can be used to enhance sexual enjoyment. Fantasy and masturbation are frequently used jointly.

Fantasy is a means by which an individual can visualize and relive past pleasant and exciting sexual experiences or create an ideal sexual experience. Older clients may be more likely to use the fantasy technique if it is suggested (especially when first introducing the technique) that they use a loved partner of the past as an object of sexual fantasy. Instruction to create an atmosphere conducive to such a fantasy is important. Low romantic lighting, dressing for the role, and flowers all may heighten sensuality. One 73-year-old said she felt very, very sexy when she wore black. Whatever is helpful for each person is appropriate. Some older clients will need to be assured that fantasy activity is normal.

Masturbation may be an acceptable alternative for some. Care must be used in introducing this topic, as some may find it offensive or shocking. Masturbation can offer release of sexual tension, and for females, encourages lubrication of the vagina. This allows intercourse with less difficulty if a partner should become available. For some, specific instruction on techniques for safe and pleasurable self-stimulation will have to be given. Others will already have a repertoire of masturbation techniques. Each individual will have to be evaluated according to his or her capability. As an example, a 70-year-old female with extensive arthritis in her hands might find direct clitoral stimulation with the hands difficult; a vibrator or soft pillow might be less taxing. Touching oneself, learning to care for and appreciate one's aging body, is positive reinforcement for one's self-esteem. For those couples who, for various reasons, cannot engage in intercourse, cooperative or mutual stimulation of each other's body is an important alternative. Promoting psychosocial freedom to enjoy masturbation for those individuals with or without partners is within the scope of practice of a primary care nurse practitioner.

Another substitute for sexual activity that might give partial gratification is affection offered by a dog, cat, or other pet. Pet care is a means of meeting intimacy needs and increasing self-concept, self-esteem, and feelings of being needed and cared about. The intent here is not to suggest that animals be used as objects of sexual activities. But for older adults who have lost many of their significant others, caring for a loving pet gives some worthwhile gratification when sexuality is viewed in its broader context.

An additional alternative is engaging in group interactional games such as back massage and circle dancing so that physical comfort and verbal caring messages can be given in a nonthreatening atmosphere. Such activities increase self-esteem and give enjoyment and pleasure. Aged persons are willing to substitute other forms of sexual expression when they are no longer able to engage in intercourse (see Figure 3-2).

Referrals

If after initial history taking, an interview, and a physical examination, the hazardous sexual event proves to be beyond the expertise of the individual primary care practitioner, an appropriate referral should be made. But temporary minor sexuality problems, especially those in-

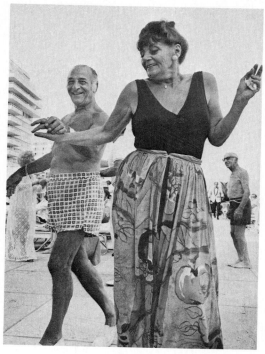

© Joan Liftin/Archive Pictures Inc.

FIGURE 3-2
Enjoying life as an older adult.

volving a need for education, can best be solved with the aid of the nurse practitioner, who has already established an interpersonal relationship with the client. When referring clients to other resources, it is wise to have as much information as possible. The practitioner should consider a number of factors before making a referral. These include the following:

1. What treatment method does the resource use?

2. What is the resource's experience with older adults?

3. What are the education and certification of the caregivers?

4. What are the resource's educational methods?

5. Costs: can the client afford it?

After referral, there should also be follow-up with regard to the sexual concern. The success of the outcome should be evaluated, with reassessment, if necessary.

Summary of Implications for Nursing Practice

There is a need for more aggressive intervention from primary care nurse practitioners in assessing the sexuality concerns of older adults. Greater effort should also be made to educate young and middle-aged adults about expected sexuality changes in later adulthood. Ideally, this education will increase their own sexual adjustment as they age. Certainly encouraging young and middle-aged adults to maintain their health and physical fitness throughout life is one of the most significant steps that can be taken to ensure lifelong healthy sexual functioning. Bonnie Prudden's book *Exer-sex* (1978) outlines an excellent fitness plan to improve sexual health.

Development of different modes and materials for sex education of older adults is also important. Vicki Schmall (1981) offers an extensive resource list of publications, media materials, and organizations concerned with aging and sexuality.

Figure 3-3 is an example of an educational pamphlet developed by nurse practitioners to educate and act as a permission-giving method to older adults. It is intended for use in various

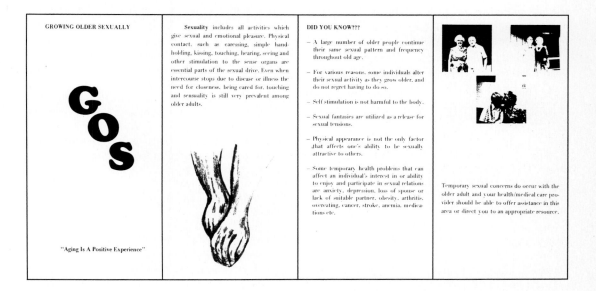

FIGURE 3-3

Growing old sexually: an example of an education/permission-giving tool developed by nurse practitioners for use with older adult clients in ambulatory care settings who might have questions and concerns about sexuality.

SOURCE: ©1981 Q. E. Utley and B. Shestowsky. Reprinted by permission.

health/medical settings in which sexuality is viewed as part of a person's total health care.

Nurse providers also have a role to play in research concerning older adults and sexuality. There are many questions that need to be addressed: What is the relationship between loss of intimacy/sexual activity and health variables? What is the relationship between developmental coping behaviors and sexual activity in the elderly? Are group interactional games the most viable alternative to the loss of one-to-one sexual activity? What is the impact of sex education during the middle years on sexual adjustment in old age? Primary care nurse practitioners have an increasingly greater role to play in sexuality counseling, education, and research with older adults.

REFERENCES

Adams, C. G. 1981. Sexuality and the older adult. In *Dissertation Abstracts International,* Vol. 41, p. 3280-A. Amherst: University of Massachusetts. Microfilm.

American Cancer Society. 1981. *Cancer facts and figures.* New York.

Barnard, M. Y., V. J. Clancy, and K. E. Krantz. 1978. *Human sexuality for health professionals.* Philadelphia: Saunders.

Belliveau, E., and L. Richter. 1970. *Understanding human sexual inadequacy.* Boston: Little, Brown.

Burnside, I. M., ed. 1975. *Sexuality and aging.* Los Angeles: University of Southern California Press.

Busse, E. W., and E. Pfeiffer, eds. 1969. *Behavior and adaptation in late life.* Boston: Little, Brown.

Butler, R. N., and M. I. Lewis. 1977. *Love and sex after sixty.* New York: Harper & Row.

Carey, P. 1975. Temporary sexual dysfunction in reversible health limitations. *Nursing Clinics of North America* 10(3):575–585.

Comfort, A. 1974. Sexuality in old age. *Journal of the American Geriatrics Society* 12(10):440–443.

Crown, S., ed. 1976. *Psychosexual problems: Psychotherapy, counseling and behavioral modification.* New York: Academic Press, Grune & Stratton.

Erikson, E. 1963. *Childhood and society.* New York: Norton.

Finkle, A. L. 1978. Genitourinary disorders of old age: Therapeutic considerations including counseling for sexual dysfunction. *Journal of the American Geriatrics Society* 26(10):453–458.

Friedman, J. G. 1979. Sexuality in older persons. *Nursing Forum* 18(1):92–101.

George, L. K. 1980. *Role transitions in later life.* Monterey, Calif.: Brooks/Cole.

Group for the Advancement of Psychiatry, Committee on Medical Education. 1974. *Assessment of sexual function: A guide to interviewing.* Washington, D.C.: Library of Congress.

Hotchner, B. 1980. Menopause and sexuality. *Topics in Clinical Nursing* 1(4):45–52.

Johnson, W. R. 1968. *Human sexual behavior and sex education.* 2d ed. Philadelphia: Lea & Febiger.

Kent, S. 1975. Continued sexual activity depends on health and availability of a partner. *Geriatrics* 30(11):142–143.

Kent, S. 1975. The intimate relationship between the urinary system and sexual function. *Geriatrics* 30(6):138–142.

Kobosa-Munro, L. 1977. Sexuality in the aging woman. *Health and Social Work* 2(4):71–86.

Laws, L. J., and P. Schwartz. 1977. *Sexual scripts: The social construction of female sexuality.* Hinsdale, Ill.: Dryden Press.

Leviton, D. 1978. The intimacy/sexual needs of terminally ill and widowed. *Death Education* 2(3):261–280.

MacRae, I., and G. Henderson. 1975. Sexuality and irreversible health limitations. *Nursing Clinics of North America* 10(3):587–597.

Masters, W. H., and V. E. Johnson. 1970. *Human sexual inadequacy.* Boston: Little, Brown.

Masters, W. H., and V. E. Johnson. 1966. *Human sexual response.* Boston: Little, Brown.

Nass, G. D., R. W. Libby, and M. P. Fisher. 1981. *Sexual choices.* Monterey, Calif.: Wadsworth.

Neugarten, B. L., ed. 1968. *Middle age and aging: A reader in social psychology.* Chicago: University of Chicago Press.

Notman, T. M., and C. C. Nadelson, eds. 1978. *The woman patient: Vol. 1. Sexual and reproductive aspects of women's health care.* New York: Plenum.

Oaks, W. W., M. A. Gerald, and I. Fisher. 1976.

Sex and the life cycle. New York: Grune & Stratton.

Palmore, E., ed. 1970. Normal aging: Reports from the Duke longitudinal study, 1955–1969. Durham, N. C.: Duke Uniersity Press.

Peterson, J., and B. Payne. 1975. *Love in the later years: The emotional, physical, sexual and social potential of the elderly.* New York: New York Associated Press.

Prudden, B. 1978. *Exer-Sex.* Stockbridge, Mass.: Aquarian Press.

Rodin, J., and I. L. Janis. 1979. The social power of health care practitioners as agents of change. *Journal of Social Issues* 35(1):62.

Rossman, I. 1975. Sexuality and the aging process: An internist's perspective. In *Sexuality and aging.* ed. I. M. Burnside. Los Angeles: University of California Press.

Rowland, K. F., and S. N. Haynes. 1978. A sexual enhancement program for elderly couples. *Journal of Sex and Marital Therapy* 4(2):91–113.

Schiff, I. 1981. The menopause and estrogen replacement. Papers. Obstetric-Gynecologic-Neonatal Nursing, Harvard Medical School, Department of Continuing Education, Boston.

Schmall, V. L. 1981. Resources: Aging and Sexuality. *Generations* Fall: 46–48.

Shomaker, D. M. 1980. Integration of physiological and sociocultural factors as a basis for sex education to the elderly. *Journal of Gerontological Nursing* 6(6):311–317.

Stahmann, R. E., and W. J. Hiebert. 1977. *Klemer's counseling in marital and sexual problems.* 2d ed. Baltimore: Waverly Press.

Troll, L., J. Israel, and K. Israel, eds. 1977. *Looking ahead: A woman's guide to the problems and joys of growing older.* Englewood Cliffs, N. J.: Prentice-Hall.

Turner, N. W. 1980. Sexual issues in separation and divorce. *Topics in Clinical Nursing* 1(4): 39–44.

Wabrek, C. J., and J. Wabrek. 1975. Sexual difficulties and the importance of the relationship. *Nursing Digest* 3(6):44–45.

Waslow, M., and M. B. Loeb. 1978. Sexuality in nursing homes. *Journal of the American Geriatrics Society* 27:73–79.

West, N. D. 1975. Sex in geriatrics: Myth or miracle? *Journal of the American Geriatrics Society* 13(12):551–552.

Whipple, B., and R. Gick. 1980. A holistic view of sexuality—education for the health professional. *Topics in Clinical Nursing* 1(4):91–98.

Woods, N. F. 1978. Human sexuality and the healthy elderly. In *Readings in gerontology,* ed. M. Brown. St. Louis: C. V. Mosby.

Woods, N. F. 1975. *Human sexuality in health and illness.* 2d ed. St. Louis: C. V. Mosby.

Yeaworth, R. C., and J. S. Friedman. 1975. Sexuality in later life. *Nursing Clinics of North America* 10(3):565–574.

Introduction

Issues of Reproduction

Contraception
Abortion
Historical and anthropological variations
Contemporary conflicts
Caregivers' involvement
Women seeking abortion
Artificial Insemination
Issues of Technology and Reproduction
DES exposure
Sterilization
In vitro fertilization
Amniocentesis
Circumcision

Issues of Eroticism

Virginity
Masturbation
Pornography
Sexual Abuse of Children

Issues of Sexual Preference

Homosexuality
Historical variations in attitudes
Individual variations
Lesbian health-care needs
Homosexual male health-care needs
Meeting homosexual health-care needs
Homosexual parents
Bisexuality
Transsexualism

Issues of Health-Care Provision

Discrimination Against Women
Sexual Abuse by Health-Care Providers
Patients' Expressions of Sexuality

Issues of Sex Research

Summary of Implications for Nursing Practice

Sexuality: Ethics and Morality

Loretta P. Higgins

Introduction

This chapter will examine some current pressing sexual issues in light of society's definitions of morality. The morality of sexual acts is not a static concept. What we believe about the morality of sexuality comes from a variety of sources, including societal mores, religion, parental values, and peer values. The mass media, including advertising components, probably play a large role in the development of value systems (Anspaugh and Dignan 1980).

We are all affected by our collective perceptions of the rightness or wrongness of certain behaviors. Sexual behavior has always been zealously cloaked in rules, regulations, and taboos. It has engaged the attention of more philosophers and theologians as a moral issue than almost any other. This is surprising since there are a great many human behaviors that could be viewed, discussed, and resolved in the context of morality. The word "morality," when mentioned without context, would surely evoke sexual connotations in the minds of many, if not most, individuals. The term "living in sin" is not usually interpreted as living in pride, living in violence, or living in bigotry (Hettlinger 1966, 25).

Because of this view of sex and sexuality, this society's ambivalence towards the subject, and because nurses as health-care providers deal with others whose views on sexuality are often different from their own, nurses need periodically to examine their own views and biases. This chapter will help readers do that.

Issues of Reproduction

Issues of reproduction, especially female reproduction, have been food for thought for philosophers and theologians for hundreds of years. These issues originated, in part, from the ways reproduction has been viewed. Woman's reproductive cycle was seen as mysterious, magical, and close to nature. Some cultures had elaborate rules governing the behavior of menstruating and parturient women. Even after science explained away a great deal of the mystery, "women's organs" continued to be discussed extensively in the medical ethics literature. It is not surprising that discussions about reproductive issues even now dominate much of the literature written in the moral, ethical, and legal realms, both in professional journals and popular magazines and newspapers. Technological advances and recent questioning of routine surgical procedures have added some new issues to these discussions.

Contraception

One issue that has been discussed for decades is contraception. Early in the 1900s, the nurse Margaret Sanger witnessed firsthand the suffering of women who, denied birth control information, either lived in the depths of poverty with large families, or died from self-inflicted abortion attempts. Sanger coined the phrase "birth control" and fought throughout her life to bring information and contraceptive devices and services to the people. She endured arrests and public humiliation but continued in her battle to change laws by publishing books and articles and by speaking to throngs of people who came to learn from her (Sanger 1971).

Change has occurred slowly. Less than 20 years ago birth control activist Bill Baird was arrested for distributing birth control devices to unmarried people. Displays of condoms and contraceptive foams in stores are relatively recent phenomena. Some religions are still opposed to the concept and practice of contraception. As a society, we have not yet reached a consensus about the rights of adolescents to have access to contraception.

Abortion

Abortion has replaced birth control as the "hot issue" of the day. The mere mention of the word causes battle lines to be drawn. It is, without doubt, one of the most discussed issues of our time. Those individuals who see themselves as "pro-choice" believe that abortion is either an amoral procedure or that withholding it is immoral. Those on the other side of the argument believe abortion is murder and, therefore, highly immoral. There are many positions between these two poles. Even to its most ardent defenders, abortion is not justified as an alternative to contraception; rather, it is seen as an alternative to completing an unplanned pregnancy or one that involves a defective fetus.

Historical and Anthropological Variations

As a deed and as an issue, abortion has been with us a long time. Devereux (1955) reported on over a hundred primitive tribes where abortions were performed for a variety of reasons and by methods limited only by the imagination. Examples of reasons for aborting were fear of pregnancy, extreme youth, political factors, improper paternity, economic factors, and mourning. The methods of abortion fell into roughly 16 categories. Mechanical techniques were quite common and included such things as jolting, jumping from high places, and wife abuse. Hard work was another method, as was applying heat or irritants to the abdomen. Some women weakened themselves by starvation or bleeding. Attacking the fetus through the abdominal wall or by instruments such as pointed sticks passed through the cervix may have been used when more conservative means failed to eject the fetus. Various herbs were sometimes used in conjunction with magic. Other times only magic was used.

In Book VII of *Politics* Aristotle wrote that abortion was acceptable before "sense and life" have begun. Neither law nor religion in Greek and Roman cultures proscribed abortion. The prohibition against abortion in the Hippocratic oath has been variously interpreted: (1) the physician should not perform abortions; (2) he or she should check with the husband first; or (3) midwives may perform abortions (Bullough and Bullough 1977, 94). In any case, the oath was not generally followed until the emergence of Christian teaching (Davis and Aroskar 1978). During the Middle Ages abortion was tolerated at least within 40 days of conception or until quickening occurred. The Catholic position was clearly stated by the latter part of the 19th century: abortion was considered murder (Bullough and Bullough 1977).

Hardin (1974) reported that in the United States there were no laws prohibiting abortion until the late 1800s, although abortion was not considered a safe procedure. Laws varied from state to state, but abortion was usually allowed only if the woman's life was in danger. Sometimes abortions were performed because of exposure to rubella during the first trimester. Perhaps a large number of dilatation and curettage procedures were abortions in disguise. Women who had the means to travel to another country or who knew the right physicians had access to abortions. Most women, however, resorted to "back alley" abortionists for "criminal abortions." These were often done in dingy, unfurnished apartments by people with questionable credentials and unsterile instruments. There is no way of knowing how many of these abortions were done, but a great many of them resulted in complications such as infection and hemorrhage.

The monumental Supreme Court decision of 1973 liberalized and equalized abortion laws. Specifically, the following decisions were made: (1) during the first trimester of the pregnancy, a woman has the right to abortion without interference by the state except to require that the abortion be performed by a physician; (2) during the second trimester and until viability of the fetus the state may not deny abortion for any reason but may stipulate standards by which abortions are performed; and (3) after viability the state may prohibit abortion except when a woman's life is endangered.

Contemporary Conflicts

The Supreme Court ruling dramatically changed the lives of many people. Facilities for abortion began to spring up all over the country and the numbers of legal abortions performed skyrocketed. However, the removal of legal sanctions against abortions did not remove opposition from those who considered it immoral. The issue of abortion is still very much alive. The political power of the antiabortionists was demonstrated in 1977 when the federal government stopped paying for abortions under Medicaid.

Currently, there are a number of bills in Congress with the purpose of limiting abortions. One bill would define fetuses as persons from conception and provide full constitutional protection for them. This would prohibit all abortions and some methods of birth control. Another bill would allow states or Congress to pass legislation restricting abortion, while yet another would provide for a speedy review of the abortion issue by the Supreme Court (Goodman 1982).

The social and political upheavals over abortion reflect the lack of consensus on the moral arguments. The arguments made on both sides of the issue rest on the concepts of autonomy, justice, rights, consent, and personhood. In the quest to prove that abortion is wrong, antiabortionists have argued that the fetus is a person from the moment of conception. To that end, scientists were called as witnesses during Congressional hearings to give their opinions about when life begins. That argument has not served to settle the issue. The people who believe in abortion as an option believe in a woman's autonomy over her own body. Even if the fetus is a person, the argument goes, in no other situation is one person totally dependent on only one person (in this case, the biological mother). In some instances the sacrifice of one person cannot be required for the welfare of another (MacRae 1974).

Another argument using consent as the central concept focuses on the fetus. If fetuses could speak for themselves, according to this argument, they would choose nonbeing rather than being born with defects or to parents who do not want them and may abuse them (Davis and Aroskar 1978).

Thomsen (1975) argues that the fetus's right to life is not absolute, that no one's right to life is absolute. Sherwin (1981) says, "The right to life does not seem to guarantee all the means necessary to support that life" (p. 30).

Wertheimer (1975) describes the "extreme conservative position" on abortion: a fetus is a full-fledged, actualized human being, an innocent human life with as much right to life as any other person. The Catholic church states that the fetus and parent have the same moral status. The antiabortionist position, in great part, is based on the protection of human life.

The moral arguments pro and con could and have filled volumes. The two camps appear no closer to reaching an agreement now than they ever have. One thing seems fairly certain: abortion will be with us until and if we find a foolproof contraceptive method acceptable to a highly motivated citizenry.

Caregivers' Involvement

Abortion is such an emotional issue, with many political, religious, cultural, and moral overtones, that no one is exempt from these influences—least of all, health-care workers. One's feelings about abortion may be so deep that he or she is not totally aware of them until they begin to affect the delivery of health care. Each nurse must work to discover, analyze, and resolve her or his feelings about this issue in order that women who seek abortion services will not be punished in any way because the nurse, doctor, or counselor is not committed to providing these services.

Health professionals must not make the paternalistic assumption that they are better judges of their patients' moral values than are the patients themselves. To limit a person's right to choose is to limit the autonomy of that person (Sherwin 1981, 25).

Nathanson and Becker (1980, 1981) reported a study that showed how physicians' attitudes could determine the availability of abortion services in any given hospital. The data demonstrated that physicians who had liberal attitudes toward abortion performed abortions regardless of whether the political environment was favorable or unfavorable. Conservative physicians, however, were more likely to perform abortions only when they were in an environment that promoted them as an important part of the gynecological services. Conservative physicians who worked in a conservative antiabortion setting were not likely to perform abortions. Therefore, the provision of abortion services in an area may depend on the risks physicians believe they are taking by providing those services.

Nurses, too, can have a positive or negative influence on abortion services. If nurses have difficulty caring for abortion clients, they may focus their hostilities on these clients and treat them in a punitive way. The nurses may complain of fatigue, frequent episodes of crying, and work-related dissatisfaction (Olson 1980).

These feelings and behaviors may be traced to conflicts these nurses are feeling, which may stem from their philosophical or religious beliefs. Abortion may clash with beliefs about women as mothers. Nurses may fear that promiscuity is becoming the norm. They may refuse to allow the boyfriend or significant other to sit on the client's bed. They may feel uncomfortable about allowing the patient too much autonomy (that is, making the abortion decision). Abortion may also cause the nurse to feel confusion about her or his role. She or he may overidentify with the fetus, may have an infertility problem, or may be a maternity nurse who has always shared concerns for mother and baby (Olson 1980).

Berger (1979) studied the attitudes of 128 nurses toward abortion and found that age and religious beliefs were most important in determining attitudes. As a group, Catholics were the most disapproving, but Catholic nurses from 20 to 29 years of age had a more favorable attitude toward abortion than did young nurses of other religions. The least approving attitudes were shown by older Catholic nurses.

How can the conflicting claims of women who have a right to abortion under the law and nurses who do not believe in abortion be settled in a manner just to both groups? One small hospital solved this problem by rotating all nurses through all departments, including the abortion unit. Some nurses protested that their religious beliefs proscribed their participation in abortion care. The issue was settled under the rubric of religious freedom and those objecting nurses were no longer required to staff the abortion unit (Davis 1980).

The Nurses Association of the American College of Obstetricians and Gynecologists (1981, 61) published a statement on abortion and sterilization that reads, in part:

> Nurses have the right to refuse to assist in the performance of abortions and/or sterilization procedures in keeping with their moral, ethical, and/or religious beliefs, except in an emergency when a patient's life is clearly endangered in which case the questioned moral issue should be disregarded.

Women Seeking Abortion

The woman seeking abortion may be affected by financial considerations, misinformation, social disapproval, and personal reasons for delaying the procedure. The ghost of the double standard in abortion services reappeared in the guise of the Hyde amendment and Supreme Court rulings that removed from the federal government the responsibility of paying for abortions through Medicaid. In June of 1983, however, the Supreme Court declared some of the regulations unconstitutional (U.S. Law Week 1983). One study showed that while about 80% of poor women who chose abortions managed to pay for them, up to one-fifth of the poor women preferring abortion had their babies. An increase in the rate of sterilization among poor women has also occurred, and it appears that women are again being harmed by self-induced or illegal attempts at abortion. Poor women are no less eager to have reproductive control. It is simply more difficult for them to gain that control (Trussell et al. 1980).

Abortion regulations that affect all women, rich or poor, are imposed in some communities by hospitals and other institutions, public health agencies, and care providers. These regulations are biased to encourage women to continue their pregnancies. In the required consent forms, early abortion may be described as a major surgical procedure, even though the death rate from a legally performed abortion is about three per 100,000 procedures, making legal abortion safer than a tonsillectomy. Abortion before 16 weeks is seven times safer than continuation of the pregnancy; abortion before 13 weeks carries the same risk as that of an antibiotic injection for gonorrhea. In addition to overstating the risks, community regulations may require that the woman be given a complete description of the current state of the embryo or fetus at the time of the requested abortion. The psychological sequelae of abortion may also be exaggerated by antiabortionists in attempts to control the number of abortions performed (Cates, Gold, and Selik 1979).

The woman seeking an abortion is seen by some as a victim of circumstances, by others as one who is taking charge of her life, and by still others as a murderer. Two groups studied were women who had repeat abortions and women who delayed abortions even though they were readily available. In a study involving 1505 women who were having abortions, with repeaters comprising 16.9% of the total (Howe, Kaplan, and English 1979), some differences were apparent between the first-timers and the repeaters. Repeaters were found to have a significantly higher average rate of intercourse, and about one-half were using contraception at the time of conception, compared to about one-third of the first-timers. The study showed that the repeaters had a greater knowledge of birth control than did first-timers and 74% of the entire sample said that they did not consider abortion to be a method of birth control. The researchers concluded that motivational deficiencies did not necessarily lead to repeat abortions. Rather, logistical problems and human error were probably the culprits.

Among public health concerns regarding abortions have been the increased morbidity and mortality rates, the greater cost, and the increased emotional stress of abortions performed after the first trimester of pregnancy. One study attempted to identify the variables that were associated with late abortions so that public health interventions could be employed to decrease the numbers (Burr and Schulz 1980). There were some statistically significant factors in abortion-delaying women such as history of irregular menstruation, level of eduction, type and number of pregnancy symptoms volunteered, and moral feelings about abortion. Age, marital status, race, prior abortion, age at menarche, and Roman Catholicism were unrelated to a late-abortion decision. The researchers concluded that the reasons for seeking an abortion after the first trimester were so influenced by highly complex individual characteristics that prediction and targeted intervention are not possible.

Adolescent women in particular have come under public scrutiny in reference to abortion. In fact, there are laws in some states requiring parental notification before an abortion is performed on a woman under 18. In the decision for or against abortion, as in others, adolescents should be encouraged to look at and weigh alternatives. It is ironic that, as interpreted in some states, the law allows the "mature" teen to choose abortion but forces the "immature" teen to continue her pregnancy. The decision to terminate a pregnancy is not one made lightly by most women. As Silber says, it is "a painful offering made toward the avoidance of suffering and the promotion of a better future" (1980, 472).

Artificial Insemination

Artificial insemination is a term familiar to many people even though there has been relatively little written about it. Artificial insemination with donor sperm (AID) is a method by which some previously infertile couples may become parents. The method is technically uncomplicated. The woman keeps a record of her basal body temperature in order to determine the occurrence of ovulation, at which time she visits her health center or physician. Semen from a donor is then injected into her vagina. The procedure usually needs to be repeated over a number of cycles. It is successful in producing a pregnancy about 57% of the time (Curie-Cohen, Luttrell, and Shapiro 1979, 588).

There were 471 respondents in a study of physicians to determine the current practice of AID in the United States (Curie-Cohen et al. 1979); 80% of the respondents reported performing artificial insemination. The primary reason (95%) for AID was husband infertility. In a small number of cases the husband was fearful of transmitting a congenital disease. Single women were inseminated by about 9.5% of the responding physicians. About 11% of the women were having the procedure done after the birth of another child by AID. The physicians indicated that they usually selected the donors by matching them to the woman's husband by hair, skin and eye colors, height, ethnic background, ABO blood types, and educational level. The donors were almost always paid for their semen. Although most of the physicians took a family history from the donors, neither in-depth screening nor biochemical testing was done. The donors were often medical students, college students, husbands of patients, hospital personnel, or friends of the physician. Most doctors reported using the same donor for only one or two pregnancies. Almost 78% had never used the same donor for more than six pregnancies. However, almost 6% of the respondents had used a single donor for 15 or more pregnancies and one had actually used one donor for 50 pregnancies.

This same study showed that about one-third of the physicians kept records on the children born or on the donors. Most declared they were opposed to legislation that would require such record-keeping. Because of the highly secretive nature of the procedure (to ensure confidentiality), the number of children born through AID can only be estimated. This study estimated that from 6,000 to 10,000 such births occur each year in the United States. From this study the authors concluded that, "Current practices reflect little concern for possibility of consanguineous matings or other effects of multiple donor use" (Curie-Cohen et al. 1979, 589).

As a result of that study, Annas (1979) made some observations and recommendations. Because, in some instances, multiple donors were used to inseminate a woman during a single cycle, there would be no way of tracing defective sperm to a particular donor in the case of a congenital anomaly. Therefore, he argued for laws that would require all children who were conceived by artificial insemination to have sealed records that would eventually be available to them. The genetic father would have no legal rights or responsibilities. In addition, Annas recommended that the donor be screened by a geneticist, uniform standards be developed for the selection of donors, permanent records be kept on donors, no mixing of sperm should be done, the number of pregnancies for any one donor be limited, there be national standards for the procedure, and the children's psychological development be studied. In the same vein, Keyserlingk (1981) raised the issue of protection of the children rather than of the parents and also recommended keeping records in order to discover defective sperm.

Because of the sensitive nature of the procedure, the strong need that participants have for secrecy, and the vague laws of many states concerning it, AID has been subjected to very little scrutiny. Some religions expressly forbid it, while for some couples it is the answer to a prayer. Many other issues are raised as well. These include identification of professions with the potential fetus/child versus couple, screening of donors and recipients, and who should perform the procedure.

Issues of Technology and Reproduction

Technology is often seen as both a blessing and a scourge. This has been especially true regarding women and reproduction. Procedures and medications that allow women reproductive freedom may also reduce women's autonomy or may cause physical harm. In such cases, the circumstances surrounding their use can be approached as moral issues.

DES Exposure

In at least one instance, that of using diethylstilbestrol (DES) to prevent miscarriages, the benefits of the drug were illusory. The drug was used for about 30 years (approximately 1940 to 1970); its use was justified on the basis of one retrospective study. DES was even used in some normal pregnancies because the woman had a history of miscarrying. A prospective study on DES indicated that it had no beneficial antiabortion effects and that the results of the first study were based on better, more frequent prenatal care, and not DES (Fuller 1978). The use of the drug was discontinued when a correlation was shown between the development of vaginal adenocarcinoma in young women and their in utero exposure to DES. Although the percentage of young women developing vaginal cancer is still relatively low, vaginal cancer in young women was virtually unheard of before DES. About 90% of exposed women do develop irregular cell growth in the vagina and some studies are showing that these women are having more spontaneous abortions than nonexposed women (see Chapter 7).

In 1978 a federal task force made recommendations for health care services for DES-exposed women. A screening program was outlined for all women 14 years of age and older. Physicians were encouraged to search their records for women who might have been exposed, but few doctors did so and military records were destroyed without any review (Wetherill 1980).

Although this DES problem is short-term because the drug is no longer used, very little organized support is available for DES-exposed women. Often, the problem has been downplayed (Wetherill 1980). Hundreds of thousands of young women have not been screened or are still prepubertal so the full impact of the problem has not yet been felt (Fuller 1978). There is evidence that men exposed in utero are also experiencing noncancerous problems of the penis and testicles, as discussed in Chapter 7. The ethical issues raised by the DES scandal are profound. Women who took DES during pregnancy often were told that the pills were vitamins. They were not told that the use of DES was empirical, nor were they given any indication that it might be harmful to them or their offspring.

Sterilization

Another issue in which use of technological advances may have moral ramifications is sterilization. Although voluntary sterilization is a safe method that has enabled many couples to limit the size of their families, it has also been used in a coercive manner, most often against women. Many women have been sterilized without their consent or knowledge. Others have been given a choice of sterilization or loss of welfare benefits. Thousands of native American women have been sterilized through the use of inadequate consent forms. In a survey of a large city in the Northeast, 51% of the Hispanic women of childbearing age had been sterilized.

Because of the often immoral uses of sterilization, federal guidelines for the procedure were published. These include the required attainment of voluntary informed consent, prohibition of threat of welfare benefit loss, and prohibition of the obtaining of consent during labor, before or after abortion, or when the client is under the influence of drugs or alcohol. Also prohibited is the use of hysterectomy as a sterilization procedure (Petchesky 1979).

In Vitro Fertilization

A fairly recent scientific feat that has been receiving much publicity and some moral questioning is *in vitro fertilization,* popularly called "test tube fertilization." The procedure is used when a woman is prevented from conceiving because of blocked fallopian tubes. An egg is retrieved from the woman, placed in a laboratory dish, and fertilized using her husband's semen. Frozen zygotes may also be used. For many women, this is their only chance to conceive. To them and their partners, in vitro fertilization is an important and wonderful discovery.

There are those who have moral disagreement with proponents of in vitro fertilization, however. Steinbacher (1980) believes that it reduces women to the level of guinea pigs. She believes it epitomizes the way women are valued — by their ability to bear children. Keyserlingk (1981) questions the need for in vitro fertilization in lieu of the many health care needs going unmet in this country. It is also a very expensive procedure, with potential for financial exploitation of the infertile. In addition, some "pro-life" individuals claim that in vitro fertilization is against the "natural order" and express concern that some of the fertilized eggs may not be returned to the woman's body but will be left to "die" in the laboratory. Thus, "wastage" of extra eggs fertilized but not implanted becomes a moral issue. Other issues concern the use of donated ova as well.

As individuals, as health-care providers, and as a people, we must, at the very least, become informed about and discuss these issues. The greatest danger is complacency and lack of animated argument.

Amniocentesis

In this procedure, amniotic fluid is withdrawn from the uterus of a pregnant woman for diagnostic purposes. It has become a common procedure in recent years. It may be used late in pregnancy to test for fetal lung maturation. Earlier in the pregnancy, usually from weeks 14 to 17, amniocentesis can discover certain conditions in the fetus such as Down's syndrome. Some women elect to have an abortion if they learn the fetus is defective. While testing for defects, technicians can also determine the sex of the fetus.

Some couples prefer not to learn about their child's gender in the amniocentesis report. Other couples have asked for an abortion after amniocentesis, not because of fetal defect, but because they would prefer a baby of the other sex. There are some strong arguments against this use of amniocentesis and abortion. Amniocentesis is a relatively scarce resource in light of the numbers of at-risk pregnancies. The sex of a child is not a disease, making abortion based on sex preference a frivolous reason for the procedure. In addition, because it is believed that the majority of people prefer males, especially for the first-born, a pronounced inequality in the sexes might occur (Fletcher 1979).

Since the Supreme Court abortion decision did not require that the woman state her reason for choosing an abortion, the discussion today focuses on the use of amniocentesis for sex selection. Fletcher (1979) proposes that such procedures be considered low priority and that all expenses should be borne by the parents.

Circumcision

Some people now view routine circumcision of male babies as a moral issue. They consider it immoral to perform a painful operation on male infants without proven medical necessity. Circumcision is surgery to remove the foreskin of the penis, leaving the glans exposed; it is usually performed within a few days after birth.

This country has the highest rate of nonreligious neonatal circumcision, at the cost of about $60 million (Lovell 1979). For the last 40 to 45 years, most newborn males in the United States have been circumcised. Consumers and health-care providers alike are beginning to question the necessity of this procedure and the literature is beginning to reflect their concern. As Grimes (1980, 108) explains: "Routine circumcision of the newborn, a controversial procedure, has ethical, medical, economic, and psychological significance for all Americans. No other operation today is performed so often for such poorly understood reasons on such unwilling patients in such unlikely settings."

Circumcision is an old custom that emerged in Africa over 5000 years ago (Grimes 1980). The first records show that it was used in Egypt, where it was required for royalty, nobility, and priests (Gibbons 1979). In some cultures it is done as a religious ritual, in others, as a rite of passage from childhood to adulthood. Nonreligious circumcision was introduced into the United States in the late 1800s (Talan 1981). Since then, the operation has become routine. Even though many prospective parents take advantage of childbirth preparation classes and become informed about pregnancy and labor, they often give little or no thought about whether to have a male child circumcised. Consequently, the decision is made after the child's birth, often by the mother alone, based on little information (Gibbons 1979).

In one study that investigated the reasons why women consented to having their sons circumcised, 35% said it was for cleanliness and health. A majority (87%) said they thought circumcision was without risk and 80% said the risks had not been explained (Lovell 1979).

Another study looked at the records of 5882 live male births to compare risks with the Gomco clamp and the Plastibell device, two commonly used circumcision instruments. The complication rate was 2%: 59 patients hemorrhaged and 23 developed local infections. There were no deaths and no transfusions were necessary. It is not good practice to circumcise a baby with hypospadias (a condition occurring about once in 267 births, in which the urinary meatus is located at a place on the penis other than the tip), because the foreskin may be necessary for plastic surgery repair. This study found that circumcision was done on six babies with unrecognized hypospadias and on two babies with recognized hypospadias. Some of the other injuries noted included complete separation of the penile skin from the mucous membrane, excessive skin removal, denuding of the entire shaft of the penis in one case, and an injury to the glans in another. The study found that the devices tested were about equal in safety (Gee and Ansel 1976).

Another study noted a significant increase in the levels of plasma cortisol 20 to 40 minutes after circumcision. Behavioral studies showed that babies who were circumcised responded differently to auditory stimuli than female newborns and uncircumcised male newborns (Grimes 1980).

The major medical reasons given for the widespread practice of circumcision are cleanliness, phimosis, and prevention of cancer of the penis. However, these reasons have been proven invalid. Good hygiene practice by uncircumcised males removes any smegma that may accumulate. *Phimosis,* or nonretractable foreskin, is common among infants—only 4% of all newborns have retractable foreskins—but the problem generally disappears with time. By the age of 6 months, 20% of all males have retractable foreskins, and this figure increases to 90% by the age of 3 (Gibbons 1979). By age 16 or 17 years, only 1% of uncircumcised males have a problem with phimosis (Grimes 1980). Regarding cancer of the penis, in Scandinavia, where males are not circumcised, the rate of cancer of the penis is one in 100,000, a rate similar to that of the United States, where the majority of males are circumcised (Gee and Ansell 1976). Bullough and Bullough (1977, 70) suspect that there is another nonmedical, and also erroneous, basis for widespread circumcision in this country: the belief that it is a cure for masturbation. Social reasons might include wanting one's child to look like most children.

Circumcision is a valid procedure in tropical areas where fungus infections are commonly a problem, as well as in desert climates where sand trapped under the foreskin can cause balanitis, an inflammation of the glans and the mucous membrane underneath it (Gee and Ansell 1976).

Even if parents in this country choose circumcision after careful consideration of these facts, it is not good practice to circumcise a newborn immediately after delivery before he has made the transition to extra-uterine physiology. Waiting up to 24 hours also gives more time for a complete and accurate assessment of the baby's health status.

Issues of Eroticism

Because we live in a sex-repressed society that is also "sex-centric," the messages that people receive about sexuality are garbled. Even though sexuality is basic to human nature, many societies have made it a problem (Hett-

linger 1966). The Bulloughs (1977) traced hostility to sex back to the ancient Greeks. The Greeks espoused a philosophy of dualism, that is, defining two natures in each person—spiritual and material. The spiritual was the higher nature and each person was to strive to perfect the spiritual while eschewing the material. Sex was, of course, material, and therefore something to overcome. Christianity adopted many of these beliefs as set forth by Plato. Augustine, an early Christian writer who before his conversion had an active sex life, became one of the major proponents of celibacy. If one could not be celibate, then marriage was a second choice. Sexual intercourse, however, should occur only for the purpose of reproduction.

We can see the effects of such a background in our own society. Because of beliefs that sexual intercourse has procreation as its only justification, any sexual behavior that does not lead to that end is considered by many to be perverted. Many states passed laws prohibiting petting practices (Hettlinger 1966), and some are still on the books. Many states have had laws defining who could use birth control. There are still laws against homosexuality that are selectively enforced.

Sexual intercourse outside of legal marriage—whether it be premarital, extramarital, or sexual activity of single, divorced, or widowed individuals—is condemned by some churches and by many individuals. Even within marriage, individuals and religious groups may also view as immoral certain nonreproductive practices, such as oral and anal sex.

In the context of sexual practices within marriage, some questions also arise concerning the rights of each spouse. Does the man have a right to his wife against her will? Can rape occur within the context of a legal marriage? In some states, courts have upheld convictions of men charged with raping their own wives (Croft 1979a, 1979b; A Revolution in Rape 1979). Does marriage mean that "anything goes"? Is consent an issue within a marriage? Does a woman contribute to a pattern of violence by participating in recurrent breakups and passionate reconciliations? (Nass, Libby, and Fisher 1981, 381).

Sadomasochism, although allegedly a practice based on mutual consent, raises moral issues for the participants as well as for society. If these practices were prosecuted in any way, issues of privacy and the right to self-determination would be raised. On the other hand, when sadomasochism trespasses the boundary of safety and injuries occur, what responsibilities does the health-care provider have, if any, toward protecting the victim? Santini, in her extensive study of such practices, concludes that although participants willingly subject themselves to practices that represent fantasies of being dominated, the victims usually suffer physical consequences (1976, 6–8).

Virginity

The concept of virginity has played an important role in moral issues throughout the centuries and many rituals have evolved around it. For example, in some cultures, a bloody sheet hung out of the window after the wedding night is considered proof that the bride was indeed a virgin. Through the years, many ingenious methods were developed to trick the new husband into believing his bride was a virgin. One method advocated by Trotula, an 11th-century woman physician, was for the already deflowered "false virgin" to place a leech on her labia the day before her wedding. Blood would then crust around the vaginal orifice, narrowing its opening, and simulate an intact hymen (O'Faolain and Martines 1973, 156).

The ideology of virginity most often pertains to women and was probably an aspect of the male's property rights. In order to retain some control, the female then uses sexuality as a bargaining element (Berger and Wenger 1973). A double standard still exists in this country in the expectation that the bride be a virgin and the groom "experienced."

Berger and Wenger suspected that the concept of virginity was a fluid one and had to be in order to be effective. Their study showed that the definitions for loss of virginity vary a great deal. There was no single female sexual behavior endorsed by every respondent of their survey as constituting loss of virginity. Most importantly, the study showed that although the concept of virginity has come down through the years as a "given," it is still complex and has many variables (p. 675).

In contrast to Western culture's affirmation of the concept of virginity, matriarchal societies placed little emphasis on an intact hymen. In societies in the Far East, girls were deflowered before puberty, because women's blood was often considered taboo and this ritual defloration spared men from having to draw women's blood (David 1972, 159).

Masturbation

Masturbation, or autoeroticism, is self-stimulation for sexual pleasure. Hands, vibrators, soft fabrics, or running water are often used for pleasurable sensations, pehaps enhanced by the reading of erotic literature or viewing of erotic pictures. The choices are almost limitless and a matter of individual preference. Such practices may or may not lead to orgasm. Even though in Western culture masturbation was once imputed to cause problems from acne to insanity, according to studies from Kinsey to the present time, it is very common. In many instances it is a healthful way of reducing sexual tension.

Nevertheless, masturbation was seen as evil, especially in Western culture, for many years. Many religions prohibited it because it involves sexual pleasure removed from reproductive functions. Prominent physicians explained "scientifically" why masturbation was harmful. Methods for curbing masturbation often involved mutilating procedures. For example, the removal or cauterization of the clitoris was used to prevent girls and women from practicing autoeroticism. Some physicians were so convinced that masturbation was the source of innumerable diseases that they formed a masturbation-prevention society and published the *Journal of Orificial Surgery*. Chastity belts for both males and females, with designs reflecting great creativity, were registered in the United States patent office. The purpose of the belts was to prevent masturbation (Bullough and Bullough 1977, 66–70).

The remnants of these attitudes and practices make masturbation a moral issue even today. Discomfort with and guilt about masturbation are still evident, and as discussed in Chapter 1, many parents are uncertain how to deal with their children's genital exploration. Among some religions and for some individuals, masturbation is considered a highly immoral practice.

As practiced by a few, masturbation can actually be dangerous. Unfortunately, creativity in the search for erotic pleasure has placed some individuals in precarious situations. Some people, mostly young males, have devised complicated methods that cause a degree of hypoxia in their bodies. It increases sexual pleasure by enhancing fantasies and producing a "high." A variety of methods have been used to achieve these ends, such as hanging devices, plastic bags, and electric current. Since death is not intended, rescue mechanisms are part of the plan. One such mechanism is the use of a stool to enable the person to stand erect and thus arrest the hanging process. When the rescue mechanism fails, death occurs. Thus the names of this occurrence: "dangerous autoerotic practice," "terminal sex," or "Kotzwarraism," after an 18th-century man who

died during such practice (Hazelwood, Burgess, and Groth 1981).

This method of dying may be mistaken as suicide or homicide when it is in reality accidental. Although it is rare at the present time (estimated at 250 deaths per year in the United States), there is concern that it will increase. More accurate statistics will become available in the future as law officials learn to recognize the signs of autoerotic death. These signs include lack of suicidal intent and evidence of a rescue mechanism, solo sexual activity, fantasy aids, and prior practices (Hazelwood et al. 1981, 130). More research needs to be done to further identify risk factors so that lifesaving interventions are available.

Fortunately, most autoerotic practices are not harmful but are very pleasurable for the individual. Sexual needs and desires are normal facets of human existence. To legislate or condone only certain practices violates the right to individual freedom to experience life in a variety of ways, as long as those ways do not violate the rights of others. As Nass, Libby, and Fisher explain, "Learning to know and enjoy our bodies intimately can help us build and maintain a solid and positive self-concept at any age. Self-pleasuring can be a rich part of our sexual lives—neither better nor worse than intercourse, just different—from the cradle to the grave." (1981, 96–97)

Pornography

Pornography and obscenity are difficult concepts to define. Pornography is visual or auditory stimuli that cause one to have erotic responses. Obscenity is visual or auditory stimuli considered offensive. The problem lies in trying to distinguish between the two in an objective manner in order to determine what is socially acceptable, because the reactions to pornography and obscenity are subjective and individual. What is pornography to one person may well be defined as obscenity by another.

Explicit sexual materials take many forms, including street pornography such as movies, live sex shows, peep shows, books, and topless bars (Van Gelder 1980, 62). Some of this material is sadistic or violent in nature: hanging, whipping, a woman in a meat grinder, a woman scissoring her labia, and women in chains or being struck by men (Van Gelder 1980, 62–64). Pornography is not confined to 42nd Street in New York or the combat zone of Boston, however. It is present on countless newsstands in the form of the classy glossies that justify their existence with articles and fiction, interspersed with full color photographs of nude persons, usually women (Walker 1980, 67). Pornography also exists in the form of comics. An analysis of these revealed that women and men were depicted as having similar carnal appetites and sexual aggression. However, the comics may be classified as male chauvinistic because male fantasies predominate. Women are pictured as prostitutes and themes such as incest, homosexuality, bondage, and seduction appear (Palmer 1979).

According to Bullough and Bullough (1977), before the print medium became common, pornography was available only to the wealthy or educated and was not considered a problem. When societies become literate and have an effective system for mass communication, pornography takes the place of prostitution as a major concern (Woodward 1978). From the 1600s to the present there have been groups that have tried to ban books or plays because of pornographic content. Prohibitions notwithstanding, production and marketing of erotica is a profitable industry.

Consumers of the over $2 billion erotic materials industry come from all socioeconomic and education levels. The main consumers, though, are urban, white, middle-class males who have had at least some higher

education (Woodward 1978). Two studies found that among adolescents, the level of exposure to pornography was low, and that its influence was not dominant. Those adolescents reflect normal patterns of psychosexual behavior (Berger et al. 1973, 307–308).

In 1957 in the Roth decision the Supreme Court ruled that material was obscene if it appealed to "prurient interests." Prurient was defined as "a sick and morbid interest in sex." The Court also decided that individual communities should set their own standards (Woodward 1978). There is controversy in the research literature as to whether or not such community standards do, in fact, exist. Brown and associates found that it appears to be possible to establish a "community standard" in small communities, that standards for judgment vary among individuals, and that these standards relate to the "degree of pornography" of the material (1978, 94).

By the 1970s some feminists became outspoken against pornography, especially the sadistic, woman-torturing pornography shown in movies and on record album covers. These women believed there was a link between ". . . male sexual fantasy and the desire to dominate, between male sexuality and male violence" (Ehrenreich, Hess, and Jacobs 1982, 64). They have organized groups to suppress pornography, while at the same time preserving the First Amendment (Morgan 1978, 78–80). Actions take the form of "browse-ins" in bookstores, conferences, pressuring firms to delete advertising that is pornographic, and organizing conferences to raise consciousness about pornography (Van Gelder 1980, 66).

Some evidence does exist in the literature that points to a relationship between violence against women and violent pornography. One study found a correlation between reported levels of arousal in men and depictions of a rape victim who described having a response of involuntary orgasm with pain (Malamuth,

Heim, and Feshbach 1980, 399–408). Some pornography appears to condone violence against women. Acts of physical abuse, rape, torture, and murder may be shown as a means of getting what one wants, as an appropriate means of handling frustration, and as being socially acceptable (Malamuth and Spinner 1980).

Many feminists disagree with the stand against pornography, however. Women as well as men enjoy pornography. One anthropologist sees it as a reflection of male dominance in our culture, not as the cause of it (Ehrenreich, Hess, and Jacobs 1982). Some encourage distinguishing between erotica and pornography in determining which materials are socially acceptable. In this distinction, pornography is sexually explicit material that is degrading and demeaning and is presented in such a way as to condone the degradation (Longino 1980). It is dehumanizing, hostile, and encourages violence (Task Force on Pornography 1981; Dworkin 1981; Griffin 1981). The roots of the word *pornography* mean "prostitution," and "female captives," implying domination of and violence against women (Steinem 1978, 54). By contrast, erotica has its root in "eros" or passionate love, imparting the ideas of choice, free will, and desire for a certain person. As Steinem explains, "Erotica is about sexuality, but pornography is about power and sex-as-weapon" (1978, 54).

Woodward (1978) believes that sexually explicit material is needed for the shy, the unattractive, the crippled, and for those in hospitals and other institutions who are unable to satisfy sexual needs in an interpersonal way. Understanding this role of erotic material, nurses may feel more comfortable with clients' use of this material in a health-care setting. On the other hand, pornography need not be seen only as a substitute. Many people with sexual partners and/or those able to satisfy sexual needs in other ways also like and enjoy erotic materials. Others feel that sexually explicit materials are necessary for sex education to be effective.

Sexual Abuse of Children

Sexual abuse of children takes many forms, from incest, to sex rings, to their use in pornographic pictures and films. Specific problems as addressed by caregivers are discussed in detail in Chapter 7. The focus here will be on the ethical arguments against such victimization of children.

Finkelhor (1979) employs important ethical arguments against sex between adults and children. This type of abuse of children is so obviously wrong to the large majority of adults that intuitive arguments are used. But some persons have debated whether these practices are intrinsically wrong. The second argument focuses on the premature sexualization of the child. Since children are not asexual, this argument, too, is not without controversy. The third argument is that this type of activity might have long-term negative effects on the child. Burgess, Goth, and McCausland (1981) postulate that there is potential for harmful long-term results. Yet so many of these children, as Dudar (1977, 80) points out in reference to child pornography, ". . . grow up with such a galaxy of problems that the picture-taking represents only one episode in a grievously blighted life." To date, there are no studies supporting the third argument.

The issue of consent is the one argument that will stand up. We are approaching the time when consent by adults will be the standard by which the morality of an act is judged. When consent is lacking, our society considers the act immoral or illegal. Consent must reflect free choice and a knowledge of what one is consenting to. Because children are not sophisticated about sex, because they are not knowledgeable about the criteria to use in judging a sexual partner, and because adults are in a position of power, children are unable to give "informed" consent. Adults and children engaged in sexual activity are not in an equal relationship (Finkelhor 1979).

Issues of Sexual Preference

Informed consent and free personal choice should be present in sexual preferences for partners of one's own sex, for partners of both sexes, or for a personal change in gender. Yet some in our society view these personal preferences as moral issues.

Homosexuality

Homosexuality means a sexual preference for a member of the same sex. The word's origin is the Greek word *homos,* meaning "the same." From antiquity, different cultures have viewed homosexuality in different ways, including homosexuals themselves.

Historical Variations in Attitudes

In ancient Greece, homosexuality was common and was associated with pederasty, a man's receiving gratification by having sexual activity with a boy. Women homosexuals were tribads. The island of Lesbos was considered the home of the tribads (Tannahill 1980).

The *Koran* does not prohibit homosexuality and among Islamic people it has been common. One reason may be because the practice of polygamy decreased the numbers of available women. The purpose of marriage was procreative so it was perhaps the need for relationships that was instrumental in encouraging male-liaisons (Bullough and Bullough 1977).

In ancient China very little sexual activity was proscribed, including homosexuality. The outlook on sexuality seemed to be totally different than that of Western culture. In fact, people who abstained from sexual activity were viewed with suspicion (Bullough and Bullough 1977).

By contrast, using the biblical story of Sodom as its basis, the Catholic church condemned homosexuality. As recently as 1976, the pope described homosexuality as shameful, infamous, and horrible (Tannahill 1980, 153). One can understand the negative outlook of our society on homosexuality if one views it in the context of the Judeo-Christian tradition which "condemns all forms of sexual expression except that between a man and a woman who are committed to a lifelong monogamous relationship and whose goal is the creation of children" (Lee 1977, 230). Undoubtedly, this negative attitude is also reflected in the irrational fear of homosexuality, or *homophobia.*

Many myths about homosexuality and homosexuals have been perpetuated in our culture. A common one is that homosexual men molest children. In reality, 90% of all sexual abuse of children is perpetrated by heterosexual men on minor males (Bachman 1981). There is also a myth about stereotypical behavior—the notion that homosexual men are effeminate and homosexual women are masculine. Wearing clothing usually associated with the other sex *(transvestism)* may or may not be associated with homosexuality (Bachman 1981). Another old, unsupported theory is that homosexual males are supposed to have weak fathers and dominant mothers. The cause or causes of homosexuality continue to elude us but present evidence indicates that any type of parent can produce homosexual offspring. Most experts now believe that the causes of homosexuality are multidimensional and individual (Kessler 1980).

Homosexuals have been and still are discriminated against and persecuted. For instance, there are civil laws still in effect that prohibit activities such as masturbation, oral-genital sex, anal-genital sex, sex between unmarried people, and sex between people of the same sex. These laws are virtually never enforced against heterosexuals but are enforced against homosexuals (Lee 1977). Homosexuals are often denied positions of responsibility and authority within our society (Richards 1979). When they do achieve such positions but have kept their sexual preferences secret, there is always the fear of being "found out" and blackmailed or fired.

Homosexuals have had to contend with the results of many early studies that concluded that these men and women had more psychopathology than heterosexuals. These studies involved clients in therapeutic settings. More recent studies using randomized populations have not supported those earlier findings (O'Leary 1979).

Nevertheless, the climate for homosexuals seems to be improving. There are probably many reasons for the changes that are occurring. One important change occurred on December 15, 1973, when the American Psychiatric Association removed homosexuality from the official list of mental disorders. Many minority groups — including homosexuals — are beginning to cast off the behavior associated with oppression and are demanding their rights as human beings and citizens. Some religious communities are showing an acceptance of homosexuality (Lee 1977). Parents of homosexuals may have difficulty accepting their children's sexual preferences and may feel guilty, believing that they are to blame. These parents are finding support and mutual understanding in groups formed for those purposes (Fairchild and Hayward 1980).

Individual Variations

Homosexual individuals are precisely that — individuals. Just as not all heterosexuals follow the same pattern of sexual functioning, neither do homosexuals. The Institute for Sex Research (also known as the Kinsey Institute) studied a large group of homosexuals, about two-thirds of whom were male and one-third female. The researchers concluded that five clusters of homosexuals could be delineated based on the way their sex lives were organized. The first group was called *close-coupled.* These people lived in relatively monogamous relationships. These respondents reported fewer sexual problems than married heterosexuals. The second group, *open-coupled,* was composed of people living with a partner but who also had sexual contacts outside the home. The third group, called *functionals,* had a very active sex life with many partners, had an active social life, were self-accepting, and were involved in the homosexual subculture. *Asexuals* comprised the fourth group. These were generally single individuals with a low level of sexual activity but who reported contentment. The *dysfunctional* group were those who regretted their homosexuality, were poorly adjusted, and were likely to be in therapy. In the past, this was the only group that was studied (Owen 1980). Women are represented to a greater extent in the first two groups than in the last three groups.

Riddle applauds the Kinsey study which, in part, says that most homosexuals are not distinguishable from heterosexuals except for the sexual part of their lives. Riddle's criticism was based on the study's conclusion that homosexuality is a rejection of heterosexuality rather than "a positive choice." She also was disappointed that most of the subjects of the study were white males (1978, 44). The study is a good beginning for further research, however.

Lesbian Health-Care Needs

As shown by the above study, lesbian women are less likely than males and no more likely than heterosexual women to engage in sexual activities with many partners (O'Leary 1979). Lesbian women have fewer health problems of the reproductive tract than do heterosexual women. Venereal diseases are rare and, while other vaginal infections such as yeast may occur, they occur less frequently. Because lesbians do not need to use contraceptives, they are not exposed to risks associated with intrauterine devices and oral contraceptives (Hornstein 1974).

There is very little documentation in health-care literature about lesbian needs. Instead, the information is circulated among women and their health centers. O'Donnell (1978) sees the need for research in this area since much information is being recirculated rather than newly generated. One noticeable point in all of the literature written about health care and lesbians is the lack of understanding these women receive in our health-care system (Campbell-Bridges 1981). The dissatisfaction they feel often keeps them from seeking care. Although some "folk" remedies may cure or palliate certain conditions, traditional treatment may be needed for some conditions. Because of the indifferent attitudes of some health-care professionals, women may not be receiving needed care.

One study polled 117 homosexual women in order to discover health-care utilization practices, their gynecologic problems, and their attitudes toward physicians. The responses showed that 38% went to private physicians for their health care, 17% used student health services, and 35% used alternative clinics. Eighty percent of the women reported that they had engaged in heterosexual acts in the past. The main gynecological problem was vaginitis, such as yeast or trichomonas. The small numbers of herpes and gonorrhea cases reported were not acquired during homosexual activities. Forty percent of the women believed that their health care would be adversely affected if they were to reveal their homosexuality to their physicians, 18% had told a physician about their sexual preference, and 49% said they would like to tell their physicians, but only seven women

said that their physicians had asked them. Sixty-three percent of the women said they would probably reveal their lesbianism if they could be sure it would not become part of their medical record. The researchers recommended that Pap screening still be done on homosexual women, that physicians consider artificial insemination of lesbians, and that physicians develop a supportive, open attitude (Johnson et al. 1981). Although these recommendations were geared toward physicians, they apply to all health-care providers, including nurses.

Homosexual Male Health-Care Needs

In contrast to female homosexuals, male homosexuals have a high incidence of problems due to sexual activity. One study of more than 4000 male homosexuals who volunteered to complete a self-administered questionnaire yielded data that are interesting, though limited in application because a nonrandom sample was used. The age range was 16 to 78 years. The study had three purposes: (1) to compare the distribution of disease from self-ranking (through questionnaires) and from clinically reported sources; (2) to predict risk factors for sexually transmissible diseases (STD); and (3) to learn about these homosexuals' reactions to the health care they received (Darrow et al. 1981).

The most common STD reported was pediculosis (pubic lice or crabs) with an incidence of almost 67%. In decreasing order were gonorrhea, nonspecific urethritis, venereal warts, scabies, syphilis, hepatitis, and herpes. The study supported previous ones that showed that homosexual men have higher rates of STD than heterosexual men or women. This is due to their having a larger number of sexual liaisons, often with strangers, and unprotected anal intercourse. The study also showed that those men who obtained health care at gay clinics went more frequently and had more positive feelings about the care they received than those who went to other institutions for health care (Darrow et al. 1981).

Because anal intercourse is a common practice among male homosexuals, symptoms of STD are often manifested as anal or colon disorders. Anorectal gonorrhea may cause burning, itching, bleeding or other discharge, and painful defecation. Many other enteric diseases such as amebiasis, giardiasis, shigellosis, and hepatitis are now recognized as STD. The term "Gay bowel syndrome" refers to a variety of intestinal problems caused by anal intercourse. Some other conditions that may result from anal intercourse are infections or ulcers that occur above the anal ring and mimic rectal carcinoma. Conditions that may be worsened or caused by anal intercourse are prolapsed hemorrhoids, fissures and fistulae, abscesses, warts, nonspecific proctitis, and anal tears. Oral-genital sex may result in gonococcal pharyngitis (Dritz 1980; Owen 1980).

The Centers for Disease Control recently announced that male homosexuals are at risk for a serious disorder called acquired immunodeficiency syndrome (AIDs), formerly known as gay-related immunodeficiency (GRID). This disorder suppresses the body's immune system and is believed responsible for a variety of problems now seen in the homosexual population. These include anemias, rare cancers such as Kaposi's sarcoma, eye damage, generalized lymphedema, and weight loss. The Centers believe that over 1000 people have been affected and 500 or so have died.

Researchers believe that a variety of organisms are probably responsible, together with other variables. There is now some question of simple contagion to other family members. A major risk factor is multiplicity of sexual partners. For example, one study showed that the median lifetime number of male partners for affected homosexual men was 1160 as opposed to 524 for male homosexuals not afflicted with AIDS. Other risk factors may be the use of sexual stimulants and illicit drugs. Many theories about the cause(s) of the disorder are forthcoming and research continues (Altman 1982).

It is clear that the male homosexual population is prey to many and varied disease processes. There are both public health and economic concerns; homosexuals must receive attention from health-care providers. Medical information about AIDS and other STD is given in Chapter 6; the following discussion concerns openness about and acceptance of homosexual preferences in health-care settings.

Meeting Homosexual Health-Care Needs

Health-care providers need to be aware that about 10% of the population, or 20 million people, are gay. It is important not to make the assumption that one's client is heterosexual. The use of gender-free terms such as partner helps in communication. Some gays keep their homosexuality a secret. "Coming out" means living with the "integration of homosexuality into one's identity." "Disclosure" means telling others about one's sexual preference (Bachman 1981).

The most important health-care need for homosexuals is acceptance. Lack of acceptance often causes gays to delay seeking health care or to stay away altogether (Maurer 1979; Caulkins 1981).

Knowledge of a patient's homosexuality may have a direct impact on the diagnosis and care the patient receives. For example, if a patient is a lesbian, ectopic pregnancy would be eliminated as a possible diagnosis when the presenting symptom is abdominal pain. One lesbian's diagnosis of venereal disease turned out to be a serious kidney problem. Throat and rectal cultures for gonorrhea must be taken as well as urethral cultures on the male homosexual (Brossart 1979).

Although in many instances it is important to know if a patient is homosexual, there may be problems in finding out and ethical issues in dispersing or recording the knowledge. One might ask if there is anything about the patient's lifestyle that might have a bearing on the present complaint. Or the patient might be asked if there is anything about her or his sexual activity that causes concern (Altshuler et al. 1980). Once the nurse has learned that the patient is gay, she or he should not disclose the information without the patient's permission, nor should pressure be put on the patient to tell his or her parents (Bachman 1981).

Pogoncheff (1979, 49) discusses the gay patient's rights in the hospital setting. Some questions the nurse should consider are: Is the patient really homosexual? (If the patient did not disclose this information.) Where did the information come from? Who knows? How is the information communicated? What are the attitudes of providers toward the patient's homosexuality? Is the patient's attitude being attributed to homosexuality rather than to personality traits or illness? What does the staff know and think about homosexuality in general?

Problems for the client are not necessarily over once disclosure has been made to the care givers. Nurses and other health-care providers must be aware of their own feelings and attitudes. Whether heterosexual, homosexual, bisexual, or celibate themselves, they must respond to homosexual clients as individuals, not to their own feelings about sexual preferences. Attitudes toward clients are expressed in many ways — facial expressions, tone of voice, manner of touching, or even avoidance of touching.

In the case of a serious illness or other situations where visiting is restricted, the "significant other" should be determined by the client, not the practitioner. Ideally, the gay client should receive legal aid to determine arrangements in cases of emergencies or serious illnesses when unable to give consent for herself or himself (Pettyjohn 1979).

A positive attitude toward sexuality by all health-care professionals would go a long way in providing humanistic, comprehensive care, no matter what the setting. These positive attitudes could be put into practice by helping all individuals to value their feelings and bodies and to understand that sexual feelings are natural at any age (Lee 1977).

Health-care providers and all individuals must be educated about homosexuality. It should be a part of every sex education program and an integral part of the curricula in professional schools for caregivers. If prejudices could be eliminated, there would be no need to have separate health care facilities so that homosexuals can feel comfortable.

Homosexual Parents

Caregivers may also serve homosexuals who are parents. Many male and female homosexuals are parents. In fact, it has been estimated that perhaps as many as 33% of lesbians are mothers. Many others would like to have children. Artificial insemination is one method a lesbian might use to become pregnant, although she may need to lie about her sexual preference to gain access to a sperm bank (O'Donnell 1978). Some lesbians use "home methods" of artificial insemination — that is, they find a man willing to donate sperm, and then inject them into their own vaginas with a turkey baster or put semen in a diaphragm (O'Donnell 1978).

There is a common fear among heterosexuals that lesbians do not make good mothers or that their children will also be homosexual. At least two studies have disputed these contentions. Hoeffer (1981) studied 20 lesbian and 20 heterosexual women and their only or oldest child. The children's peers seemed to have a great deal more influence on their choices of toys and activities than did their mothers.

Both groups of mothers were similar in their encouragement of sex-role behavior. Another study showed that lesbian and heterosexual mothers were very much alike in their child-care practices (Kirkpatrick, Smith, and Roy 1981).

Gay fathers are faced with problems also. They are men with two identities at the opposite ends on a scale of social acceptance. Because of his fathering role a gay man may have difficulty establishing a relationship with another man. He must be able to function in both a heterosexual and a homosexual sphere in to order to gain self-acceptance as a gay father (Bozett 1981). Caregivers who are themselves heterosexual must acknowledge homosexual parents as individuals whose personal sexual preferences are both acceptable and irrelevant to their role as parents.

Bisexuality

Bisexuality or *ambisexuality* is another way people have of expressing their sexuality. It means sexual attraction to people of both sexes and engaging in sexual activity with people of either sex. Some experts believe there is no such phenomenon, that bisexuals simply have not discovered who they are and what they like (Orlando 1978). Most bisexuals reject this stereotype, however. Since the "sexual revolution" many people are trying things out and perhaps experimenting with new forms of sexual expression. It is estimated that 15% to 20% of the population consider themselves to be bisexual (Thomas 1980).

One group of researchers administered a questionnaire to 138 male and 58 female second-year medical students in order to learn more about bisexuality. About two-thirds of the men and women reported that during puberty they felt some sexual attraction to members of the same sex. Forty-five percent of the males and 48% of the females reported

they were currently aware of having those feelings (McConaghy et al. 1979).

Orlando (1978) discussed unique problems of the bisexual woman. She expressed the feeling that often heterosexual women were not comfortable with her. She thought men were sometimes interested in her out of curiosity. Also, she is discriminated against by both heterosexuals and homosexuals. While feeling the sting of homophobia, she nevertheless is not welcome in the gay community. Caregivers who are heterosexuals or homosexuals cannot let their own preferences pose similar barriers in health-care services.

Transsexualism

Transsexuals are individuals who feel that they have been born with the body of the wrong sex. They have a compulsion to live, dress, and behave as a member of the opposite sex. Surgery to physically transform one sex to the other was reported as early as 1931. The procedure became known in this country in 1953 when Christine Jorgensen publicized her sex-change surgery that was performed in Denmark. In 1967 Johns Hopkins legitimized transsexual surgery by formally opening a center to do surgery of this type (Raymond 1979, 22). Most transsexual surgery involves conversion from male to female.

The surgery involved is extensive and is performed over a period of time in stages. Before surgery is undertaken, however, counseling is done, the individual lives as a member of the opposite sex for a period of time, and hormones are given to enhance secondary sexual characteristics of the desired sex (such as breast development, body contours, and facial and body hair). This takes one to two years or more of hormone therapy.

There are numerous moral, legal, and political issues surrounding this therapeutic surgery for "gender dysphoria." Raymond

(1979, xviii) believes that the basic cause of transsexualism is "a society that produces sex-role stereotyping"—that is, one that does not allow expression of self that is gender-free. For example, why should women be "permitted" to be both nurturing and to wear "men's" attire, but not men? For the interested reader, Raymond's book does a good job of analyzing transsexualism in a moral-political context.

In our increasingly medicalized society, is transsexual surgery one more unnecessary technological achievement or is it a truly needed procedure of great help to those who choose it? It is expensive, taking the time of teams of professionals. Could this time and money be spent in ways more beneficial to all of the population, or at least to a larger portion of society? These are important questions that each citizen and health-care professional must come to terms with. Meanwhile, the procedures are being performed at the request of those who feel that to be honestly who they are, they must present themselves publicly as the other sex.

There are few follow-up studies of transsexuals. Once these individuals change their sex, they seem to desire anonymity and are not readily available as subjects for research. Hunt and Hampson (1980) were able to study 17 male-to-female transsexuals after surgery. Their data showed no changes in the subjects' levels of psychopathology from the preoperative levels. There were moderate gains in interpersonal relationships and economic functioning. The area in which the largest gains occurred were in sexual satisfaction and acceptance by family members. Not one of the subjects had any doubts about the surgery. The study noted that 24% of the group expressed a "driven need for further surgical procedures" (p. 436). The authors concluded that transsexual surgery is palliative, not curative. Its aim should be to promote better adjustment rather than to correct underlying psychological problems. The researchers recommended that transsexuals live and work in the new role prior to surgery, and that they be carefully selected preoperatively on the basis of ego strength and adjustment during the trial period.

In the quest for the cause or causes of homosexuality and an understanding of transsexualism many hypotheses have been created and tested. Although these two expressions of sexuality are often lumped together, it is important to recognize that they are completely different phenomena. One study tested the hypothesis that transsexualism is a defense against homosexuality. That is, the transsexual man can label the sexual experiences he has with another man heterosexual rather than homosexual (Hellman et al. 1981). It has been observed that many transsexuals are Catholic but that Catholics make up proportionately less of the homosexual population. Therefore, it was thought that transsexualism might be a defense against the Catholic prohibition of homosexuality. However, the study by Hellman and colleagues did not support those hypotheses.

Pattison and Pattison (1980) reported on a study involving 11 men who said they had changed from homosexuality to heterosexuality through a religious experience. Two subsequent letters proposed explanations. The first postulated that reaction formation may have occurred, because the men were committed to the therapy group, the crisis center, and their peers (Hetrick and Martin 1981). The second criticism of the study viewed it as an example of heterosexual bias in psychotherapy (Morin 1981). It is important to recognize that although behavior may change, basic sexual preference may remain the same.

Issues of Health-Care Provision

In addition to encountering ramifications of the issues previously discussed, health-care providers may be directly involved with sexual issues in health-care provision. Issues discussed here are discrimination against women, sexual abuse by health-care providers, and sexual involvement of clients with care providers or visitors.

Discrimination Against Women

Because over 90% of physicians are men and 75% of other health-care personnel are women, and because women's health complaints are often related to their reproductive tracts, it is no surprise that women often have complaints about the health-care system. Some examples of the dehumanization of women can still be seen in the use of the lithotomy position for childbirth, the virtual obliteration until very recently of the field of midwifery, and the feelings of women that their complaints are not taken seriously (Thompson and Thompson 1980).

The ways in which health-care providers have treated women's reproductive systems have often put women at risk. Unsafe or questionably safe contraceptive practices, the large number of unnecessary hysterectomies, and denying women equal treatment because of menstruation and menopause — often on the basis of unproven medical "research" — leave no doubt that reform is essential (Notman and Nadelson 1978).

One example of paternalism that negatively influences the health care of women is the custom whereby physicians must write an "order" for a Reach to Recovery volunteer to see a woman who has had a mastectomy. These volunteers work through the American Cancer Society and are women who have had mastectomies. They visit women in the hospital who have recently undergone a mastectomy procedure for the purpose of giving them information about prostheses and exercise. One study revealed that women who saw a Reach to Recovery volunteer during their mastectomy postoperative recovery had higher levels of knowledge about their own hand and arm care and about breast cancer than women who had not seen a volunteer. Other benefits were their better self-breast-exam technique and greater range of motion in the affected arm. But perhaps one of the most important benefits of these visits was that the patient could see a woman who had had the same type of surgery dressed in street clothes and going about her daily activities. The researcher recommended that nurses take more initiative in suggesting that women be visited by Reach to Recovery volunteers. She also suggested that all postmastectomy patients be given the opportunity to see a volunteer (Stecchi 1980).

There is resistance to the Reach to Recovery program from physicians, however. That resistance seems unreasonable since it is not a costly program, it is sponsored by the American Cancer Society, and it is a woman-to-woman program. The issue here seems to be one of controlling the woman's access to information (Haskins 1980).

Sexual Abuse by Health-Care Providers

Another problem that demonstrates the woman's vulnerability as a patient is the sexually abusive physician. Although the relationship between the patient and the health-care provider should be founded on trust, there are times when the patient's best interests are set aside and she (females most often encounter this situation) becomes an object of pleasure to her physician. Physician abuse may occur in a variety of settings, but psychiatric and gynecological patients seem to be most vulnerable.

Burgess (1981) studied 16 women who were victims of sexual exploitation by a gynecologist. For this study, sexual misconduct by physicians was defined as ". . . intentional manipulation of a female's genitals under the guise of conducting an internal gynecological examination—manual manipulation that in some cases resulted in orgasm" (p. 1336). The women were molested during an eight-year span by a physician who publicly admitted his guilt. The women were between 23 and 37 years of age; all were married. The women described their examinations as lengthy, lasting 20 to 30 minutes. There was misuse of the physician's hands (rubbing the clitoris, for example); the nurse was absent; and an excess of lubricant was used. The patients felt that something was wrong but felt powerless. Ten women described feelings of sexual arousal, eight described orgasm, and eight described physical discomfort. All of the women reported that they felt upset, confused, dirty, humiliated, degraded, and embarrassed. The women felt that no one would believe them. As Burgess explains, ". . . when the accused in pressured sexual situations is a person in higher authority than the accuser, numbers of complaints are usually required to convince the interviewer that the accusation may be true" (pp. 1339–1340).

The women, after developing a network, sought legal resolution, a process that took four years. The physician continued in gynecological practice during that time. He was then allowed to keep his license and commence study of anesthesiology.

In a study of "erotic" practitioners, Kardener (1976) found that physicians who engaged in nonerotic behavior such as hugging, kissing, or affectionate touching of patients were more likely to engage in erotic behavior. The freer the physician was in demonstrating affectionate "nonerotic" behavior, the more statistically likely he was to become erotic with his clients.

Ethical issues are also raised about erotic contact in therapy settings. Some psychiatrists and psychologists and occasionally sex therapists have been accused of sexual contact with their clients. Sexual relations between client

and therapist are never justified and serve only to exploit the client (Redilick 1977). The American Psychoanalytic Association recommends three courses of action to be followed when a therapist engages in sexual relations with a client: (1) teminate analysis with the patient in question, (2) refer the patient to another analyst, and (3) seek further analysis for self while awaiting disciplinary action by peers (Redilick 1977, 150).

What is the nurse to do if a patient confides that a physician has made sexual advances? Readers of *RN* magazine answered that the nurse should make a careful assessment by asking the patient what the doctor did and what she said. The nurse should not reassure the patient when the nurse has no control over the situation. The nurse must also be careful not to compromise the doctor's reputation or the patient's rights. The information should be documented and the supervisor informed. The respondents also suggested that a nurse always accompany the physician to the patient's bedside (The Sexually Harrassed Patient 1979).

Patients' Expressions of Sexuality

Another sex-related issue for the health-care provider is that of the sexually seductive patient. Chapter 5 describes some common sexual acting-out behaviors nurses encounter, under "Assessment of Cues." Rather than react with anger, the caregiver needs to look beyond the behavior to the underlying problem. Frank (1980) says the patient may be seeking a warm, safe relationship, and admonishes the caregiver to "confront it kindly." On the other hand, some believe that sexually seductive patients are rare and that male physicians focus on this idea because of their discomfort with female clients.

When seductive behavior does occur, the caregiver may need to help the patient direct his or her sexual energies into socially accepted methods. The nurse may help the patient substitute or sublimate if that seems appropriate. Masturbation may be encouraged to relieve sexual tension. The nurse must be sensitive to the male patient's feelings when she or he discovers evidence of semen (Hampton 1979). In some cases, the patient may be worried about sexual function and act out of fear. Seductive behaviors may be a cry for help; the nurse can help the patient in obtaining counseling and information about his or her sexual future.

Even in our health-care system, we need to remember that the presence of sexual desires is normal. When possible and when the patient's condition warrants, conjugal visits might be considered. Rather than being shocked to find a partner lying in bed next to her/his patient and gossiping about it at the nurses' station, the nurse might close the door and hang up a "do not disturb" sign.

Issues of Sex Research

Our Western culture has been so uncomfortable with sexuality that any studies of the subject have, in the past, been greeted with shock and indignation. Freud's work on sexuality clashed with the rigid standards of religious groups and the general tenor of the times. Both world wars loosened the rigidity somewhat and some written materials became available. The publication by Kinsey of his interview-based studies in the late 1940s stimulated much controversy as well as shock and indignation over the findings that many supposedly taboo behaviors were actually quite common. When Masters and Johnson published work in the 1960s based on laboratory observations of physiologic responses of humans during sexual activity, the shock

ripples seemed a bit milder, although controversy over their techniques and results still abounded.

Because Hite believed that female sexuality was still seen as a response to male sexuality, she did a survey study to find out women's attitudes on sexuality and received 3000 nonrandomized responses from a questionnaire in a magazine. Over 100,000 married women responded to a sexual patterns questionnaire in *Redbook* magazine (Tavris and Sadd 1975). Friday (1973, 1975, 1980) has published three books on sexual fantasies based on personal accounts volunteered by men and women. As our attitudes toward sexuality become less puritanical and more open, the reactions to such studies of sexuality will probably follow the patterns of reactions to any scientific study rather than focusing on opinions of the rightness or wrongness of the individual behaviors disclosed. For example, controversy exists about the lack of broad representation of the population in Friday's samples, and accusations have been leveled that her studies are little more than pornography, rather than research. The Blumstein and Pepper study on American Couples, published in 1983, suggests that a wave of conservatism is occurring (Brody 1983). Since the sample was nonrandomized and did not include minority groups, however, it is difficult to generalize to the society as a whole.

For now, though, sex research itself—especially that using research subjects for observation or experimentation rather than merely questionnaire responses—raises questions about ethics. Nagging questions prompted a book that dealt, in part, with the morality of sex research (Masters, Johnson, and Kolodny 1977). Many people disagree with the very idea of any sex research; others want to be sure that consent issues are carefully attended to. If, as mentioned previously in this chapter, our society is going in the direction where the norm for morality is consenting adults, then sex research should not be a problem.

A type of research tangentially related to sexuality that continues to raise storms of protest is centered on males of the XYY genotype, thought by some researchers to be unusually violence-prone. This genotype occurs only rarely. One study of 4400 consecutive newborns found 11 males of this genotype. These children were evaluated at 1 year of age and at 2½ years of age against normal controls and were found to be slightly slower in a few developmental areas (Leonard et al. 1974). Because some researchers believed that these children could profit from early intervention if their type was known, early diagnosis of XYY was seen as important (Franzke 1975).

Others continue to be against such disclosure. They argue that leaps linking XYY males with violence and crime have been made without scientific basis. Critics also contend that researchers leaped into XYY studies without a knowledge of the extent of the aberration in society. Often studies were done on prison populations. The only sure knowledge at present about XYY males is that they are 2 to 4 inches taller than average and are subfertile (Steinfels and Levine 1980).

At the present time, funding for sex research from private and government sources is almost nonexistent. Controversy continues over the ethics of such research, the issue of "informed consent" when the research design is observational, rights to privacy and confidentiality, difficulties with human subjects committees, and disagreement as to what constitutes harm to a subject. The social benefits of sex research are also under scrutiny. And, as Nass, Libby, and Fisher point out, since most funded research is supported by the U.S. Department of Health and Human Services and most private foundations are as conservative as HHS, sex researchers may continue to be faced with a bleak economic future (1981, A-10,11).

Through the years inadequate research designs have spawned untruths and ignorance that take even more years to correct. Until we get random sample designs we will continue to have "truths" based on volunteer populations. There is no way to assess how representative these findings are. Sex researchers must be particularly careful because sexuality remains a sensitive subject for scientific research and a controversial one in terms of funding and ethical issues surrounding methodology. The participation of nurses in research in sexuality is essential.

Summary of Implications for Nursing Practice

Because of a long history of sexual repression there is much ambivalence and guilt in our society concerning sexuality. Health-care providers are not immune to these feelings. But, as professionals, we must at least become aware that not all our patients agree with our personal views. It helps to have an understanding of how our values were formed. Patients need our support and an attitude of acceptance. Because the value given to sexuality has traditionally been based on the ability to reproduce, some groups are ridiculed when their members desire or express sexual needs. The elderly are particularly susceptible to this ridicule. Health professionals can take the lead in asserting that sexuality is a basic aspect of each of us as human beings. To what degree we choose to express our sexuality, as long as we don't harm others, is an individual choice.

REFERENCES

Altman, L. K. 1982. New homosexual disorder worries health officials. *New York Times,* 11 May.

Altshuler, K., C. Burchell, E. K. Jerome, D. R., Kessler, F. Owen, W. D. Manahan, and E. D. Peske. 1980. When sexual orientation is in doubt. *Patient Care* 14(15):58–59, 63–66, 68–69, 72–73, 77–86.

Annas, G. J. 1979. Artificial insemination: Beyond the best interests of the donor. *Hastings Center Report* 9(4):14–15, 43.

Anspaugh, D. J., and M. Dignan. 1980. Religion, the church and sexuality — can they be compatible? *Health Values: Achieving High Level Wellness* 4:71–74.

Bachman, R. 1981. Homosexuality: The cost of being different. *Canadian Nurse* 77(2):20–23.

Berger, A. S., W. Simon, and J. H. Gagnon. 1973. Youth and pornography in social context. *Archives of Social Behavior* 2(4):279–308.

Berger, D. G., and M. G. Wenger. 1973. The ideology of virginity. *Journal of Marriage and the Family* 35:666–676.

Berger, J. M. 1979. The relationship of age to nurses' attitudes toward abortion. *Journal of Obstetric, Gynecologic, and Neonatal Nursing* 8:231–233.

Bozett, F. W. 1981. Gay fathers: Evolution of the gay-father identity. *American Journal of Orthopsychiatry* 51:552–559.

Brody, J. E. 1983. Major study on couples looks at jobs and money as well as sex. *New York Times,* 4 October C1.

Brossart, J. 1979. The gay patient: What you should be doing. *RN* 42(4):50–52.

Brown, C., J. Anderson, L. Burggrat, and N. Thompson. 1978. Community standards, conservatism, and judgments of pornography. *The Journal of Sex Research* 14(2):81–95.

Bullough, V. L., and B. Bullough. 1977. *Sin, sickness, and sanity: A history of sexual attitudes.* New York: New American Library.

Burgess, A. W. 1981. Physician sexual misconduct and patients' responses. *American Journal of Psychiatry* 138:1335–1342.

Burgess, A. W., A. W. Groth, and N. P. McCausland. 1981. Child sex initiation rings. *American Journal of Orthopsychiatry* 51:110–110.

Burr, W. A., and K. F. Schulz. 1980. Delayed abortion in area of easy accessibility. *Journal of the American Medical Association* 244:44–48.

Campbell-Bridges, M. 1981. Homosexuality and the medical model. *Issues in Health Care of Women* 3(5–6):307–319.

Cates, W., J. Gold, and R. M. Selik. 1979. Regulation of abortion services — for better or worse? *The New England Journal of Medicine* 301:720–723.

Caulkins, S. 1981. The male homosexual client. *Issues in Health Care of Women* 3(5–6):321–340.

Croft, G. 1979a. Mass. Man is Convicted in Rape of Estranged Wife. *Boston Globe* 22 Sept.

Croft, G. 1979b. Three years in rape of wife. *Boston Globe* 25 Sept.

Curie-Cohen, M., L. Luttrell, and S. Shapiro. 1979. Current practice of artificial insemination by donor in the United States. *New England Journal of Medicine* 300(11):585–590.

Darrow, W. W., D. Barrett, K. Jay, and A. Young. 1981. The gay report on sexually transmitted diseases. *American Journal of Public Health.* 71:1004–1011.

Davis, A. J. 1980. Competing ethical claims in abortion. *American Journal of Nursing* 80:1359.

Davis, A. J., and M. A. Aroskar. 1978. *Ethical dilemmas and nursing practice.* New York: Appleton-Century-Crofts.

Devereux, G. 1955. *A study of abortion in primitive societies.* New York: Julian Press.

Dritz, S. K. 1980. Medical aspects of homosexuality. *New England Journal of Medicine* 302:463–464.

Dudar, H. 1977. America discovers child pornography. *Ms.*, Aug.

Dworkin, A. 1981. *Pornography: Men possessing women.* New York: Putnam/Perigree.

Ehrenreich, B., E. Hess, and G. Jacobs. 1982. A report on the sex crisis. *Ms.*, Mar.

Fairchild, B., and N. Hayward. 1980. My child is a homosexual. *Family Health* 12(6):38, 48.

Finkelhor, D. 1979. What's wrong with sex between adults and children? Ethics and the problem of sexual abuse. *American Journal of Orthopsychiatry* 49:692–697.

Fletcher, J. C. 1979. Ethics and amniocentesis for fetal sex identification. *New England Journal of Medicine* 301:550–553.

Franks, R. D. 1980. The seductive patient. *American Family Physician* 22(2):111–114.

Franzke, A. W. 1975. Telling parents about XYY

sons. *New England Journal of Medicine* 293:100–101.

Friday, N. 1975. *Forbidden flowers: More women's sexual fantasies.* New York: Pocket Books.

Friday, N. 1980. *Men in love: Men's sexual fantasies: The triumph of love over rage.* New York: Dell.

Friday, N. 1973. *My secret garden: Women's sexual fantasies.* New York: Pocket Books.

Fuller, A. F. 1978. The DES syndrome and clear cell adenocarcinoma in young women. *Cancer Nursing* 1(2):201–205.

Gee, W. F., and J. S. Ansell. 1976. Neonatal circumcision: A ten-year overview: With comparison of the Gomco clamp and the Plastibell device. *Pediatrics* 58:824–827.

Gibbons, M. B. 1979. Why circumcise? *Pediatric Nursing* 5(4):9–12.

Goodman, E. 1982. Sen. Hatfield's antiabortion bill makes him member of the club. *Boston Globe,* 4 May, 15.

Griffin, S. 1981. *Pornography and silence: Culture's revenge against nature.* New York: Harper & Row.

Grimes, D. A. 1980. Routine circumcision reconsidered. *American Journal of Nursing* 80:108–109.

Hampton, P. 1979. Coping with the male patient's sexuality. *Nursing Forum* 18:304–310.

Handsfield, H. H. 1981. Sexually transmitted diseases in homosexual men. *American Journal of Public Health* 71:989–990.

Hardin, G. 1974. The evil of mandatory motherhood. *Psychology Today* 8(6):42.

Haskins, B. B. 1980. Gynocracy?: Who should advise women's lives? *Bioethics Quarterly* 2:245–246.

Hazelwood, R. R., A. W. Burgess, and N. Groth. 1981. Death during autoerotic practices. *Social Science and Medicine* 15E:129–133.

Hellman, R. E., R. Green, J. L. Gray, and K. Williams. 1981. Childhood sexual identity, childhood religiosity, and 'homophobia' as influences in the development of transsexualism, homosexuality, and heterosexuality. *Archives of General Psychiatry* 38:910–915.

Hetrick, E. S., and A. D. Martin. 1981. Letter. *American Journal of Psychiatry.* 138:1510–1511.

Hettlinger, R. F. 1966. *Living with sex: The student's dilemma.* New York: Seabury Press.

Hite, S. 1976. *The Hite report.* New York: Dell.

Hoeffer, B. 1981. Children's acquisition of sex-role behavior in lesbian-mother families. *American Journal of Orthopsychiatry.* 51:536–544.

Hornstein, F. 1974. *Lesbian health care.* Los Angeles: Feminist Women's Health Center.

Howe, B., H. R. Kaplan, and C. English. 1979. Repeat abortions: Blaming the victims. *American Journal of Public Health* 69:1242–1246.

Hunt, D. D., and J. L. Hampson. 1980. Follow-up of 17 biologic male transsexuals after sex-reassignment surgery. *American Journal of Psychiatry* 137:432–438.

Johnson, S. R., S. M. Guenther, D. W. Laube, and W. C. Keettel. 1981. Factors influencing lesbian gynecologic care: A preliminary study. *American Journal of Obstetrics and Gynecology* 140:20–25.

Kaiser, B. L., and I. H. Kaiser. 1974. The challenge of the women's movement to American gynecology. *American Journal of Obstetrics and Gynecology* 120:653–661.

Kardener, S. H., M. Fuller, and I. N. Mensk. 1976. Characteristics of "erotic" practitioners. *American Journal of Psychiatry* 133:1324–1325.

Kessler, D. R. 1980. What causes homosexuality? *Patient Care* 14(15):53, 56.

Keyserlingk, E. W. 1981. Artificial insemination and *in vitro* fertilization. *Bioethics Quarterly* 3:35–49.

Kirkpatrick, M., C. Smith, and R. Roy. Lesbian mothers and their children: A comparitive survey. *American Journal of Orthopsychiatry.* 1981. 51:545–551.

Lee, R. D. 1977. Homosexuality: An integral part of human sexuality. In *The sexual and gender development of young children: The role of the educator,* ed. E. K. Oremland and J. D. Oremland. Cambridge, Mass.: Ballinger.

Leonard, M. F., G. Landy, F. H. Riddle, and H. A. Lubs. 1974. Early development of children with abnormalities of the sex chromosomes: A prospective study. *Pediatrics* 54:208–212.

Longino, H. 1980. Pornography, oppression and freedom: A closer look. In *Take back the night: Women on pornography,* ed. L. Lederer. New York: Morrow Quill.

Lovell, J. E., and J. Cox. 1979. Maternal attitudes toward circumcision. *The Journal of Family Practice* 9:811–813.

MacRae, J. 1974. A feminist view of abortion. In

Women and religion, ed. J. Plaskow and J. A. Romero. Missoula, Mont.: Scholars' Press.

Malamuth, N., N. Heim, and S. Feshbach. 1980. Sexual responsiveness of college students to rape depictions. *Journal of Perspectives in Social Psychology* 38(3):399–408.

Malamuth, N., and B. Spinner. 1980. A longitudinal content analysis of sexual violence in the best-selling erotic magazines. *Journal of Sex Research,* vol. 16.

Masters, W. H., V. E. Johnson, and R. C. Kolodny. 1977. *Ethical issues in sex therapy and research.* Boston: Little, Brown.

Masters, W. H., and V. E. Johnson. 1966. *Human Sexual Response.* Boston: Little, Brown.

Maurer, T. B. 1979. Health care and the gay community. *Nursing Dimensions* 2(1):83–85.

McConaghy, N., M. S. Armstrong, P. C. Birrell, and N. Buhrick. 1979. The incidence of bisexual feelings and opposite sex behavior in medical students. *The Journal of Nervous and Mental Disease* 167:685–688.

Morgan, R. 1978. How to run the pornographers out of town (and preserve the First Amendment). *Ms.,* 7(5).

Morin, S. F. 1981. Letter. *American Journal of Psychiatry* 138:1511.

Mudd, E. H. 1977. The historical background of ethical considerations in sex research and sex therapy. In *Ethical issues in sex therapy and research,* ed. W. H. Masters, V. E. Johnson, and R. C. Kolodny. Boston: Little, Brown.

Nass, G. D., R. W. Libby, and M. P. Fisher. 1981. *Sexual choices.* Monterey, Calif.: Wadsworth.

Nathanson, C. A., and M. H. Becker. 1980. Obstetricians' attitudes and hospital abortion services. *Family Planning Perspectives* 12:26–32.

Nathanson, C. A., and M. H. Becker. 1981. Professional norms, personal attitudes, and medical practice: The case of abortion. *Journal of Health and Social Behavior* 22:198–211.

Notman, M. T., and C. C. Nadelson. 1978. Women as patients and experimental subjects. In *Encyclopedia of Bioethics,* ed. W. T. Reich, vol. 4. New York: Free Press.

Nurses Association of the American College of Obstetricians and Gynecologists (NAACOG). 1981. *Standards for obstetric, gynecologic and neonatal nursing.* 2d ed. Washington, D. C.

O'Donnell, M. 1978. Lesbian health care: Issues and literature. *Science for the People* May/June:8–19.

Olson, M. 1980. Helping staff nurses care for women seeking saline abortions. *Journal of Obstetric, Gynecologic, and Neonatal Nursing* 9:170–173.

O'Faolain, J., and L. Martines, eds. 1973. *Not in God's image.* Glasgow, Great Britain: William Collins.

O'Leary, V. 1979. Lesbianism. *Nursing Dimensions* 2(2):78–82.

Orlando. 1978. Bisexuality: A choice not an echo. *Ms.,* Oct.

Owen, W. F. 1980. The clinical approach to the homosexual patient. *Annals of Internal Medicine* 93:90–92.

Owen, W. F. 1980. Sexually transmitted diseases and traumatic problems in homosexual men. *Annals of Internal Medicine* 92:805–808.

Palmer, C. E. 1979. Pornographic comics: A content analysis. *The Journal of Sex Research* 15(4):285–298.

Pattison, E. M., and M. L. Pattison. 1980. "Ex-gays": Religiously mediated change in homosexuals. *American Journal of Psychiatry* 137:1553–1562.

Petchesky, R. P. 1979. Reproduction, ethics, and public policy: The federal sterilization regulations. *Hastings Center Report* 9(5):29–41.

Pettyjohn, R. D. 1979. Health care of the gay individual. *Nursing Forum* 18:366–393.

Pogoncheff, E. 1979. The gay patient: What not to do. *RN* 42(4):46–50.

Raymond, J. G. 1979. *The transsexual empire: The making of the she-male.* Boston: Beacon Press.

Redilick, R. 1977. The ethics of sex therapy. In *Ethical issues in sex therapy and research,* ed. W. H. Masters, V. E. Johnson, and R. C. Kolodny. Boston: Little, Brown.

A revolution in rape. 1979. *Time,* 2 April, 50.

Richards, S. 1979. Homosexuality: Victims of society. *Nursing Mirror* 149(18):28–30.

Riddle, D. I. 1978. Kinsey's answer to Anita Bryant. *Ms.,* Sept., 43–44.

Sanger, M. [1938]1971. *Margaret Sanger: An autobiography.* New York: Dover.

Santini, R. 1976. *The secret fire: A new view of women and passion.* Chicago: Playboy Press.

The sexually harrassed patient. 1979. *RN* 42(12):83–86.

Sherwin, S. 1981. The concept of person in the context of abortion. *Bioethics Quarterly* 3:21 – 34.

Silber, T. 1980. Abortion in adolescence: The ethical dimension. *Adolescence* 15:461 – 474.

Stecchi, J. H. 1980. The effects of the Reach to Recovery program on the quality of life and rehabilitation of mastectomy patients. *Bioethics Quarterly* 2:237 – 244.

Steinbacher, R. S. 1980. Ethical issues in human reproduction technology: Analysis by women. *Women & Health* 5(2):100 – 101.

Steinem, G. 1978. Erotica and pornography, a clear and present difference. *Ms.,* 7(5).

Steinfels, M. O., and C. Levine. 1980. The XYY controversy: Researching violence and genetics. *Hastings Center Report* 10:1 – 32 (supplement).

Talan, J. 1981. Male circumcision: Unnecessary surgery? *Ms.,* April.

Tannahill, R. 1980. *Sex in history.* New York: Stein & Day.

Task Force on Pornography at the University of Connecticut. 1981. Pornography and violence against women, issues and answers. University of Connecticut. Mimeo.

Tavris, C., and S. Sadd. 1975. *The Redbook report on female sexuality.* New York: Delacorte.

Thomas, S. P. 1980. Bisexuality: A sexual orientation of great diversity. *Journal of Psychiatric Nursing and Mental Health Services* 18(4):19 – 27.

Thompson, J. E., and H. O. Thompson. 1980. The ethics of being a female patient and a female care provider in a male-dominated health-illness system. *Issues in Health Care of Women* 2(3):25 – 54.

Thomson, J. J. 1975. A defense of abortion. In *Moral problems: A collection of philosophical essays.* 2d ed., ed. J. Rachels. New York: Harper & Row.

Trussell, J., J. Menken, B. L. Lindheim, and B. Vaughan. 1980. The impact of restricting Medicaid financing for abortion. *Family Planning Perspectives* 12:120 – 130.

The United States Law Week. 51LW4767. No. 81-746 & 81-1172.

Van Gelder, L. 1980. When women confront street porn. *Ms.,* 8(8).

Walker, A. 1980. When women confront porn at home. *Ms.,* 8(8).

Wertheimer, R. 1975. Understanding the abortion argument. In *Moral problems: A collection of philosophical essays.* 2d ed., ed. J. Rachels. New York: Harper & Row.

Wetherill, P. S. 1980. DES exposure: A continuing disaster. *Women & Health* 5(2):91 – 93.

Woodward, C. A. 1978. Understanding pornography consumption. *Journal of Psychiatric Nursing* 16(11):36 – 38.

Introduction

Preparing for Sexual Assessment and Intervention

    Understanding the Barriers
    Becoming Competent with Sexual Issues
    Facilitating One's Own Sexual Comfort
    Preparing Clients for Sexual Dialogue
    Recognizing Cultural Influences

Sexual Assessment

    Risks to Sexual Health
    The Sexual History
    Assessment of Cues
    Physical/Sexual Examination Considerations
        Assuring informed consent
        Reducing anxiety
        Assuring privacy
        Providing for physical comfort and safety advocacy
    Physical/Sexual Examination of the Male
    Physical/Sexual Examination of the Female
    The Sexological Examination
    Diagnostic Testing

Planning Strategies for Sexual Health Promotion

    Sex Education
    Sexual Counseling
    Sex Therapy
    Requirements of Sex Educators, Counselors, and Therapists
    Advocacy

Summary of Implications for Nursing Practice

Assessment: Sexuality and Nursing Care

Ronna E. Krozy

Introduction

Every individual is a sexual being from conception until death. Unfortunately, professional health-care providers have long avoided or inadequately dealt with the sexual health-care needs and concerns of clients and the consumer public as a whole.

The dilemma that many providers have traditionally found themselves in results from being products of a society that has considered sex a taboo subject, while at the same time expected nurses to examine clients, perform intrusive procedures, and collect personal data. Consequently, clients were often depersonalized and their sexual concerns largely ignored.

Today, reluctance, embarrassment, and anxiety are giving way to responsiveness on the part of clients and nurses alike. Consumers are becoming more assertive in seeking opportunities to increase their knowledge, discuss their sexual problems, validate their understanding, and share concerns that affect their sexual health and lifestyle. Nurses often hear comments such as these: "My husband isn't interested in sex since his prostate surgery." "I thought you couldn't get pregnant if you were breastfeeding." "Is it true that estrogen therapy makes you more likely to get cancer?" Other concerns are often masked in more "socially acceptable" dialogue: "All this talk about sex after 60 is so foolish!"

Nurses are becoming increasingly cognizant of clients' sexual needs and more skillful in their approach to sexual health care. Few nurses are educationally prepared to provide intensive sex therapy, but many are in a position to provide anticipatory guidance, understanding, and an environment conducive to open communication. At the very least, a nurse can refer a client to an appropriate resource. This may be as simple as asking a colleague to speak with a client or as informal as suggesting appropriate resources, agencies, or services.

Within the scope of their practice, nurses often come in contact with clients (individuals, families, or groups) whose sexual well-being may be threatened and who may need their assistance. These clients may include pregnant adolescents, infertile couples, homosexuals with STD, clients with sexually compromising surgery or illness, rape victims, or parents concerned with their child's masturbation. In each instance, practitioners may be confronted with sexual issues that challenge both their knowledge and their values. Yet, if caregivers believe that nursing is a holistic science that treats the total person, they will need to include sexuality in promoting the physical, emotional, and spiritual well-being of the client. Many nurses, however, still find it difficult, if not impossible, to address this particular area. This chapter will discuss sexual assessment procedures, with suggestions for easing discomfort of both practitioner and client, and will also describe strategies for promoting sexual health.

Preparing for Sexual Assessment and Intervention

For nurses to be of help to clients with sexual concerns, nurses must first understand the traditional barriers that prevented recognition of these concerns. They must also become knowledgeable about and comfortable with sexual issues and become comfortable with their own sexuality. Clients, too, may need thoughtful preparation before entering into sexual dialogue with the caregiver. And in offering sexual assessment, counseling, and education, nurses must recognize that cultural heritages may influence their clients' responses — and their own.

In developing the ease and communication skills necessary for sexual dialogue with clients, nurses should also recognize tht therapeutic communication differs from social communication in both goals and methods. *Therapeutic communication* may be described as interaction directed toward encouraging a client's expression of concerns, needs, attitudes, values, and beliefs in order to facilitate problem identification and resolution. Therapeutic communication is *nondirective* when the client is instrumental in focusing the interaction, *directive* when the nurse assists the client to focus the interaction. The nurse rarely facilitates or employs an "either-or" approach; more often, a mix of the two types of therapeutic communication is used.

Understanding the Barriers

It wasn't long ago that a client's sexuality was not even *considered* in planning nursing care, much less assessed. Even nurses who were highly knowledgeable about reproductive sexuality failed to assess or counsel the nonreproductive aspects of the client's sexual life. One factor responsible for this omission was the limited information on sexology, the scientific study of human sexuality.

Sexual themes have appeared since earliest times in art, religion, and literature, but most early works did not have a scientific approach and might even be considered pornographic. (They did, however, serve a purpose in providing sex education.) DeLora and Warren

(1977) note that sexuality in the 18th century was viewed by doctors as an illness, in the 19th century as a psychological phenomenon, and in the 20th century as a sociological phenomenon encompassing both the normal and the abnormal. As noted in Chapter 1, contributions by Freud, Ellis, Kinsey, and others helped to legitimize the professional study of sexuality. In the mid-1960s, Masters and Johnson described the physiology of the sexual response cycle, facilitating the integration of biological, physiological, psychological, and sociological dimensions of sexuality. The use of this new information was not incorporated into the nursing literature until 1970 when the November issue of *Nursing Outlook* dealt with the topic. Since that time, the literature suggests that "human sexuality has become an accepted part of total health care [and] nurses have a responsibility to promote sexual health in their practice" (Mims and Swenson 1978, 121).

Not all nurses, however, deal with their client's sexuality and many barriers continue to exist. For example, some nurses believe that a client's sex life is his or her own business, that it is too personal an issue to discuss, and that if the client had a sexual problem or desired information, he or she would let the nurse know.

Some nurses feel that discussing sex is somehow improper or inappropriate for them and that it is an area better left to the physician, psychiatrist, or spiritual adviser. There is also the notion of nursing as pure and asexual, helped by symbolic reinforcers: "angel of mercy," "mother surrogate," the white uniform, and the Nightingale pledge to "pass my life in purity." Paradoxically, some nurses fear that if they discuss sex clients may consider them promiscuous or believe the movie portrayals of nurses since "nurses have seen it all."

Another barrier is the idea that certain people (the aged, handicapped, or terminally ill) are not sexual and therefore sexuality need not be considered. On the contrary, sexuality is not merely something which people do. Rather, there are distinct differences between an individual's sexual identity and needs and the individual's sexual activity. We are all sexual beings, whether or not we are sexually active.

Lack of knowledge also impedes nurses from dealing with sexuality. One study by Fontaine (1976) found that most faculty members considered their basic educational preparation in human sexuality to be fairly or very inadequate. Even today, a number of nursing schools do not include comprehensive courses in sex education but confine the content to the study of reproduction. Some educators assume that the best place to teach sexuality is in the maternity nursing course. Instead, sexuality should be taught within the theoretical framework of the nursing process, at the beginning of the nursing sequence, as it constitutes part of the complete health history.

Even when the nurse is considerably knowledgeable, sexual assessment or intervention will be difficult if the nurse is personally uncomfortable about discussing this subject with others. This is supported by Fontaine's (1976) findings that faculty members reported far less ability to discuss sexuality with clients than their self-rated level of sexual knowledge. If nurses are to facilitate optimal sexual health and functioning in their clients, they will need to resolve their own sexual issues, acquire factual information, and develop the skill to question, counsel, or educate their clients or refer them to qualified resources. Nurses, however, should take pride in the fact that clients are often more willing to share their intimate concerns with a nurse than another professional. Nurses are often seen as compassionate and trusted allies, and as knowledgeable resources. It is up to them to take advantage of this fortuitous position in helping to prevent or uncover and resolve sexual problems.

Becoming Competent with Sexual Issues

In order to become competent in dealing with sexual issues, there are two important prerequisites: sexual self-comfort and sexual knowledge. In their sexual health model, Mims and Swenson (1978) suggest that nurses may possess four levels of competence in promoting sexual health. The first level, life experience, contains both destructive and intuitively helpful behaviors. These arise from culture, myth, and taboo. The second, or basic, level incorporates the assessment part of the nursing process and is dependent on the nurse's awareness and basic knowledge. At this level, the practitioner can gather information. The intermediate level utilizes the planning, intervention, and evaluation aspects of the nursing process; the practitioner provides factual information and encourages clients to discuss sexuality at length. The fourth, most advanced level requires extensive preparation, for it is at this level that practitioner offers sex therapy or comprehensive counseling and conducts research.

Coming to terms with one's sexuality is often a difficult task for nurses. Many have been raised in a society proscribing sexual discussion, education, or research, and educated in curricula that largely ignored sexuality. Nurses and other health professionals can facilitate their own sexual self-comfort by comparing the following characteristics with their own feelings and then learning the techniques that will bring about these characteristics:

1. *The nurse should acknowledge that she or he, like the client, is a sexual being, and should be aware of how her or his behavior impacts on or is affected by the client.* Hohmann (1972) notes that the psychosexual adjustment of clients with spinal cord injury often depends on the way their male and female caretakers interact with them. For example, the female nurse may unconsciously act in a provocative manner or male nurses may dis-

cuss sexual exploits without considering the client's reaction. It is considered poor nursing practice to resolve one's sexual issues or meet one's sexual needs through the client. Clients should not be burdened by the nurse's sexuality. Health professionals need to be aware of their own sexual reactions to patients and avoid behaving in any way that could lead to acting out.

2. *Ideally, the nurse should be a sexually healthy individual in order to work with clients holistically.* Crosby (1976) contends that sexual health requires three processes: (1) sexual self-awareness (being in touch with our sexual responsiveness, feelings, and genitals), (2) sexual self-acceptance (valuing our sexual organs and feelings as we value the rest of our body and emotions), and (3) sexual self-possession (the ability to integrate our genitals with our mind, spirit, and body).

3. *The nurse should possess positive self-regard or esteem.* Crosby (1976) sees this quality as self-love. He believes that self-love is the prerequisite to loving another, but it is not to be confused with narcissism, a form of self-infatuation associated with immaturity. Thus, to accept ourselves for what we are as total beings promotes our ability to view others in the same way.

The sexually self-comfortable individual has analyzed her or his value system and is aware of its effect on her or his beliefs, practices, and attitudes. In like fashion, the competent nurse holds an accurate perception of the religious, sociocultural, and personal tenets that guide the client. By acknowledging that people have the right to choose their own sexual values, the nurse is able to remain nonjudgmental and open, unthreatened and unthreatening, when faced with the client's sexual preferences. This attitude of openness also allows the nurse to accept the client unconditionally.

Crosby (1976) considers the ability to self-disclose a characteristic of sexual self-comfort. This can only be accomplished through full acceptance and trust of one's own feelings and experiences. He points out, however, that competence in sexual intervention does not require experiencing "everything under the sun." Rather, it is not just the knowledge caregivers possess, but also the way in which their sexuality is integrated into their experience that permits them to share aspects of themselves for therapeutic purposes. However, self-disclosure should be used only if the client will benefit.

4. *The nurse should be able to discuss sexuality in a factual, honest, confident way with individuals who are in their early, middle, or senior years.* This demands good communication techniques as well as an understanding of the scope of sexuality and normal growth and development. For many nurses, it may require altering longstanding misconceptions about sex in childhood, or sex and aging.

5. *The nurse should possess up-to-date, scientific information regarding sexuality.* Some of the areas with which the nurse must be familiar are male and female anatomy and physiology, sexual dysfunctions—their causes and treatments, reproduction, the continuum of normal sexual behavior, human sexual response, sex education methodology, sexual deviations and variations, and new research findings. Books, such as this one, formal course work, and continuing education in the field will increase the nurse's knowledge.

Facilitating One's Own Sexual Comfort

We can promote our own self-awareness and sexual self-comfort by using the techniques of values clarification and desensitization. Simon (1974) states that *values clarification* is a process which allows us to become aware of and analyze our feelings, attitudes, and behaviors, confront inconsistencies, and decide what is meaningful. This technique also helps us to establish common grounds when we are communicating and to understand how particular terminology is being used. One exercise which is useful and fun is to define the word "promiscuous," inviting friends or professional peers to do the same, and then comparing definitions. The difficulty that may be encountered serves to demonstrate how sexual values differ, even among people who appear to share similar beliefs.

Another exercise is to develop a list of subjects related to sexuality such as masturbation, abortion, sex education, nonmarital intercourse, or oral-genital sex. These can be written in the left-hand margin of a piece of paper. Then, on the top of the paper column headings can be written: "OK for me," "Not OK for me," "OK for others," "Not OK for others," "Comments." For each subject, we can check off our feelings and then go back and think about why these choices were made. This analysis is written in the "Comments" column. Another approach is to change the column headings to correspond with age categories (young child, teenager, . . . senior) or setting (nursing home, hospital, day-care center). The important point is to consider whether the attitudes arose as a result of personal experience, something we read, religion, family teaching, and/or other influences.

Once we have gained insight into our own values and their roots, we can begin to appreciate the meaning of sexual values in others. Doing so is the first step in desensitization.

Desensitization is an experiential learning process whereby an individual develops comfort through deliberate repeated exposures to and analysis of situations that produce anxiety. The purpose of sexual desensitization is self-enlightenment and freeing the person who wishes to engage in sexual assessment, teaching, or counseling. Several methods are used.

Role-playing or group discussion on topics such as communicating one's sexual needs, or group feedback after viewing or reading sexually explicit materials are examples of desensitization exercises. Workshops that focus on sexual attitude restructuring may be held by academic institutions or health facilities where sexual problems are treated. Desensitization groups ideally should consist of males and females so that each group can share its own perspectives. There should be a skilled group leader who is prepared to deal with emotional issues that might emerge. *Values in Sexuality* by Morrison and Price (1974) describes additional desensitization exercises.

Another technique to enhance sexual self-comfort is *inoculation*. This technique allows the individual to prepare a defense against a future threat. As it applies to sexuality, inoculation would help the nurse to develop appropriate behavioral responses (both verbal and nonverbal) to such situations as being asked for a date by a client, being touched in an intimate way, or finding a client masturbating or nude. One inoculation exercise is for nurses to write a list of situations that might catch them off guard. For each situation, caregivers write how they would normally feel and react: "I'd be really angry — I'd slap his/her hand." Then each caregiver considers how her or his reaction could be changed to be more therapeutic: "I'm upset by what you did (or said) but I'd like to talk about it."

When nurses have gained comfort and knowledge in the topic of sexuality, they are ready to address clients' issues.

Preparing Clients for Sexual Dialogue

To gain the client's cooperation and facilitate openness, the caregiver should prepare the client for sexual dialogue (assessment, counseling, or education). The following strategies should be helpful.

The client should be informed early in the relationship that the nurse will be asking for information that might be sensitive or personal. The nurse should let the client know that this will help uncover any problems that might need intervention or raise questions that the nurse can assist in answering.

The purpose of asking the sexual questions should be determined. The caregiver should only ask for information that will be useful in establishing a nursing diagnosis or indicating that a problem exists. Generally, the sexual portion of the health history should be of similar length as other areas. When a client's major problem involves a sexual dysfunction or when the client's condition has a great potential for disrupting his or her sexuality, a more detailed and comprehensive sexual history would be justified.

A sexual history should not be omitted merely because the client is single, elderly, or disabled. Neither should assumptions be made about the client's sexual needs, interests, levels of activity, or even sexual orientation. Brossart (1979) suggests that in assessing a client, gender pronouns should be avoided and terms like partner or mate used rather than husband or wife. If the caregiver does not ask questions that are applicable to the client's real-life situation or that allow the client to respond honestly, the client may be forced to answer incompletely or not at all. Brossart also suggests that unexpected answers be considered in a sensitive way. Gay women, for example, are often in a bind when they admit they are sexually active and use no birth control, but haven't revealed their sexual preference. Finally, the caregiver should ask the client if he or she is sexually active or celibate. If the client is sexually active, he or she can be asked in a straightforward but sensitive way whether it is with the opposite or the same sex. The nurse's ability to ask this question without demonstrating disapproval should help the client to answer.

Should the client express surprise at being asked sexual questions in general or a specific question, the nurse may wish to reinforce that assumptions cannot be made about clients' sexual behavior, given the wide range of ways in which people express their sexuality. At the same time, however, the client should not be forced to talk about sex. It may be quite difficult for a client to reveal sexual information because of guilt, anxiety, shame, or fear of disapproval. Social or cultural proscriptions may bar sexual discussions. Or, the difficulty may ensue because the nurse is of the opposite sex or perceived by the client as too young (or too old) to understand. When the client appears uneasy about a particular question, the nurse should ask whether it would be preferable to bring it up at a later point. Clients have the right to refuse to discuss any or all aspects of their sexuality.

There is no one appropriate time to introduce the topic of sexuality, but it is usually better addressed after the nurse and client have had an opportunity to establish dialogue. This usually occurs during the latter portion of an interview. Some nurses find the sexual history flows naturally as part of the systems review of reproductive or genitourinary function or as part of the family/social history. When a health history is not completed at one time, as often occurs in community nursing, the sexual history may be acquired over a span of time.

When asking for sexual information, it is best to start with those questions that are least sensitive and work up to those that are more sensitive. A female, for example, might be more comfortable with questions moving from menstruation to pregnancy to genital problems to sexual satisfaction. A more direct line of questioning is often applied to the male but this does not mean that the male client may not feel threatened or embarrassed. The male, however, may be more inclined to joke or be sarcastic. Asking about the ideal rather than the real is a good technique to help the client respond. For example, it may be easier for the client to describe how his or her relationship (sex life, degree of sexual activity, and so on) differs from what was expected or what is desired.

Terminology that the client will understand should be used. If the client uses unsophisticated "street" language, the nurse should not demonstrate shock or disapproval, as that may block further communication. At the same time, the nurse should use language that she or he is comfortable with, explaining any terms that may be confusing.

Caregivers should ask questions that require substantive answers and let the client know that they are willing and able to talk about sex. Semmens and Semmens (1978) note that professionals often ask sexual questions requiring a "yes" or "no" because subconsciously ". . . they do not want detailed information that exposes their own frustrations and sexual attitudes" (p. 35). See the suggested guidelines. Open leads for communication should be provided. The nurse might state, for example, that many men or women have concerns about their sexual function after having an accident, illness, or operation like the client's. Then the nurse can ask what the client's concerns are. Another approach is to cite examples of the most often asked questions and to follow up by asking whether the client has any of these questions. It should be kept in mind that clients frequently will not ask for sexual information or initiate conversation without perceiving that it is permissible to do so. Moreover, nurses should not assume that once they have discussed a sexual issue, all will be revealed or resolved. The nurse may need to provide an ongoing discussion in order to help the client develop trust or comfort in exposing his or her problems.

Suggested Communication Guidelines for the Nurse

1. Introduce sexuality initially in subtle nonthreatening ways with clients. This can be in the form of "permission giving," that is, letting the client know that it's OK to talk about sexual concerns. For example: A history is usually taken when the client is admitted to the hospital. Along with the standard "Have you been in a hospital before?" or "What medication are you taking at home?" You might include "Many people find that illness influences relationships. Have you found a change in your sexual relationships?" Or during a clinic visit, "Women often remark on how many emotional and physical issues they encounter. Has your pregnancy made a difference in your sexual relationship?" True, these may be answered with a simple yes or no (or not at all), but the nurse has opened a door.

2. State your purpose for questioning or offering guidance. Don't be vague. "This medication often affects the ability to achieve or maintain an erection. Have you had this problem?"

3. Don't assume the client's level of or lack of knowledge. Assess what he or she knows and understands. "What do you understand about how the diaphragm works as a contraceptive?"

4. Minimize client anxiety: Promote an environment conducive to discussion. Provide privacy and comfort, and minimize distractions. Sit at eye level, maintain eye contact, and sit close enough without invading the client's personal space.

5. A client may be very sensitive or threatened by certain topics. If you meet resistance, change the subject and return to it later if it seems appropriate. Don't challenge the client, demanding rationale or answers.

6. Start discussions with an idea of time available and allow sufficient time for the interactions or make arrangements for later discussions. Rapport and trust are *not* established when the nurse appears rushed, distracted, or bored.

7. Assure confidentiality of discussions and records and *MAINTAIN THAT CONFIDENTIALITY.* If a referral is to be made, obtain client's permission *first.* If information is to be shared with professional colleagues, clients should know this.

8. Recognize signs of client anxiety: tapping foot, frowning, avoiding eye contact, heavy smoking. Give permission to stop discussion. "You seem anxious about our discussion; if you'd like to stop I can come back this afternoon."

9. *Minimize anxiety* for clients by appropriately timing discussions. The client may be more vulnerable at certain times. For example, don't ask in the middle of a vaginal exam, "How has your pregnancy affected your sexual relationship with your partner?"

10. Use vocabulary the client understands. Nurses don't have to use the same words as the client, but they do need to clarify meanings so both are on the same wave length. Avoid slang, medical jargon, abstract terms, and unnecessarily long or wordy questions or explanations.

11. Nurses will profit by being attentive, active listeners. Showing interest encourages client descriptions and clarification: "yes"—"go on"—"I see."

12. Avoid questions that can be answered with simply yes or no, such as "Are your menstrual periods painful?" Rather, use open-ended questions: "Ms. Smith, will you describe any discomfort you may have experienced with your menstrual periods." In this way you

encourage description of a problem or concern.

13. Answer direct questions and offer information when the client requests or when the need arises, but avoid incomplete or premature explanations. This may decrease the client's problem-solving abilities and may increase anxiety.

14. Acknowledge when you don't have an answer to a factual question, but offer to seek the answer and *DO IT.*

15. Personal questions directed to the nurse — "What do you use as a birth control method?" — can be redirected to the client: "Is there some reason you wish to know?" Personal questions can be answered honestly: "I don't care to share that but I am interested in why you ask."

16. To encourage further clarification or elaboration:

   • Rephrase or reflect on client's statement: "Your vaginal discharge is getting heavier?"

   • Make observations; share your perceptions: "You seem to be very anxious about using the IUD."

   • Assess the client's value system, attitudes, and beliefs: "Can you describe how you felt when the doctor told you about your herpes infection?"

17. Don't probe or pursue a particular topic with a client out of curiosity: "Why do you want to have anal sex with your girlfriend?"

18. Avoid common barriers to communication:

   • Giving advice: "Believe me, I'd never take the pill."

   • Disapproval: "You're too young to have your tubes tied."

   • Trite expressions: "I know just how you feel."

   • False reassurance: "Just take this medication and everything will be OK."

19. Do not misinterpret client's understanding or agreement by his or her head nodding or verbal comments. This is often a client's response to an individual perceived as an authority figure, a cultural expression commonly used to show respect.

Developed by Roberta M. Orne.

The nurse's approach, whether in assessment or intervention, should be matter-of-fact, with a focus on practices acceptable to the client. For example, a nurse might state that most authorities view masturbation as a healthy release of sexual tension. A follow-up question requesting the client's opinion is one means of uncovering the client's value system. Nurses must remember, however, that their definition of normal, acceptable behavior and the client's definition may be vastly different. Hogan (1980) suggests that some people are intolerant of *any* behavior which differs from their own and may view individuals as being perverted or abnormal when they practice (or advocate practicing) various acts. Knowing the ethical and moral beliefs of the client is an important component of planned intervention, particularly when a change in the client's usual sexual activity is required.

Consideration must be given to the atmosphere in which the interview is to take place. The client will be more relaxed in a quiet, private location while comfortably positioned. The nurse should be sure that the interview will proceed without interruption or distraction. Whenever possible, a mutually acceptable time should be arranged. Burgess (1981) advises that the nurse's physical comfort is also important, as hunger, thirst, fatigue, or preoccupation can decrease the nurse's effectiveness as a listener.

It is important to be aware of the client's need for personal space. The nurse should inquire whether the client feels comfortable with the distance between them or ask the client to place the chair at a point where he or she feels at ease.

Eye contact should be maintained, without staring at the client, and attention should be paid to what is being said. Nurses should also be aware of their own nonverbal responses. Humans are expressive beings who often communicate messages unconsciously with their eyes, facial expressions, or body movements. Caregivers must learn to listen carefully, to use silence in a constructive way, and to be comfortable with silence when the client needs time to search for the words to express thoughts or feelings (Hogan 1981). The nurse should assure the client that any information shared will be treated as confidential, and keep that commitment.

Finally, caregivers will enhance a client's comfort in dealing with his or her sexual issues by recognizing their own discomfort and gracefully declining from any discussion that causes them discomfort. If a nurse is truly uncomfortable with the topic of sexuality, she or he should refer the client to another health professional who is competent in that area. A statement such as, "I think Alice Samuels would be an excellent resource person to discuss that issue with. May I set up an appointment for the two of you to talk?" can be employed with the least amount of embarrassment. Referral is preferable to pretending acceptance of the client's lifestyle or feigning the ability to discuss sexual issues. Personal discomfort will be evident in body language (blushing, averted eyes, quivering voice, or stiffness), nursing care (avoidance of or deliberately minimizing touching), or the way the client's significant others are dealt with.

Recognizing Cultural Influences

In all stages of the nursing process, beginning with assessment, a common oversight of some nurses is failure to acknowledge the influence of a client's cultural heritage. All too often, nurses label clients "noncompliant" or "uncooperative" when in actuality these clients are unwilling to violate their cultural beliefs, or misunderstand or misinterpret treatments or care, especially if solutions are unilaterally planned by the nurse.

Cultural influence is most noticed when clients are reluctant or fail to participate in their own health care. Nurses are often frustrated when clients fail to keep appointments, neglect to follow treatments, or disregard directions. This may be because they lack the "cause and effect" understanding behind the practice of sexual health maintenance. Attempts should be made to link health care to existing beliefs and practices within the culture. This is important in order to promote health and avoid client anger, stress, uncertainty, insecurity, and ambivalence.

Some cultures highly value reproduction; contraception may be unacceptable or perceived as a threat to sexual self-concept. Taboos exist in some cultures about touching the female genitalia and breasts, as in proscriptions against vaginal exams by men or before marriage. In some cultures, strong beliefs desexualize women who are mothers and discourage sexual expression except the obvious expression of pregnancy.

The nurse can be both sensitive to and supportive of cultural values and beliefs unless they are extremely detrimental to the client's health. The nurse's awareness and flexibility can increase clients' trust, rapport, and compliance.

Sexual Assessment

As part of the nursing process, *sexual assessment* is the gathering of subjective and objective information related to a client's sexual beliefs, attitudes, experiences, behaviors, needs, resources, and health status. The client may be an individual, couple, family, group, or community. The purpose of a sexual assessment is to establish a nursing diagnosis and a plan of intervention based on the diagnosis and the client's goals and resources.

Sexual assessment includes the identification of risk factors that could impede sexual health or evidence of sexual disruption, taking a sexual history from the client and/or significant others, observation of indirect verbal or nonverbal sexual messages, physical examination, and laboratory testing.

Risks to Sexual Health

Through each stage of life, individuals may be exposed to internal and external risks that threaten their sexual well-being. Disruptions in sexual function may result from biophysical impairments or trauma. More often it is the conflict among traditional beliefs, changing norms, and new scientific knowledge that creates barriers to sexual expression or results in sexual dysfunction. The term *sexual dysfunction* refers to an actual impairment in one or more phases of the human sexual response cycle (Kaplan 1974) described in Chapter 2. Sexual dysfunction can result from such common risk factors as sexual trauma, performance anxiety, negative conditioning, or sexual ignorance.

In order to prevent, eliminate, or minimize crises in sexuality, nurses need to be aware of the more common risks and problems that occur from infancy through the senior years. This knowledge will enable the nurse to plan direct intervention such as counseling, education, or guidance or indirect intervention by referral or advocacy.

Table 5-1 demonstrates some of the sexual risks and problem indicators through the life cycle. Those appropriate based on the age of the client should be considered when taking a health history and doing a physical examination.

Sexual History

The sexual history may be taken in the course of the complete health history once the client feels comfortable. There are several approaches to gathering sexual data: the client completes a self-administered questionnaire, the nurse conducts a semi-structured interview on general areas, or a specific structured interview is carried out.

This chapter includes a comprehensive self-administered questionnaire. The acronym CARITAS was developed to serve as a tool in recalling the areas to be assessed (Krozy 1981, 176):

Concern: What is the client's definition of the real or potential concern? What is the client's goal? What is the nurse's concern?
Attitudes: What attitudes, beliefs, and values are operating? What are the client's attitudes toward him/herself; toward sexual expression and practice?
Relationship: What is the type or quality of the client's relationship (marriage,

TABLE 5-1 *Sexual Risks and Problem Indicators Throughout Life*

Biophysiological Risks	Psychosocial Risks	Cognitive Risks	Religious and Legal Risks	Environmental Risks	Problem Indicators
INFANCY					
Hormonal error	Disruption of oral pleasure	Parental knowledge of sexual knowledge	Sexuality seen as basically immoral		Excessive crying or lassitude
Anomaly of genitalia	Negative feedback for genital exploration				
Physical deformity	Parental disappointment with sex of child				
Gender misdiagnosis	Parental negative attitudes toward sex due to personal or religious beliefs				
Gender reassignment					
Intrauterine acquisition of STD					
EARLY CHILDHOOD					
Genital corrective surgery	Negative association of genitals	Incorrect terminology for genitals and functions taught		Lack of parent or sibling of opposite sex	Uses only slang terms for sexual parts and functions (does not know correct terms)
Genital injury/infection	Punishment for genital exploration	Observation/listening to parental sexual activity without explanation			Dressed to look like opposite sex (this may also be related to culture, fashion, intent of parents)
Hormonal replacement	Sexual trauma through abuse, rape, incest, pornography				Presence of STD
	Threat of mutilation or being incomplete				

Extreme sanction against nudity Hostile response to accidental viewing of nudity			Masturbatory fear or guilt Excessive masturbation (to the extent of interfering with and taking the place of other appropriate activities —as assessed for each individual)
LATE CHILDHOOD Genital trauma, surgery, etc. Hormonal imbalance Physical deformities Harsh punishment for sexual curiosity Shame or embarrassment associated with sexual functions and organs Sexual trauma, exploitation—pornography, incest	Exposure to and misinterpretation of pornographic material Thwarting of sexual curiosity, questions unanswered Parental lying about sexual functions (for example, the stork)	Unsupervised play (with dangerous items likely to cause injury or infection or play that represents exploitation of one child by another, creating fear, anxiety, guilt)	Masturbatory fear and guilt Excessive masturbation (taking the place of or interfering with other age-appropriate activities) Unacceptable sexual activity between children (this *may* be hetero/homosexual, incestuous, SM) Rejection of same-sex playmates or play-activity Signs of genital trauma, STD

TABLE 5-1 *(Continued)*

ADOLESCENCE

Biophysiological Risks	Psychosocial Risks	Cognitive Risks	Religious and Legal Risks	Environmental Risks	Problem Indicators
Sensory and/or motor disability	Physical impairment	Absence of sex education in home, school, or religious instiution	Lack of consensus regarding sexual rights of teenagers	Unchaperoned homes and teen gatherings	Poor body image
Pregnancy	Parental marital discord	"Street learning"	Uncertain boundaries between religious/social groups and state	Institutionalized living	Low self-esteem
STD	Peer pressure toward sexual activity	Pornography	Lack of standards in rape prosecutions	Lack of opportunity to socialize with opposite sex	Masturbatory guilt or excessiveness
Sexual trauma	Rigid sex roles	Professional ignorance of sexual developmental needs of healthy/impaired adolescents		Newly established independent living	Sexual attitudes that create guilt, conflict, anxiety
Obesity/extreme thinness	Sexual trauma, exploitation— through pornography, prostitution, sexual slavery				Inability to communicate sexually
Alcohol and drug usage					Cross-dressing
Depression					Disgust at own gender or genitals
Use of contraceptives					Homophobia
					Fetishism
					Homosexuality (when not a comfortable, accepted lifestyle)
					Multiple sexual partners
					Pregnancy
					Prostitution
					STD
					Sexual dysfunction
					Sexual violence

122

ADULTHOOD

Sensory or motor disability	Unwanted pregnancy	Lack of knowledge of sexual facts	Laws governing sex behavior between consenting adults	Institutionalized living	Poor body image
Mutilative surgery	Sexual trauma	Professional ignorance of sexual developmental needs of healthy/impaired adults	Discrepant legal and scientific definitions of various sexual acts	Lack of privacy	Low self-esteem
Loss of reproductive integrity	Marital discord		Lack of definition of obscenity	Lack of opportunity to socialize	Sexual dysfunction
Contraceptive usage (pill, IUD)	Loss/nonavailability of sexual partner		Discrepant personal and religious values about sexuality	Isolation	Sexual guilt/anxiety
Licit/illicit drug usage: antihypertensives, alcohol, antidepressants, etc.	Preoccupation				Inability to communicate sexual needs
Menopause	Boredom				Transsexualism
Body insult—chronic					Transvestitism
Disease, injury					Homosexuality (when not a comfortable, integrated lifestyle)
					Fetishism
					Multiple or extramarital sexual partners (may or may not be a "problem")
					STD
					Multiple abortions
					Sexual disinterest
					Celibacy (when it is not a preferred lifestyle)
					Criminal acts

TABLE 5-1 *(Continued)*

Biophysiological Risks	Psychosocial Risks	Cognitive Risks	Religious and Legal Risks	Environmental Risks	Problem Indicators
SENIOR ADULTHOOD					
Hormonal decrease	Social taboos/proscription against sexual activity	Belief in myths against sexual activity in old age	Lack of elder abuse or neglect laws	Institutionalized living	Feelings of unattractiveness
Genital disease or surgery	Family hostility toward dating or remarriage	Lack of knowledge of normal aging process		Deliberate separation of sexes	Sexual dysfunction (including Widower's syndrome)
Generalized poor health	Punishment or derision at any sexual expression	Lack of preparation for aging		Lack of privacy	Masturbatory guilt
Chronic diseases: cardiovascular, neurologic, respiratory, metabolic, musculoskeletal	Sexual assault, trauma	Lack of teaching about sexual activity and various diseases		Disproportionate ratio of aged males to females	Sexual fears and guilt
Fatigue		Professional ignorance about normal developmental needs of healthy/impaired senior adults		Isolation	Sexualization of other body functions—fecal or urinary incontinence, requests for frequent enemas
Pain				Lack of transportation or finances	Sexual frustration
Drug therapies				Lack of opportunity to socialize	Use of prostitution (if client is uncomfortable with this alternative)
Deliberate overmedication for sexual "acting out"					Unnecessary sexual abstinence
					Depression
					Suicidal attempt

124

homosexual, celibate, loving, estranged, . . .)? Who else needs to be
involved and at what point?

Illness: What effect does the client's
condition (physical, emotional, surgical,
or drug treatment) have on his/her
sexuality? What interventions could
counteract that effect?

Trust: Trust is one of the most important
aspects in resolving sexual problems.
Does the client have enough trust in the
significant others (physician, nurse,
partner) to be open to help?

Awareness: How aware is the client of the
dynamics of sexuality? What does the
client know? What should the client
know and what must the client (and
family) be taught?

Sensuality: What techniques, environments, or experiences have improved or
hindered sexual pleasure or sexual
expression?

A Self-Administered Sexual History

(A written statement should be included that assures the client(s) that all information shared will be kept in strictest confidence by the health-care provider.)

Part I. General information

Name _____ Age _____

Marital status: 1) never married _____ 2) married _____ 3) divorced _____ 4) widowed _____
   5) separated _____

Present or former occupation _____

Work status: 1) full-time _____ 2) part-time _____ 3) retired _____

Living arrangements:

   1) alone _____

   2) with spouse only _____

   3) with spouse and family _____

   4) with family, no spouse _____

   5) with friend of same sex _____

   6) with friend of opposite sex _____

   7) other _____

Highest education completed:

   1) 8th grade or less _____

   2) some high school _____

   3) high school graduate _____

   4) some college _____

   5) four or more years college _____

Religious preference: 1) Protestant _____ 2) Catholic _____ 3) Jewish _____ 4) none _____
   5) other _____

Frequency of attending place of worship (approximate):

   1) one or more times/week _____

   2) about twice a month _____

   3) once every 2-3 months _____

   4) twice a year _____

   5) once a year or less _____

   6) never _____

Do you consider yourself to be: very religious _____ somewhat religious _____ not religious _____

Ethnic identity: 1) American _____   2) Irish _____   3) Italian _____   4) French _____
      5) Hispanic _____   6) Afro _____   7) Asian _____   8) Other _____

Number of children: 1) none _____   2) 1–2 _____   3) 3–4 _____   4) 5–6 _____
      5) 7 or more _____

Part II. Developmental history: Women

A. Menstruation

Age at first period _____ *Date last period* _____

Do you consider your periods regular _____ *or irregular* _____ *Number of days flow* _____

Do you use tampons? _____ *pads?* _____ *both?* _____ *Number of tampons/pads per day* _____

Degree of pain with periods: 1) none _____ 2) mild _____ 3) moderate _____ 4) severe _____

What do you do for menstrual pain (that is, bedrest, medication, hot water bottle)? _____
_____

Do you experience premenstrual symptoms? _____ **If yes, explain** _____
_____ No _____

Do you take any medications for premenstrual symptoms? _____

Are you experiencing symptoms of menopause? If yes, explain _____
_____ No _____

Have your menstrual periods stopped completely? If yes, since when? _____
_____ No _____

Problems with menopause _____

Medications _____

B. Pregnancy and contraception

Number of pregnancies: 1) none _____   2) 1–2 _____   3) 3–4 _____   4) 5–6 _____
      5) 7 or more _____

Number of children born: 1) none _____   2) 1–2 _____   3) 3–4 _____   4) 5–6 _____
      5) 7 or more

Number of miscarriages: 1) none _____   2) 1–2 _____   3) 3–4 _____   4) 5–6 _____
      5) 7 or more

Number of abortions: 1) none _____ 2) 1–2 _____ 3) 3–4 _____ 4) 5–6 _____ 5) 7 or
      more _____

Number of adopted children: 1) none_____   2) 1–2 _____   3) 3–4 _____   4) 5–6 _____
      5) 7 or more

Number of stepchildren: 1) none _____   2) 1–2 _____   3) 3–4 _____   4) 5–6 _____
5) 7 or more
Did you have difficulty becoming pregnant? **If yes, explain** _____
_____

Type of delivery: vaginal _____   cesarean _____   both _____
Do you currently use any method(s) of birth control? **If yes, describe** _____
_____ **No** _____

When did you last use this method? _____
Is this method satisfactory? **Yes** _____   **If no, explain** _____
_____

Do you have any questions or concerns about your method or some other method of birth control? _____
_____

C. Sexual health history

How often do you have a Pap smear? _____
Was it ever abnormal? **Yes** _____   **No** _____
What was the diagnosis? _____
What was done? _____
Do you practice breast self-examination? **Yes** _____   **No** _____
If yes, how often? _____
Have you ever had breast or gynecological surgery? **If yes, explain** _____
_____ **No** _____

Has this surgery caused problems? _____
Have you ever had vaginal itching, redness, odor, or discharge? **If yes, diagnosis** _____
Treatment _____ **No** _____
How often have you had these symptoms? _____
Have you had an infection of the urinary bladder or urethra? **If yes, cause** _____
_____

Treatment _____
How often? _____
Have you ever had a sexually transmitted (venereal) disease? **If yes, diagnosis** _____
Treatment _____
How many times? _____
Were you ever treated for a uterine, ovarian, or tubal infection? **If yes, explain** _____
Do you douche? _____   **How often?** _____   **Why?** _____
Type of douche solution _____
Do you use vaginal deodorant sprays or suppositories? **Yes** _____   **No** _____

Please check any of the following conditions which you might have:

_____   lack of sexual interest

_____   difficulty becoming sexually aroused

_____   difficulty with lubrication

_____   painful intercourse

_____   difficulty reaching orgasm (climax)

_____   inability to reach orgasm

_____   other? _____

Part III. Developmental history: Men

Do you have difficulty urinating (that is, frequency, pain, or blood in urine)? If yes, explain _____

_____ No _____

Have you been treated for a urinary tract infection? If yes, cause _____

_____

Treatment _____

How often? _____

Have you had problems with your prostate? If yes, explain _____

_____ No _____

Are you circumcised? Yes _____   No _____   If no, have you ever had difficulty retracting foreskin, irritation, other _____

Have you sustained an injury to the testicles or penis? If yes, explain _____

_____ No _____

Have you ever had genital surgery? If yes, why? _____

_____ No _____

Have you ever been treated for a sexually transmitted (venereal) disease? If yes, diagnosis _____

_____ No _____

Treatment _____ No _____

Have you ever practiced testicular self-examination? If yes, when _____

_____ No _____

Please check any of the following conditions which you might have:

_____   lack of sexual interest

_____   difficulty becoming sexually aroused

_____   difficulty getting an erection

_____   difficulty maintaining an erection

_____   difficulty ejaculating

_____   ejaculating too quickly

_____   painful intercourse

_____   other? _____

Part IV. Sexual history: All individuals

Please answer all questions by filling in the information or circling the appropriate response. If you are not sure of an answer (for example, a medication name), put a question mark (?) in the blank.

When did you first learn about how your body functions? _____

From whom? _____

When did you first learn about how the opposite sex's body functions? _____

_____

From whom? _____

How old were you when you experienced your first sexual activity? _____

Nature of activity _____

Your reaction to it _____

How often did you observe your parents showing affection (hugs, kisses, etc.) toward each other? Very often _____ sometimes _____ never _____

Do you consider yourself to be

_____ exclusively heterosexual

_____ mostly heterosexual

_____ bisexual

_____ mostly homosexual

_____ exclusively homosexual

Do you consider your sexual preference to be a problem? If yes, explain _____

How would you compare your partner's sexual interest to your own? greater interest _____ same _____ less interest _____ not applicable _____

How affectionate were your parents toward you? very affectionate _____ somewhat affectionate _____ not affectionate _____

How attractive do you consider yourself? very attractive _____ somewhat attractive _____ not attractive _____

Masturbation is a healthy release of sexual tension. I agree _____ disagree _____ uncertain _____

In the past six months, approximately *how often have you engaged in some form of sexual activity?* 1) several times/week _____   2) once/week _____   3) 2–3 times/month _____   4) once in 2–3 months _____ 5) once in 4–6 months _____ 7) never _____

How satisfied are you with the frequency *of your sexual activity?* very satisfied _____ somewhat satisfied _____ dissatisfied _____

How satisfied are you with the quality *of your sexual activity?* very satisfied _____ somewhat satisfied _____ dissatisfied _____

If you could change something in your sexual activity, what would that be? _____

_____

How satisfied is your partner with your sexual performance? very satisfied _____ somewhat satisfied _____ dissatisfied _____ don't know _____ not applicable _____

How satisfied is your partner with his/her own sexual performance? very satisfied _____ somewhat satisfied _____ dissatisfied _____ don't know _____ not applicable _____

What would your partner change in his/her sex life? _____

_____

_____

How easily do you communicate your sexual needs to your partner? very easily _____ somewhat _____ not at all _____ not applicable _____

How easily does your partner communicate his/her sexual needs to you? very easily _____ somewhat _____ not at all _____ not applicable _____ .

Please check whether you or your partner have any of the following conditions:

Condition	You	Partner
Diabetes	_____	_____
Respiratory disease	_____	_____
Heart disease	_____	_____
High blood pressure	_____	_____
Medication: _____		
Problem drinking	_____	_____
Daily amount and kind: _____		
Depression	_____	_____
Medication: _____		
Overweight	_____	_____
Anemia	_____	_____
Parkinson's disease	_____	_____
Stroke/spinal cord injury	_____	_____
Arthritis	_____	_____
Other		

_____

_____

Have you ever experienced a sexual trauma? If yes, what happened and when? _____

_____

How resolved? _____

_____

Do you have any questions about your own or your partner's sexuality which you would like answered by a health professional? _____

_____

An additional resource for developing components of a sexual history that covers each age group and is highly comprehensive is, *Assessment of Sexual Function: A Guide to Interviewing,* published by the Group for the Advancement of Psychiatry (1973).

Assessment of Cues

In addition to assessing sexuality through formalized data collection, the health professional must be skillful in identifying cues. Cues are verbal and nonverbal masked messages people may send out when they have sexual problems that have not been overtly addressed. People may complain of vague problems (Glover 1977) or make such statements as, "I'm not the man (or woman) I used to be," or "My spouse doesn't pay much attention to me these days." Adolescents often ask for help indirectly by saying, "I have a friend who . . . ."

Another cue related to a client's sexual needs is inappropriate sexual behavior or sexual "acting out." According to Woods (1979) one who flirts with a member of the opposite sex may be trying to prove that he or she is sexually attractive. To gain control or attention, individuals may expose their genitals. Males whose sexual self-image is threatened may act out by touching a female nurse's breasts or making risqué remarks. Hostility and anger may also be expressed in this way. As indicated in Chapter 4, nurses must learn to recognize the messages these acts convey: concern about sexuality, lack of appropriate sexual outlets, or a need to explore sexual concerns.

In the elderly, sexual acting out is usually a cry for help (Oberleder 1976). Often, older people are deprived of the closeness and touching that all of us need, and attempt to meet this need inappropriately. Holding a client's hand is a positive and acceptable way to provide a sense of caring as well as preventing sexual passes. Oberleder (1976) notes that *sexual regression,* "the pathological and unconscious sexualization of body functions such as eating, urinating, and defecation" (p. 329), may result from sensory and sexual deprivation. When deprived of the sensations of moisture, warmth, smoothness, and softness, the individual may resort to "messing." The strategy for nursing intervention would be substitution, using warm baths, back rubs, and soft items, such as a furry toy or blanket. Sexual regression may also be prevented by adequate preparation and sensitive handling of clients during an examination of the genitalia. Additional cues carrying sexual messages include frequent requests for enemas, pulling out urinary catheters, and removing condom drainage.

In children, various cues should alert professionals to the possibility of sexual trauma. Burgess and Holmstrom (1975) observe that children suffering from sexual trauma may present it by "staying inside more frequently, not wanting to go to school, crying with no provocation . . . excessive (bathing), or a sudden onset of bedwetting" (p. 557). Other clues parents might report are the child's staying out all night, walking home nude, accumulating gifts, or drawing a picture suggestive of sexual acts or trauma that emphasize genitals or depict fear or threats.

Physical/Sexual Examination Considerations

The next phase of sexual assessment is the gathering of objective data through examination of the genitalia and related structures and through diagnostic testing. The physical examination is conducted in order to establish baseline clinical data as part of a routine health check-up, to diagnose a specific disease, or as a prerequisite to sex therapy. The latter, often termed the *sexological exam,* is aimed at uncovering any organic etiology causing a sexual dysfunction, as well as assessing levels of sexual responsiveness and partner interactions. The sexological exam and diagnostic testing will be discussed in later sections.

For the physical/sexual examination, depending on the nurse's skill and educational preparation, she or he may either assist the examiner or conduct the examination. In either instance, an essential nursing measure is to adequately prepare the client. Effective preparation will facilitate informed consent, client cooperation, and a reduction in the anxiety that frequently occurs with examination of the sexual organs.

Assuring Informed Consent

It is the client's right to know and the health professional's responsibility to explain each aspect of the sexual examination. Terms that the client can understand should be used. Clients need to know the nature of the exam, whether there might be any discomfort, why the exam is being done, and if there is any risk involved. A writtten explanation of common procedures can be helpful in educating clients or raising any questions they might have. Written materials, particularly instructions, are often more effective than oral explanations, as they allow the individual to review and absorb the information when he or she is feeling less stressed.

Clients should also be familiar with the health professionals involved in their care. If a client does not already know the person who will be performing the examination, the person should introduce herself or himself or be introduced. The professional's credentials should also be mentioned ("I'm Kathy Jones, a certified nurse-midwife").

Informed consent may also necessitate that the health professional secure permission from a parent or legal guardian of the client. It is imperative to be familiar with any legal regulations or restrictions that exist (for example, providing treatment to a minor).

Reducing Anxiety

Anyone who has had a thorough physical/sexual exam — even a health professional — knows how easy it is to feel uncomfortable or embarrassed. One woman, with legs in stirrups, commented, "They say position is everything in life, but I don't think this is what they had in mind." And one gentleman quipped during a sigmoidoscopy, "I can't imagine how 'some people' could actually enjoy this." These individuals were able to cope with their uneasiness through humor, a common method for dealing with anxiety-producing situations.

Anxiety prior to or during a physical examination may result from real or anticipated pain, embarrassment (particularly when the examiner is of the opposite sex), ignorance of the procedure, past sexual trauma, past negative experience during a sexual exam, or fear of the findings (that is, STD, pregnancy, cancer). Males may consider the rectal exam particularly distasteful because of its association with homosexual activity.

A very young child may fear mutilation or perceive a parent's anxiety. A child needs a caregiver who is particularly sensitive in order to prevent long-lasting sexual maladjustment.

Anxiety or anger may also arise if the practitioner conducts the exam in a brusque, insensitive manner. During a gynecological exam, for example, a warmed speculum, an unhurried approach, and an explanation of what is going on at the foot of the examining table can be very reassuring. A mirror and a lighted transparent speculum are helpful, allowing the client to watch the examination.

Anxiety may be manifested as blushing, giggling, handwringing, silence, chattering, or looking away while talking. Occasionally a client may demonstrate an extreme anxiety reaction with profuse perspiration, palpitations, nausea, vomiting, muscle tension, dizziness, or fainting. In such instances, it is wise to postpone the examination until a later time when a mild sedative may be prescribed for this type of client. Rarely, the exam may need to be performed under anesthesia. For example, women being treated for vaginismus, an involuntary contraction of the muscles surrounding the vaginal orifice, may need to be anesthetized to facilitate a pelvic exam (Kolodny et al. 1979).

When the client demonstrates signs of anxiety, the nurse can help the client to relax by acknowledging, "You seem to be anxious or tense." This acknowledgment should be followed by a question to determine the cause of the client's uneasiness.

An effective anxiety-reducing technique was demonstrated by one nurse/practitioner. An adolescent, visibly nervous, was about to have her first pelvic exam for a vaginal discharge. Rather than just talking about the exam, the nurse hiked up her uniform, hopped onto the table and, with underwear "flapping in the breeze," placed her feet in the stirrups. "This is the way women are examined," she explained. "It's not terrific, but we all have to go through it." The young woman chuckled, surely thinking, "If it's okay for her, it's okay for me." This same innovative nurse received permission to "sensitize" young male interns during their obstetrics rotation by having them "experience" the lithotomy position. Unfortunately, they were not required to undress.

Assuring Privacy

The concept of privacy includes respect for the individual's modesty, as well as for confidentiality. Every effort should be made to see that the examination is performed in an area that offers maximum privacy. A private room with a door and a sink is best. When this is not possible, the area should be closed off from the eyes and ears of others.

Prior to the examination, the client should be instructed about which clothing to remove and where the clothes can be placed. A hospital gown and coverlet should be provided and the client told whether to fasten the gown in the front or back. Sufficient time should be allowed for undressing, as well as redressing, and the client should indicate readiness by verbal response to a knock before anyone enters the room.

Examination supplies should be present before the exam begins to decrease unnecessary interruptions or intrusions.

Whenever possible, examining tables should be placed with the foot of the table away from the entrance of the room. Requiring others to knock on the door and request permission to enter, as well as placing an "In use" sign on the door, are also good privacy measures.

Discussions about personal data or physical findings should be conducted discreetly and in a private location between those directly involved with the client's care. It is particularly important to protect the client's right to privacy in a clinic setting where allied health workers may be part of the client's community. Gossip among health professionals is not professional.

Providing for Physical Comfort and Safety

Prior to the examination, the client should be instructed to void, saving a specimen for the laboratory, if indicated.

The client should be protected from becoming chilled by adjusting the room temperature, if possible, or covering the client with something more than a paper sheet.

Every effort should be made to prevent the

client from falling while getting on or off the table. If the client is weak or shaky, he or she should be assisted into the examining position. In helping a female into the lithotomy position, the nurse's hands should be placed under the client's buttocks, and the client assisted in moving to the table's edge.

If the examining table is flat, a small pillow wrapped in disposable paper placed under the client's head may provide more comfort.

For the female pelvic exam, a woman may be allowed to wear her shoes. This may prevent the discomfort arising from pressure of the stirrups on the feet. An effective "homemade" device is placing padded oven mitts over the stirrups. Knee supports have been reported to be more comfortable than heel stirrups (Kolodny et al. 1979).

As noted earlier, the speculum should be slightly warmed — never hot. The examiner should consider using a smaller-sized speculum if the client is virginal, nulliparous, or elderly.

For the proctologic exam in the knee-chest position, comfort may be increased by using a thin padding under the knees and a small pillow under the head. Most often, knee-chest position is achieved by side-lying.

The examination lamp can become very hot and should be kept at a safe distance from the client's skin.

As the examination proceeds, the client should be told what is going to be done and what equipment will be used. Ample water-soluble lubricant should be applied to a speculum or gloved finger. Lubricant should not be used, however, when a Pap test is to be taken because it could distort the cytology, or when a culture is to be taken because the lubricant might be bactericidal (Ulene and Matousek 1976).

The examiner should proceed slowly and gently. Exerting slight pressure on the inside of the thigh will prevent startling the patient when his or her genitalia are touched. The examiner should state whatever it is that he or she is about to do.

To facilitate relaxation of the muscles, the client can be instructed to take deep breaths. Holding the client's hand and reassuring him or her in a soothing voice is often welcome. If discomfort is present, the examiner should stop or slow the procedure until the client can gain control and reiterate any discussion of what will occur, as appropriate.

After the examination is over, the client should be given a washcloth and towel or perineal wipes to remove any lubricant or bodily secretions before dressing.

Advocacy

Client advocacy is an important function for health-care professionals. It includes (1) protecting clients from physical or emotional harm, (2) conveying their needs or concerns to other health providers, (3) explaining their health care to them, and (4) helping them to understand and exercise their rights. Each of these areas has implications for the client undergoing physical/sexual examination.

A client must be protected from repeated unnecessary pelvic examination for the sole purpose of student experience. Often the recipient of this practice has been a poor, minority female receiving public assistance and clinic care. A client has the right to refuse to submit to a pelvic examination, even when it is deemed medically necessary.

Protection must be afforded to individuals who are particularly vulnerable: the very young or old, the sexually inexperienced or inactive, the rape victim, or the individual with sensory impairment. Informing the examiner that it is the client's first examination of this type or that the client's perineum is extremely sensitive will alert the examiner to special needs. As noted in Chapter 7, the rape victim may be bruised, frightened, and in shock, yet the need for a thorough examination and accurate recording is crucial. Needless to say, extreme gentleness and empathy are required. Another protective measure is providing a chaperone to any woman undergoing pelvic exam by a male examiner.

Physical/Sexual Examination of the Male

First, inspection of the external genitalia is conducted to determine the presence of pathological conditions or abnormalities that could interfere with optimal sexual function. The examiner assesses the testes and scrotum for tenderness, redness, disproportionate size, presence of a tumor, hydrocele, or varicocele. The examiner might wish to teach the client, particularly the young male, about testicular self-exam at this time (see Figure 5-1).

The penis is examined for localized lesions or lesions surrounding the urinary meatus, evidence of discharge, redness, pain, hypo- or hyperspadias, scar tissue resulting from corrective surgery, evidence of trauma, and the condition of the prepuce and glans penis in the uncircumcized male.

The pubic hair should be inspected for the presence of pediculosis, scabies, tinea cruris, or venereal warts.

The rectal examination, particularly for the male, is an important but often neglected part of the physical. Nass, Libby, and Fisher (1981) suggest that this omission may result from the unconscious fears and negative associations held by the physician. Yet the early detection of rectal, colon, and prostatic cancers, which cause a high rate of male mortality, and of benign prostatic hypertrophy, require manual palpation from within the rectum. A fecal smear for occult blood is also obtainable in this way and should be tested. Figure 5-2 explains the rectal examination in the male.

For males approaching 50, a *sigmoidoscopy* should constitute part of the regular physical examination. The sigmoidoscope, a slender, flexible, lighted fiberoptic tube, permits extensive visualization of the colon for detection of nonpalpable tumors or pathology (see

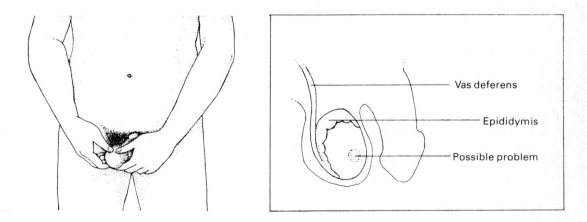

FIGURE 5-1
Testicular self-examination.

SOURCE: From *Sexual Choices,* 2nd ed., by G. D. Nass, R. W. Libby, and M. P. Fisher. Copyright © 1984, 1981 by Wadsworth, Inc. Reprinted by permission of the publisher, Wadsworth Health Sciences, Monterey, California.

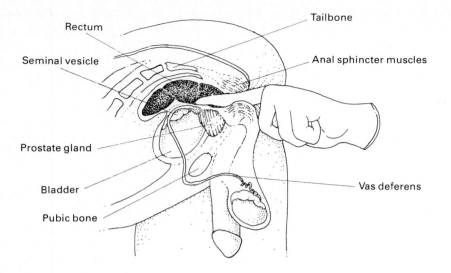

Rectum

Seminal vesicle

Prostate gland

Bladder

Pubic bone

Tailbone

Anal sphincter muscles

Vas deferens

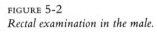

FIGURE 5-2
Rectal examination in the male.

SOURCE: From *Sexual Choices,* 2nd ed., by G. D. Nass, R. W. Libby, and M. P. Fisher.
Copyright © 1984, 1981 by Wadsworth, Inc. Reprinted by permission of the publisher,
Wadsworth Health Sciences, Monterey, California.

Table 5-2 for a summary of the American Cancer Society's recommendations for cancer-related examinations).

Visual examination of the perineum and perianal area may demonstrate hemorrhoids, lesions, and signs of inflammation, infection, or trauma. Rectal discharge should be tested for sexually transmitted disease, particularly if the client has engaged in rectal intercourse.

The male's overall appearance and development should be assessed. Underdevelopment of the musculature, flabbiness, or sparsity of pubic, axillary, or facial hair may suggest a hormonal imbalance. Presence of gynecomastia or any mass should be noted. Breast cancer has been found in 1% of males.

For more detailed instruction on the male examination, Cohen (1979) gives programmed instructions.

Physical/Sexual Examination of the Female

The female examination consists of visual and manual inspection of the breasts, genitalia, abdomen, and rectum. A Pap smear and other laboratory tests are included as necessary.

Both breasts are observed for disproportionate size, abnormal shape, dimpling, redness, lesions, bruising, discharge, or crusting of the nipples.

Breast palpation is undertaken to determine the presence of abnormal masses suggestive of malignancy, cystic disease, tuberculosis lesion, or abcess. Each breast is palpated in concentric circles or spokes of a wheel beginning at the outer aspect and including the areola. The nipple is gently pressed between thumb and forefinger in a lateral and top-to-bottom motion to express any discharge. A small pillow or folded towel under the shoulder of the examined side elevates the anterior chest wall for better palpation. The subaxillary nodes are also palpated.

The examiner may wish to teach the client breast self-examination (BSE) at this time or to observe the client's performance if she currently practices BSE (see Figure 5-3). The client should be encouraged to practice BSE monthly, one week after menstruation, and written instructions should be given for reinforcement. The woman who is postmenopausal should be instructed to choose the same time each month. Pamphlets in English and other languages are available free from the American Cancer Society and the National Cancer Institute.

When teaching BSE, keep in mind that clients are often anxious about touching and/or exposing themselves and even viewing films of bare breasts. Some of this anxiety can be allayed through the use of the older Betsey breast model or a newer and smaller, single, simulated breast. Each model has hidden lumps. Another method for teaching BSE is to have the demonstrator or client perform the exam wearing a leotard without a bra. A third approach is to teach males about breast examination, as it is not uncommon that a mate has discovered a breast lump during sex play.

Visual inspection of the labia, clitoris, and vaginal orifice is undertaken to detect signs of irritation or trauma, lesions caused by herpes or other organisms, venereal warts, scabies, pubic lice, discharge, swelling, clitoral adhesions, or leukoplakia. Foul odor to discharge is an indication of a microorganism. In the postpartum woman, it is essential to treat any infection as well as check the condition of the episiotomy. Palpation of the labia may uncover a cyst of the Bartholin's glands or the Skene's glands.

Visualization of the interior vagina and cervix is accomplished with a *speculum*. The *speculum*, which separates the anterior and posterior vaginal walls, is not adjusted to its open position until comfortably in place. Insertion is facilitated by placing the well-lubricated speculum in a vertical position and rotating it to the horizontal position. A speculum and examining light permit observation for lesions, lacerations, inflammation, polyps, or discharge, as well as the string of an intrauterine device (IUD). The Pap test is also obtained in this way. Figure 5-4A demonstrates the pelvic examination using the speculum.

A *Pap smear* is a cytological examination of cells found in the cervix and vaginal fluid. It is used to identify precancerous and cancerous cells. The specimen is obtained by gently scraping the squamocolumnar surface of the cervix with a wooden spatula and swabbing the vaginal pool. Each specimen is clearly identified, spread thinly on a slide, sprayed or immersed with a chemical fixative, and sent for analysis. A Pap smear may be used to identify abnormal cytology of other areas as well as noncancerous abnormalities in the cervix.

A Pap smear is an essential part of the female exam. Through education of the public about this simple and painless test and the need for early diagnosis and treatment, the incidence of cervical cancer mortality has decreased significantly. Based upon extensive study, the American Cancer Society has developed new guidelines regarding the frequency of Pap testing. These recommendations are shown in Table 5-2.

Before the speculum is removed for bimanual pelvic examination, the client should be offered an opportunity to view her cervix in a mirror. Many women have no idea what their "insides" look like or exactly how their sexual organs function. This is an important prerequisite to sexual health.

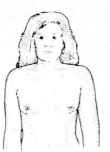

A. Stand with arms down.

B. Lean forward.

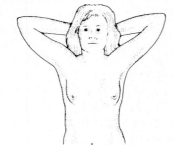

C. Raise arms overhead and press hands behind your head.

D. Place hands on hips and tighten chest and arm muscles by pressing firmly inward.

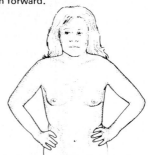

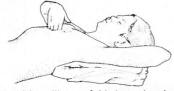

E. Lie with a pillow or folded towel under your left shoulder. Place your left arm above your head. With your right hand, feel the inner half of your left breast from top to bottom and from nipple to breastbone.

F. Feel the outer half from bottom to top and from the nipple to the side of the chest.

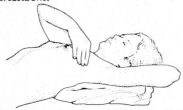

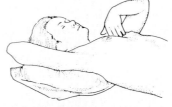

G. Pay special attention to the area between the breast and armpit itself.

H. Now, place the pillow or folded towel under your right shoulder. Repeat the same process for your right breast using the palm of your left hand.

FIGURE 5-3
Breast self-examination.

TABLE 5-2   *Summary of ACS Recommendations for the Early Detection of Cancer in Asymptomatic Persons*

Test or Procedure	Population		
	Sex	Age	Frequency
Sigmoidoscopy	M & F	over 50	every 3–5 years; after 2 negative exams 1 year apart
Stool guaiac slide test	M & F	over 50	every year
Digital rectal examination	M & F	over 40	every year
Pap test	F	20–65; under 20, if sexually active	at least every 3 years*; after 2 negative exams 1 year apart
Pelvic examination	F	20–40 over 40	every 3 years; every year
Endometrial tissue sample	F	at menopause women at high risk[1]	at menopause
Breast self-examination	F	over 20	every month
Breast physical examination	F	20–40 over 40	every 3 years every year
Mammography	F	between 35–40 under 50 over 50	baseline consult personal physician every year (especially for women at high risk)
Chest x-ray			not recommended
Sputum cytology			not recommended
Health counseling and cancer check up[2]	M & F M & F	over 20 over 40	every 3 years every year

[1] History of infertility, obesity, failure of ovulation, abnormal uterine bleeding, or estrogen therapy.
[2] To include examination for cancers of the thyroid, testicles, prostate, ovaries, lymph nodes, oral region, and skin.
* The American College of Obstetricians and Gynecologists recommends annual Pap smears.
SOURCE American Cancer Society. 1980. Guidelines for the cancer-related check-up: Recommendations and rationales, in CA-A *Cancer Journal for Clinicians* 30(4):231. Reprinted by permission.

The *bimanual pelvic examination* is conducted by applying pressure above the symphysis pubis with one or two fingers inserted in the vagina. It is extremely important that the client's bladder is empty because a full bladder can interfere with palpating the uterus, give a false impression of pregnancy or a mass, or obscure a mass. The client with a full bladder may also be uncomfortable and unable to relax during the exam.

The purpose of the bimanual examination is to palpate the uterus and cervix for size, shape, consistency, position, and mobility. Softening of the cervix is a sign of pregnancy. The structures lying laterally to the uterus, in the adnexal areas, include the fallopian tubes, ovaries, and supporting ligaments. In normal individuals, the tubes and ligaments are generally nonpalpable. Figure 5-4B illustrates the bimanual pelvic examination.

The *rectovaginal examination* is performed to palpate the rectovaginal septum, posterior cul-de-sac, uterosacral ligaments, and posterior portion of the pelvis. It also facilitates securing a stool specimen for occult blood and palpation of any lower masses.

The client is often anxious about this portion of the examination because of the uncomfortable sensations experienced. It should not be painful. Reassurance of the importance of this procedure and recommending relaxation techniques will help to make the client more comfortable.

A sigmoidoscopy is also recommended for women 50 and older (see Table 5-2). For detailed instruction on the female pelvic examination, see Cohen (1978a, 1978b), and Hawkins and Higgins (1982).

The Sexological Examination

The sexological examination differs from the physical/sexual examination in several ways. The purpose of the sexological exam is to determine an organic basis for any problem directly related to sexual pleasuring or reproduction and to determine responsiveness and communication between partners. The "client" is most often a couple, requiring that

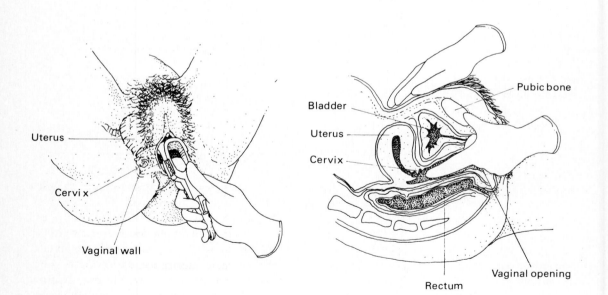

A. Speculum Exam

Uterus

Cervix

Vaginal wall

B. Bimanual Pelvic Exam

Pubic bone

Bladder

Uterus

Cervix

Vaginal opening

Rectum

FIGURE 5-4
Pelvic examination in the female.

SOURCE: From *Sexual Choices,* 2nd ed., by G. D. Nass, R. W. Libby, and M. P. Fisher. Copyright © 1984, 1981 by Wadsworth, Inc. Reprinted by permission of the publisher, Wadsworth Health Sciences, Monterey, California.

both parties undergo a thorough historical and physical assessment.

According to Kolodny et al. (1979), the sexological exam, assessing biologic and psychosocial data, prevents unnecessary psychotherapy when a sexual dysfunction is primarily organic; allows for evaluating improvement during sex therapy; facilitates a therapeutic plan based on the client's physical health status and personal values; and "provides a data base from which many questions related to sexual anatomy and physiology may be asked" (p. 360).

A conjoint medical examination, in which both parties are examined in each other's presence, commonly precedes or is part of sex therapy. The examination, which may be performed by a physician sex therapist and cotherapist of the opposite sex, often promotes communication between partners, uncovers inhibitions and allows correction of misinformation (Kaplan 1974). Not all sex therapy teams have a physician cotherapist, however, in which case a consultation referral to a gynecologist or urologist may be necessary.

Semmens and Semmens (1979) note that during the examination of the male, the squeeze technique (or more currently, the "8-step" or "stop-start" technique) for premature ejaculation and other areas of sexual responsivity, including the male nipples, may be demonstrated. When examining the female, the external and internal genitalia are demonstrated. Particular attention is paid to the structure and function of the clitoris in female pleasuring and the methods for clitoral stimulation. Evaluation of vaginal muscle tone is determined and the female may be taught Kegel exercises — conscious tightening of the abdominal and perineal muscles.

Semmens and Semmens further note that both clients should be offered the opportunity to examine each other. Each partner is asked to communicate the degree of sensitivity of the various parts of the sexual anatomy. Perineal

scar tissue, for example, can interfere with the vaginal nerve supply and turgor and may be responsible for sexual disinterest and unresponsiveness.

Kaplan (1974) notes that as part of the sexological exam, some therapists assess their client's sexual responsiveness by stimulating the client's body and genitals themselves or by actual observation of the partner's sexual interactions. This is in contrast to the format of Masters and Johnson, and most other therapists, who primarily rely on their clients' verbal reports. Kaplan cautions:

> The trend toward explicit participation of the therapist in [the] patient's sexual experiences in the treatment of sexual dysfunctions has been exploited by a number of opportunistic "therapists" who engage in sexual activities with their patients and/or conduct group sex experiences and provide specially trained "sex-therapist"-prostitutes for this purpose. The ethics of some of these practices are highly questionable, and the effectiveness . . . has not been demonstrated. (p. 204)

Diagnostic Testing

The etiology of sexual dysfunction may be biological, interpersonal, or emotional. Currently, most sexual dysfunctions are thought to have a psychological basis. However, numerous acute and chronic illnesses may cause dysfunction by blocking desire or excitement, affecting male erection and ejaculation, or affecting female lubrication and orgasm. The exact percentage of organically based problems is not yet known and much more research is needed. Most of the research has been conducted with males and far less is known about organic dysfunction in women. (For a detailed list of physical factors in sexual dysfunction of males, see Kaplan 1974, 80–85 and Kolodny et al. 1979, 376–377.)

The term *diagnostic testing* generally refers to laboratory analysis of biological products but may also include x-ray or exploratory surgical procedures. Types of assessments that may be useful are listed in Table 5-3. The purpose of these tests is to determine the presence of various conditions such as diabetes, venereal diseases, liver dysfunction, anemia, prostatic carcinoma, Paget's disease, renal disease, or hormonal insufficiency.

Diagnostic testing may also be performed as part of an infertility workup. Friedman (1981) describes such procedures as basal body temperature graph, the Huhner test (to determine whether sperm can swim in the cervical mucus), a thyroid radioisotope assay (to determine hypothyroidism), and a 24-hour urine for 17 ketosteroids (to test adrenal function).

An x-ray may be taken to determine tubal patency (hysterosalpingogram) or this may be done by laparoscopy (an internal inspection of the tubes through a small abdominal incision using a lighted scope). For the male, diagnosis chiefly involves semen analyses. These are described in Chapter 7. Finally, diagnostic testing may include mammography. Table 5-2 describes the new recommendations for this test.

Planning Strategies for Sexual Health Promotion

Planning helps to establish realistic, achievable treatment goals that are mutually defined and given priorities by the client and the health professional. A plan for care is derived

TABLE 5-3*   *Diagnostic Tests and Procedures: Sexual Health Assessment*

Woman	Both	Man
Pap smear	CBC	Serum testosterone cystoscopy
Vaginal cultures and smears	Urinalysis — routine and microscopic	
Serum hormones: estrogens, progesterone, prolactin	Urine culture	
Maturation index	Blood serology — STD	
Cervical culture	Thyroid studies	
Laparoscopy	Kidney function studies	
Mammography	Liver function studies	
	Blood electrolytes	
	FBS	
	Hemoglobin A1C	
	Triglycerides	
	GC cultures — cervix, urethra, nasopharynx, anus	

* The reader is referred to several references on laboratory tests for complete descriptions (Byrne et al. 1981; Widmann 1979; Wallach 1978; Tilkian and Conover 1975; Strand and Elmer 1980).

from the sexual history and physical exam, based upon the nursing diagnosis and guided by a multidisciplinary theoretical framework. Planning includes the specification of goals in behavioral terms, the methodology for intervention, and the personal resources or outside supports needed to attain the goals.

The following questions are useful in developing the care plan:

1. Is the assessment data sufficient to establish/support the nursing or medical diagnosis?

2. What is the nature of the sexual problem?

3. What are the client's immediate and long-term future goals?

4. Is the treatment plan or intervention strategy acceptable to the client (and significant other[s])?

5. What resources are available or lacking in order to reach the goal?

6. Does the plan outline the behavioral outcomes desired, the degree of behavioral change required, the amount of time, and the conditions under which the behavioral change is to take place?

7. Is the evaluation process spelled out in the plan?

8. What barriers are likely to impede the goal?

9. What is the best method to reach the goal?

The goal of nursing intervention is to help the client achieve optimal sexual health through primary, secondary, or tertiary strategies.

Primary preventive intervention (pre-crisis) is aimed at promoting sexual health through such strategies as early sex education, anticipatory guidance, parent effectiveness training, and providing positive role models. *Crisis intervention* is aimed at early diagnosis and treatment of sexual problems that could lead to

sexual dysfunction. Education, counseling (individual, couple, or group), or medical management might be instituted. *Tertiary preventive intervention* (post-crisis) would be used to intervene with a long-standing sexual dysfunction or problem or to assist the client to adapt to an irreversible condition. Tertiary modes would incorporate education, counseling, and/or sex therapy, as well as medical or surgical treatment (for example, implantation of a penile prosthesis).

Healthy sexual functioning may also be promoted by advocacy and self-help. Advocacy should be instituted at any time a client's sexual rights are being compromised while sexual self-help—the possession of appropriate knowledge and skill to promote one's own maximum sexual health and defend one's own sexual rights—should be the ultimate goal of any intervention.

In order to plan an intervention strategy, it is necessary for the caregiver to understand the objectives of the various intervention strategies and to assess his or her own level of competence.

Sex Education

Sex education is a process of teaching and learning, imparting factual information, and assisting individuals to develop attitudes and behaviors for coping with sexual issues (Schiller 1973). Burt and Meeks consider sex education as "education for love" (1975, 1).

Kirkendall (1965) cites the goals of sex education as sexual self-knowledge, positive sexual attitudes, sex without fear, awareness of rights and responsibilities, sexual enjoyment, development of morality, protection from exploitation, social reform, and conditions promoting sexual creativity and effectiveness. *The Report of the Commission on Obscenity and Pornography* (1970) suggests that sex education consider pluralism of values, age, and circumstances, and incorporate multidisciplinary cooperation and input, special preparation of teachers, and imaginative teaching methodologies such as educational television.

Schulz (1979) echoes the beliefs of many sex educators that "every person has the right to receive sexual information and to consider accepting sexuality for pleasure as well as for reproduction" (p. 481). As indicated in Chapter 1, however, resistance does occur because of the belief that sex education is best taught at home or church or that it causes promiscuity. Yet most authors concur that sex education creates informed decision-making and responsible behavior and may alter vicarious and erroneous "locker room" learning. Resistance to sex education may also reflect a lack of professional expertise in dealing with sexual learning needs of populations formerly not considered (such as the retarded client).

Schiller (1973) defines eight areas of involvement for the sex educator:

1. Laying the foundation for introducing a sex education program into a school, agency, or institution
2. Teaching sex education in various settings (that is, workshop, academic program)
3. Curriculum development
4. Use of various teaching strategies
5. Program evaluation
6. Group leadership, counseling, and referral
7. Teaching sex education to various groups (that is, parents, adolescents, disabled)
8. Coordinating sex education in academic institutions or geographical areas

Sexual Counseling

Masters and Johnson (1978a) view counseling as an educational and advisement process, incorporating biophysiological and psychoso-cial factors, without psychotherapy. Clark (1978) defines counseling as a process that does not give advice to the client but "teaches the client how to discover things about himself" (p. 44). In either approach, sexual counseling is aimed at helping people resolve personal and interpersonal problems related to sexuality.

Sex counselors function in various ways (Schiller, 1973):

1. Individual, couple, and group counseling around sexual dysfunctions
2. Team membership in case studies of sexual problems
3. Sex education, advisement, or consultation
4. Consultation to various disciplines for specialized problems

Sex Therapy

Sex therapy is a form of psychotherapy integrating biomedical and psychosocial factors (Masters and Johnson 1978a). The format advocated by Masters and Johnson (Masters 1978) utilizes *conjoint* or couple therapy, with the relationship considered the "client." This form of active treatment prescribes specific tasks that must be carried out in a systematic sequence. One of these tasks is *sensate focus,* a method aimed at enhancing communication, lowering anxiety, increasing sensory awareness, and changing maladaptive patterns of sexual behavior (Masters 1978). Deep-seated personality disorders and psychopathology need not be present for a sexual dysfunction to occur. Masters and Johnson (1976) feel that physical problems are responsible for sexual dysfunction in approximately 5% of cases, with a larger but undetermined number arising from metabolic origin.

There are a number of approaches used in sex therapy. Masters and Johnson use male and female co-therapists to decrease the effects of transference/countertransference. A group therapy structure may be used for individuals with similar problems (Schneidman and McGuire 1976) or mixed dysfunctions (Leiblum, Rosen, and Pierce 1976). Hartman and Fithian (1974) and Kaplan (1974) have developed comprehensive sex therapy approaches. Some therapy techniques appear in Chapter 7.

Sex therapists carry out the following functions (Masters and Johnson 1976):

1. Sexual history taking and education, in line with the couple's goals
2. Facilitating better communication through sensate focus and verbalizing
3. Providing feedback to help analyze and communicate feelings
4. Evaluating outcomes
5. Providing continuous follow-up
6. Peer review

Requirements of Sex Educators, Counselors, and Therapists

Professionals who are involved with sexual issues must possess sexual self-comfort, respect for clients, and personal integrity. They require skills in communication and leadership. Their knowledge of biopsychosocial and legal aspects of sexuality must be current and they need to retain their competency through continuous learning, supervision, and self-evaluation.

To assume the role of sex counselor or therapist, one should at least attain a master's degree. While nurses will undoubtedly develop competence in counseling clients (and many sexual problems have been found amenable to nursing intervention) it is important for nurses to recognize when the client's needs exceed their level of expertise and require referral.

The American Association of Sex Educators, Counselors and Therapists (AASECT) currently certifies specialists. AASECT's regulations are specific and stringent. For example, as of July 1, 1981, the requirements to be an AASECT-certified sex therapist included the following: a doctoral degree and two years' experience or a master's degree and three years' experience; extensive knowledge from reproduction to research methodology; counseling theory and practice; 100 individual or 150 group hours of supervised training with an AASECT-approved trainer; a workshop in sexual attitude restructuring; and personal and professional references.

Most states do not have regulations regarding sex therapists. Before referring a client, a nurse should be fully cognizant of whether an individual is a qualified and reputable therapist.

Advocacy

An advocate speaks in behalf of a person or cause. It may become an essential nursing function to pressure agencies into modifying policies or to educate clients in ways to overcome needless restrictions (Lockhart 1975, 328).

Advocacy as it relates to sexual health promotion means that the sexual rights of an individual will be acknowledged and respected through the action of another individual. As indicated earlier, the health professional's role in sexual advocacy includes protecting clients' privacy and modesty, preventing excessive genital examination, and protecting clients (particularly the young, old, and poor) from being "seen" by numbers of interns.

Many groups of individuals are considered sexually oppressed (Johnson 1975; Gochros and Gochros 1977). Johnson (1975) states that health professionals may deal with the sexual interests and activities of people with identifiable handicaps in three ways: to rigidly control or eliminate sexuality, to accept or allow it, or to consciously cultivate sexual potential. This latter approach — whereby impaired individuals are assisted to understand, adjust, and enjoy their sexuality according to desire and opportunity — is advocacy.

Advocacy also involves challenging policies that would separate married couples in nursing homes, forbid any physical contact between consenting adults, allow the use of medications or punishment to stem sexual needs, or dehumanize people in any way.

As an advocate a nurse might ask that a physician consider the sexual functioning of a client before conducting radical surgery or prescribing certain medications. For example, the nurse could suggest that a stoma be placed in a position which both the health professional and client have decided would not interfere with wearing usual clothing or engaging in intercourse. Or the nurse might suggest the use of an antihypertensive medication with little effect on sexual potency.

At the community level, a nurse may wish to promote sexual health through political action. Some of the areas include advocacy on behalf of self-determination in issues involving sexuality, institution of sex education in schools, prevention of discrimination due to sexual preference, or assurance of education for pregnant adolescents.

An important role is to promote sexual self-help skills and knowledge in consumers. Health professionals should be aware of some of the better popular books on the market in order to recommend them to clients (Barbach 1976; Boston Women's Health Collective 1976, 1978; Galton 1979) and should encourage the practice of breast, testicular, and even vaginal self-exam.

Nurses and other health professionals are becoming more involved in assuring human sexual rights. In 1978, the American Nurses' Association Council of Advanced Practitioners in Psychiatric and Mental Health Nursing passed a resolution endorsing the civil rights of gay persons and encouraging health professionals to develop an awareness

---

Bill of Rights to Guarantee Sexual Freedom

- The right to express yourself as a sexual being.

- The right to be self-confident and self-directing in regard to your sexuality.

- The right to become the person you would like to be.

- The right to select and be with a sex partner of your choice, whether it be of the same sex or of the opposite sex.

- The right to be aware of the influence your sexuality can have on someone else and to use it in a constructive and therapeutic manner.

- The right to encourage your peer group members to function as sexual beings.

- The right to assist others in asserting and expressing their sexuality.

- The right to be accepting and tolerant of another's sexual attitudes and preferences.

- The right to assist men and women of all ages to recognize their sexuality as an integral part of their personality, inherited at conception, molded and tempered by environment, sustained by health, threatened by disease, and reversed by choice.

of gay culture. Linbania Jacobson's Bill of Rights to Guarantee Sexual Freedom (1974) provides a valuable basis for promoting sexual health.

Summary of Implications for Nursing Practice

Nurses are becoming increasingly aware of the importance of sexuality in the lives of their clients. They are becoming knowledgeable about the many internal and external factors which can create sexual disruption and they are learning to take an active role in sexual assessment, education, and counseling.

There are many reasons why nursing can have an influential role in sexual health promotion. Because of the close nature of the nurse/client relationship, clients often feel more comfortable sharing their intimate concerns with the nurse or asking them sexual questions.

Nurses practice in diverse settings, with individuals of every age, socioeconomic, and cultural group. Nurses thus have the opportunity to provide early sex education to children or anticipatory guidance to parents; to help adolescents make responsible choices in their sexual behavior; to identify people at risk for sexual dysfunction; to assist, as well as protect, clients undergoing a physical/sexual examination; to educate or counsel clients whose sexual well-being is threatened; or to refer clients to competent therapists when the client's needs surpass the nurse's skill.

Nurses can be influential as advocates to eliminate policies or conditions which sexually exploit, dehumanize, or traumatize individuals. They can also facilitate the consumer's understanding and practice of positive sexual health behaviors by teaching self-help skills.

With greater freedom to discuss sexuality, more people may seek professional help for sexual problems. This may encourage more nurses to acquire the advanced education required to become a certified sex counselor or therapist.

In most instances, however, the majority of their clients' sexual issues will not require sex therapy. Rather, they will be amenable to effective nursing intervention. What is necessary is knowledge, integrity, sexual self-comfort, and sensitivity on the part of the nurse.

REFERENCES

American Cancer Society. 1980. Guidelines for cancer-related checkup: Recommendations and rationale. *Ca-A Cancer Journal for Clinicians* 30(4).

Barbach, L. G. 1975. *For yourself: The fulfillment of female sexuality.* New York: New American Library.

Barnard, M. U., B. J. Clancy, and K. E. Krantz. 1978. *Human sexuality for health professionals.* Philadelphia: Saunders.

Boston Women's Health Collective. 1976. *Our bodies, ourselves.* 2d ed. New York: Simon & Schuster.

Boston Women's Health Collective. 1978. *Ourselves and our children.* New York: Random House.

Brossart, J. 1979. The gay patient: What you *should* be doing. *RN* 42:50–52.

Burgess, A. W. 1981. *Psychiatric nursing in the hospital and the community.* 3d ed. Englewood Cliffs, N. J.: Prentice-Hall.

Burgess, A. W., and L. L. Holmstrom. 1975. Sexual trauma of children and adolescents: Pressure, sex, and secrecy. *Nursing Clinics of North America* 10(3):551–563.

Burt, J. J., and L. B. Meeks. 1975. *Education for sexuality.* 2d ed. Philadelphia: Saunders.

Byrne, C. J., D. F. Saxton, P. K. Relikan, and P. M. Nugent. 1981. *Laboratory tests: Implications for nurses and allied health professionals.* Menlo Park, Calif.: Addison-Wesley.

Clover, B. H. 1977. Sex counseling of the elderly. *Hospital Practice.* 12:101–113.

Cohen, S. 1978. Patient assessment: Examination of the female pelvis: Part 1. *American Journal of Nursing* 101:1–26.

Cohen, S. 1978. Patient assessment: Examination of the female pelvis: Part II. *American Journal of Nursing* 11:1–28.

Cohen, S. 1979. Patient assessment: Examination of the male genitalia. *American Journal of Nursing* 4:689–712.

Commission on Obscenity and Pornography. 1970. *The report of the commission on obscenity and pornography.* New York: Bantam.

Crosby, J. F. 1976. Is the medium the message? The nurse-midwife as a counselor in sexuality. *Journal of Nurse-Midwifery* 21(1):5–12.

DeLora, J. S., and C. A. B. Warren. 1977. *Understanding sexual interaction.* Boston: Houghton Mifflin.

Elder, M. S. 1970. Unmet challenge—nurse counseling on sexuality. *Nursing Outlook* 18(11):38–40.

Fontaine, K. L. 1976. Human sexuality: Faculty knowledge and attitudes. *Nursing Outlook* 24(3):174–176.

Friedman, B. F. 1981. The infertility workup. *American Journal of Nursing* 11:2040–2046.

Galton, L. 1979. *The complete medical, fitness and health guide for men.* New York: Simon & Schuster.

Gochros, H., and J. Gochros. 1977. *The sexually oppressed.* New York: Association Press.

Group for the Advancement of Psychiatry, Committee on Medical Education. 1973. *Assessment of sexual function: A guide to interviewing,* vol. 8, report 88. New York.

Hartman, W. E., and M. A. Fithian. 1974. *Treatment of sexual dysfunction.* New York: Jason Aronson.

Hawkins, J. W., and L. P. Higgins. 1982. *Health care of women: Gynecologic assessment.* Monterey, Calif.: Wadsworth.

Hogan, R. M. 1980. Nursing and human sexuality. *Nursing Times,* 24 July, 1296–1300.

Hohmann, G. W. 1972. Considerations in management of psychosexual readjustment in the spinal cord injured male. *Rehabilitation Psychology,* 19:50–58.

Hyde, J. S. 1979. *Understanding human sexuality.* New York: McGraw-Hill.

Jacobson, L. 1974. Illness and human sexuality. *Nursing Outlook* 22(1):50–53.

Johnson, W. R. 1975. *Sex education and counseling of special groups.* Springfield, Ill.: Thomas.

Kaplan, H. S. 1974. *The new sex therapy.* New York: Brunner/Mazel.

Kirkendall, L. A. 1965. *Sex education.* SIECUS study guide no. 1. New York. SIECUS.

Kolodny, R. C., W. H. Masters, V. E. Johnson, and M. A. Biggs. 1979. *Textbook of human sexuality for nurses.* Boston: Little, Brown.

Krizinofski, M. T. 1973. Human sexuality and nursing practice. *Nursing Clinics of North America* 8(4):673–681.

Krozy, R. 1981. Human sexuality. In *Psychiatric Nursing in the hospital and the community.* 3d ed., ed. A. W. Burgess. Englewood Cliffs, N. J.: Prentice-Hall.

Leach, A. M. 1978. The client who arouses feelings about sexual identity. In *Comprehensive psychiatric nursing,* ed. J. Haber, et al., 357–370. New York: McGraw-Hill.

Leiblum, S. R., R. C. Rosen, and D. Pierce. 1976. Group treatment format: Mixed sexual dysfunctions. *Archives of Sexual Behavior* 5:313–322.

Lockhart, C. A. 1975. Community nursing services in the home. In *Community health nursing: Patterns and practice,* ed. S. E. Archer and R. Fleshman. North Scituate, Mass.: Duxbury Press.

Masters, W. H. 1978. Sex therapy: Concepts and format. Paper presented at *Seminar on Human Sexuality,* 6–7 November, at Masters and Johnson Institute, Boston.

Masters, W. H., and V. E. Johnson. 1978. Ethics guidelines for sex therapists, sex counselors, and sex researchers. St. Louis: The Reproductive Biology Research Foundation. Mimeo.

Masters. W. H., and V. E. Johnson. 1966. *Human sexual response.* Boston: Little, Brown.

Masters, W. H., and V. E. Johnson. 1976. Principles of the new sex therapy. *American Journal of Psychiatry* 133(5):548–554.

Mims, F. H., and M. Swenson. 1978. A model to promote sexual health care. *Nursing Outlook* 26(2):121–125.

Morrison, E. S., and M. U. Price. 1974. *Values in sexuality.* New York: Hart.

Nass, G. D., R. W. Libby, and M. P. Fisher. 1981. *Sexual choices.* Monterey, Calif.: Wadsworth.

Oberleder, M. 1976. Managing problem behavior of elderly patients. *Hospital and Community Psychiatry.* 27:325–330.

Robineault, I. P. 1978. *Sex, society and the disabled: A developmental inquiry into roles, reactions and responsibilities.* Hagerstown, Md.: Harper & Row.

Schiller, P. 1973. *Creative approach to sex education and counseling.* New York: Association Press.

Schneidman, B., and L. McGuire. 1976. Group therapy for nonorgasmic women: Two age levels. *Archives of Sexual Behavior* 5:239–248.

Schulz, D. A. 1979. *Human sexuality.* Englewood Cliffs, N. J.: Prentice-Hall.

Semmens, J. P., and F. J. Semmens. 1978. The sexual history and physical examination. In *Human sexuality for health professionals,* ed. M. U. Barnard, B. J. Clancy, and K. E. Krantz. Philadelphia: Saunders.

Simon, S. B. 1974. *Meeting yourself halfway.* Niles, Ill.: Argus Communications.

Solnick, R. L., ed. 1978. *Sexuality and aging.* rev. ed. Los Angeles: University of Southern California, Ethel Percy Andrus Gerontology Center.

Strand, M. M., and L. A. Elmer. 1980. *Clinical laboratory tests: A manual for nurses.* 2d ed. St. Louis: C. V. Mosby.

Tilkian, S. M., and M. H. Conover. 1975. *Clinical implications of laboratory tests.* St. Louis: C. V. Mosby.

Ulene, A., and I. Matousek. 1974. Module: Pelvic examination: Submodule: Examination procedures. OMNI (OB/GYN Modular Instruction). Raritan, N. J.: Ortho Pharmaceutical Company, Department of Educational Services.

Wallach, J. 1978. *Interpretation of diagnostic tests.* 3d ed. Boston: Little, Brown.

Widmann, F. H. 1979. *Clinical interpretation of laboratory tests.* 8th ed. Philadelphia: Davis.

Woods, N. F. 1979. *Human Sexuality in health and illness,* 2nd ed. St. Louis: C. V. Mosby.

Introduction

Pregnancy and the Postpartum

Pregnancy and Sexuality
    Perceptions of the problem
    Biophysical reactions
    Suggested nursing interventions for problem-solving with clients
Postpartum Sexuality
    Perceptions and biophysical reactions
    Suggested nursing interventions for problem-solving with clients

The Menopausal Experience

The Female Menopause
    Biophysical reactions
The Male Climacteric
    Biophysical reactions
Perceptions of the Problem: Men and Women
Suggested Nursing Interventions for Problem-Solving with Clients

The Nurse and the Client Experiencing Dysmenorrhea or Premenstrual Syndrome

Dysmenorrhea
Premenstrual Syndrome
Suggested Nursing Interventions for Problem-Solving with Clients

Reproductive Choice

The Nurse and the Client Who Chooses Contraception

Perceptions of the Problem
Problem-Solving
Ineffective Methods

The Nurse and the Client Who Chooses Abortion

Perceptions of the Problem
Problem-Solving

The Nurse and the Client Experiencing a Sexually Transmissible Disease

Perceptions of the Problem
Suggested Health Teaching for Primary Prevention
Suggested Health Teaching to Reduce the Hazardous Event, Prevent Recurrence, and Avoid Crisis

CHAPTER 6

Human Sexuality and Nursing Interventions: Pre-Crisis

Roberta M. Orne

Introduction

As sexual beings throughout life, we humans experience many predictable developmental events and common situational events that have an impact on our sexuality. Some people experience these changes as problems. While hazardous events and somatic insults may or may not produce disequilibrium, they will most likely require new problem-solving abilities and adaptation. Thus, there is the potential for increased vulnerability to crisis.

The nurse's goal in pre-crisis intervention is to help individuals and/or their families to avoid crisis. The conceptual framework of the crisis theory model equips the nurse to:

- Assess perceptions of real or potential hazardous events, effects of body insult, and developmental stage.
- Identify client/family problems, needs, and strengths.
- Solve problems with clients/families and plan strategies to counter the negative effects of the insult and gain new knowledge, insight, and/or skills.
- Intervene by assisting clients/families to maximize existing internal and external resources, mobilize those needed to reach realistic solutions, and reduce the hazard or restore equilibrium.
- Evaluate the process, outcomes, and need

for revision in assessment, planning, or intervention.

This approach to professional practice has a client-centered, rather than the more traditional problem-centered, focus. The nurse assumes the role of client advocate and encourages active client/family participation. There are several problems the nurse commonly encounters in this role. Clients whose value system or cultural background differs widely from that of the nurse may choose solutions that conflict with those viewed as "more appropriate" by the provider. Other clients may choose to abdicate altogether an active role in problem-solving, preferring to be passive recipients of the nurse's plans.

Perhaps the single most important factor affecting successful collaborative problem-solving is communication. Chapter 5 discussed a variety of general skills and techniques needed for effective and comfortable communication between client and care providers about sexual concerns. This chapter will explore potentially hazardous events frequently encountered during the life span and will provide specific suggestions for problem-solving that can be encouraged by the caregiver.

Pregnancy and the Postpartum

Pregnancy, birth, and the postpartum period can readily be identified as developmental events that have the potential to disrupt the equilibrium of the fetus, the woman, her partner, and significant others in her life.

Pregnancy and Sexuality

Pregnancy may or may not be associated with sexual problems, but it inevitably brings about certain changes in one's sex life.

Perceptions of the Problem

The suspicion or fact of pregnancy may be perceived as a threat, loss, or challenge to sexual integrity. Biophysical changes are often the first clue or confirmation that a pregnancy exists. Enlarged, tender breasts, more prominent nipples, lethargy, fatigue, and queasiness are signs that the body's adaptation process is well underway. Pregnancy often arouses mixed emotions about sexuality and lovemaking. Ambivalence and some negative feelings are often experienced by the woman and/or her partner, especially in the first trimester.

Some women perceive pregnancy with a heightened sense of femininity, an enhanced sexual self-image, and increased feelings of sensuality (see Figure 6-1). Many say they gain a new awareness of their bodies and freedom from worry about contraception. Others feel anxious, defensive, or unhappy about their changing bodies. They may relate this feeling to a real or potential loss of independence and lifestyle, a sexual relationship, or role. Sexual self-esteem can be threatened by innuendos that transmit the message, "thin is sexy but pregnant is fat, awkward, and asexual."

Attitudes toward sexuality during pregnancy are affected by the age of the partners. In 1980, 95% of all births in the United States were to women 34 and younger. Between 1980 and 1990, it is projected that births to women ages 35 to 44 will increase by 37% and that by 1990 46% of births will occur to women 35 and older (Adams, Oakley, and Marks 1982, 493–494). The woman who delays childbearing in order to establish her identity and career often brings to the pregnancy a stable relationship and a sense of self acquired through maturation. These factors will affect how the woman feels about her body, her baby, and her sexuality.

Men experience a wide variety of feelings about a partner's pregnancy. Enhanced sexual self-esteem may be perceived if the pregnancy is valued or perceived as proof of masculinity.

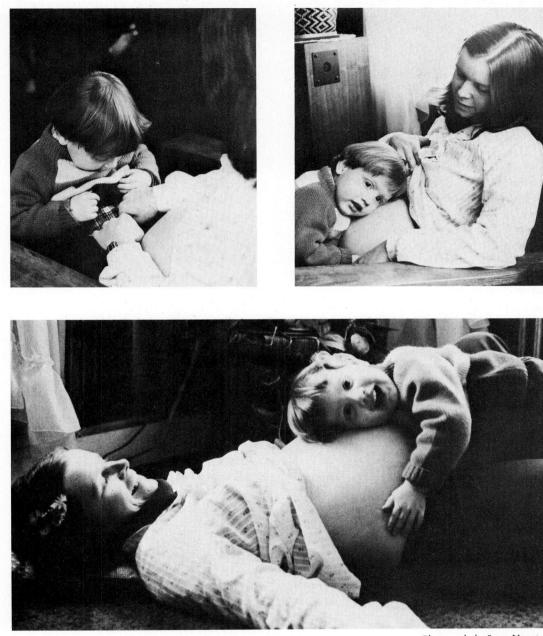

Photographs by Susan Newman.

FIGURE 6-1
A pregnant woman and her son enjoy the pregnancy.

The man's sense of sexual integrity may be threatened if intimacy and lovemaking are avoided, thought to be physically dangerous to the fetus or partner, or if negative feelings exist about the partner's changing appearance and emotions. Perceptions about future parenthood are also influenced by the man's feelings for and identity with his own father or father figure.

Cultural taboos, misunderstanding, and fear also influence sexual problem-solving during pregnancy (Kitzinger 1979). Until recently, medical advice often reinforced anxiety by cautioning abstinence from sexual intercourse during the four to six weeks before birth and up to three months postpartum. Some couples decrease or avoid sexual intimacy during much of pregnancy. This may be due to the woman's discomfort or fatigue, or to fear of rupturing the membranes, stimulating premature labor, or compromising fetal safety, to name but a few reasons. Today caregivers have considerably more knowledge from research studies on which to base anticipatory guidance, health teaching, and counseling.

Biophysical Reactions

A woman's physical discomfort can play a major role in determining intimacy patterns. Fatigue, breast discomfort, and nausea can diminish enthusiasm for lovemaking, primarily during the first trimester. The greatly enlarged uterus of the third trimester can be a "mechanical problem" for sexual intimacy.

There seems to be no "typical" sexual pattern during pregnancy. Masters and Johnson's (1966) research indicates a decrease in libido and frequency of sexual activity during the first and third trimesters and an increase in the second trimester. Some studies generally support these findings, while others (Kyndely 1978) found that couples report little or no change in how they experience or express sexuality during pregnancy. Bing and Coleman's findings (1977) include both of the above patterns plus two others; some couples report a steady increase in libido and others a steady decline.

Women often experience heightened sexual tension and more intense orgasms during pregnancy. These can be related to the increased pregnancy-induced pelvic vascularity and venous engorgement. An additional result of increased vascularity is more rapid lubrication, which occurs by the end of the first trimester. Masturbation, many report, stimulates more intensive uterine contractions than intercourse. Orgasms while pregnant may not relieve pelvic vasocongestion, which is often perceived as residual sexual tension. The resolution phase of the pregnant woman's sexual response may last as long as 45 minutes for the multipara and up to 15 minutes for the nullipara.

The uterus can be highly irritable as pregnancy advances to term. Some women experience painful orgasmic and postorgasmic uterine contractions similar to those of labor. This is thought to be related to increased intrauterine pressure. Occasionally a woman will report tonic orgasmic spasms lasting as long as a minute. Reports indicate that although fetal heart rate is temporarily slowed when this occurs, there is usually no evidence of fetal distress.

Research studies have thus far failed to show a strong correlation between orgasm and premature labor. A prematurely ripe cervix, however, may induce the onset of labor following orgasmic intercourse or masturbation. Prostaglandins, present in seminal fluid, may be associated but there is little documented evidence as yet.

Naeye's (1979) data suggest that frequency of intercourse in the month prior to delivery may increase the risk of amniotic fluid infection, affecting both fetal and neonatal mortality. The exact causes for this association are not yet clear.

Although there is some controversy over the safety of lovemaking during pregnancy, most evidence suggests it is unlikely that intercourse and orgasm will cause premature labor or premature rupture of the membranes. If the uterine cervix is closed and the amniotic membranes intact, the fetus is well cushioned. Most professionals now encourage intimacy and lovemaking throughout the normal pregnancy. However, potential risk for spontaneous abortion, infection, and premature birth does exist if there is a history of habitual abortions, vaginal bleeding or pain, abdominal pain, ruptured membranes, premature cervical dilation, uterine abnormalities, or spotting during the first trimester. Obstacles, real or imagined, can greatly increase vulnerability to crisis.

Suggested Nursing Interventions for Problem-Solving with Clients

1. Discomfort during intercourse may be overcome by experimenting with various coital positions. The male-superior position, which permits deep penile penetration, can put pressure on the enlarged uterus and breasts and is often uncomfortable, especially near term. Lying side-by-side or rear-entry are options. Another more comfortable position is one in which the couple face each other while the woman positions herself with both knees drawn up and over either side of the side-lying male. The woman is able to control penetration in the female-superior position by placing her hand on the shaft of the penis.

2. Nurses often need to "give permission" to encourage discussing sexuality during pregnancy. Women should be encouraged to bring partners to prenatal visits. This often stimulates dialogue between the couple as well as identifying individual concerns. Prepared childbirth and parenting classes are other avenues for integrating pregnancy and sexuality.

3. Couples should be aware that oral sex during pregnancy can be potentially dangerous if air is blown into the vagina. If this happens, air is forced between the membranes and the uterine wall and enters the maternal vascular bed through the placental lakes, causing an air embolism. An air embolism may also result from douching, a practice usually contraindicated during pregnancy. Increased pelvic and genital vascularity and peripheral vessel dilation heighten the woman's risk to an embolus in pregnancy and the early postpartum.

4. Also, note suggestions listed in *Postpartum Sexuality* that may be appropriate to pregnancy. For example, Kegel (pelvic floor) exercises will help to build pubococcygeal muscle tone for delivery.

Postpartum Sexuality

The period following childbirth typically brings a new set of changes—physical, psychological, and interpersonal—that may affect sexual expression.

Perceptions and Biophysical Reactions

Interest in sexual intimacy and resumption of intercourse varies with each individual and couple following pregnancy and birth. Many couples report that sex can be "less than ideal." Both women and their partners frequently report decreased libido, sexual arousal, and response, for a number of reasons: fatigue, vaginal discharge, anxiety and tension, fear of pregnancy, vaginal irritation during or after coitus, lack of confidence in birth control method, breast sensitivity and/or physical discomfort (especially at the vaginal introitus if lubrication is insufficient).

Significant decreases in estrogen and progesterone levels following delivery will partially explain changes in libido and sexual and orgasmic response that may last for several months. Decreased vaginal lubrication, perceived as a tightening and dryness of the vagina, is common during the first six weeks to six months. Lubrication also tends to take longer, vaginal distension is less marked, vasocongestion of the labia is delayed into the plateau stage, and orgasmic contractions are often less intense.

Fear of injury to an episiotomy or abdominal cesarean incision may cause a couple to delay sexual intimacy for an unnecessarily long time. In most women, surgical incisions heal in two to four weeks. Many health-care providers say that intercourse can usually be safely resumed at this time if bleeding has stopped.

On the other hand, some couples say their interest in sex is very high following a birth. For women, this interest may be related to vasocongestion of the postpartum pelvis, perceived as heightened sexual tension. Some women report they become initially orgasmic after giving birth and others say they have more intense and satisfying orgasms following the first pregnancy. Factors that can contribute to enhanced sexual desire and response are breastfeeding, positive attitudes of partners, and a high degree of previous sexual intimacy.

Breastfeeding evokes a wide variety of feelings in both men and women. The nursing woman may experience highly sensual feelings similar to those of coital arousal, but some women are not erotically stimulated by the infant's suckling. Men may express jealousy about sensuous feelings their partners experience during breastfeeding. Guilt, anger and frustration may be felt by either partner when there is a lack of understanding about the normally pleasurable, and often sensual, response to nursing. Similarities do exist between coital response and breastfeeding: uterine contractions occur, nipples become more vascular and erect, there is close skin-to-skin contact, and orgasm has been experienced by some nursing women.

Many factors influence the emotions aroused during breastfeeding; however, cultural aspects are rarely considered. Since cultural attitudes about breastfeeding and female sexuality are intimately related, basic social issues may be involved in individual perception — conflicts over male versus female sexual roles, sex for pleasure versus sex for procreation, and the breast as a source of sexual pleasure versus a source of infant nourishment.

Riordan and Rapp found that the dominant North American attitude regarding erotic pleasures of nursing is primarily one of silence. They note that if specific sensual feelings are even discussed, it is usually with hesitation, embarrassment, and in privacy (1980, 110). Thus, while some women express positive attitudes about sensual feelings, others feel guilty or fear they are abnormal; some reject breastfeeding altogether.

Suggested Nursing Interventions for Problem-Solving with Clients

1. Kegel (pelvic floor) exercises for the postpartum woman should be strongly encouraged. The caregiver should emphasize that gluteal and pelvic floor exercises, when appropriately done, will (1) strengthen the pubococcygeus (PC) muscle, (2) slim the buttocks, (3) improve circulation to the pelvis and perineum and stimulate healing of an episiotomy, lacerations, and hemorrhoids, and (4) improve vaginal tone and sexual sensation. A gradual buildup to 100 Kegels a day would

be ideal. These should be encouraged as a lifetime sexual health-care practice. These instructions should be given:

a. Contract muscles (as though stopping and starting mid-stream urinating or stopping a bowel movement).

b. Hold for three seconds. Relax for three seconds.

c. Repeat these three-second contract-relax exercises ten times, twice a day at first and gradually build up time. These can usually be started on first day postpartum.

Note: If exercise is too strenuous, the PC muscle can become sore. If this happens, the woman can be advised to either stop doing the exercise for one or two days until this temporary tenderness disappears and then resume it, or reduce the number of times done per day and then gradually increase. To test the effectiveness of this exercise, the woman can lie down, insert one finger into the vagina and feel for tightening when contracting the PC muscle.

2. A water-soluble gel (such as K-Y jelly) or an unscented contraceptive foam, cream, or jelly or saliva will increase normally decreased vaginal lubrication during sexual arousal. Water-soluble jelly is sterile, soothing, and relatively odorless. It will feel cold on the skin, so it should be applied with fingers in and around the vagina before intercourse. Safflower, coconut, or baby oil or cocoa butter can also be used. These last longer than water-soluble jelly and don't dry up.

3. Individual couples need to be reassured about the variety of ways, other than intercourse, that sexual pleasure can be expressed. There is not a "right or wrong way" of expressing love or caring when sensitivity for the partner is shown. Touching, holding, and massaging may be pleasurable. The use of vibrators and incorporation of mutual masturbation into lovemaking are viable alternatives, but such suggestions may increase anxiety for some.

4. The female-superior or side-by-side positions for intercourse make it easier to control the depth of penile thrusting and pressure on the perineum and abdomen. A variety of positions can be experimented with to find the most satisfying ones.

5. During coital arousal and orgasm the breastfeeding woman may find her milk will "let down" and breasts begin to leak or spurt milk. This is due to the release of oxytocin. Some find this pleasurable. Other women may want to avoid this leakage by nursing the baby prior to intercourse or by wearing a bra.

6. Group support systems can be of value for a new parent, to share concerns and information and to explore alternatives. Many communities have new parent groups, frequently an extension of prepared childbirth classes. LaLeche League offers small informal group support and excellent literature for the breastfeeding woman and her partner.

7. Breastfeeding may delay menstruation and ovulation. This delay is due, in part, to high levels of serum prolactin, which block pituitary gonadotrophin release. However, breastfeeding is not considered a reliably effective method of birth control. In this culture, prolonged infant sucking at the breast rarely occurs and breast milk is rarely the sole source of infant nutrition. Lactation-induced infertility is therefore extremely unpredictable. Ovulation can occur during lactation and often precedes the first menstrual period. Non-nursing women usually resume menstrual periods within six to 12 weeks postpartum but for lactating

women, the timing of this return to menstruation is more unpredictable. These early periods may be anovulatory but this should not be assumed. Other contraceptive methods must be used to ensure protection.

8. Because little is known about the effects of contraceptive drugs on the infant and breast milk, the use of birth control pills and medicated IUDs during lactation is controversial. Their use is not recommended by most health-care providers. For non-nursing women, oral contraceptives are usually not started for four to six weeks because they have the potential to increase thromboembolic and circulation risks.

9. Other contraceptive methods: IUDs are commonly inserted four to six weeks following a birth or at the time of the first or second menstrual period. Martin (1978, 178) reports that "pregnancy, expulsion, and removal rates are highest for IUDs inserted within two to four weeks postpartum." Earlier insertion can also increase the risk of uterine perforation. Following a cesarean birth, two to three months should be allowed before IUD insertion. Diaphragms will need to be checked or refitted at the postpartum exam. Changes in size of the vaginal vault can occur following pregnancy and birth or abortion. Condoms and vaginal spermicides are recommended for interim use and are highly effective as a regular method of choice. Obviously, any guidance should be based on individual readiness, need, and motivation.

10. Suggested readings for clients (see References and Bibliography for more sources):
    • *Making Love During Pregnancy* by Bing and Coleman
    • *The Pregnancy After 30 Workbook* edited by Brewer

The nursing intervention process for pregnant and postpartum sexuality is outlined in Table 6-1.

The Menopausal Experience

Recently, increased interest, research, and media attention have been directed to the middle years. Consequently, both the consumer public and health-care providers have begun to be more aware and knowledgeable about men and women's mid-life sexual health concerns.

The Female Menopause

Historically, there has been little said or written on the positive side about the female menopausal experience. "Menopause was considered one of the most stressful experiences in a woman's life" (Dyer 1979). In fact, sexuality of the menopausal woman was most often described in terms of atrophy and dysfunction, loss of fertility and femininity, and disinterest in sex. It was insinuated that after menopause women would fade quietly into sexless old age; unfortunately, some passively did just that. Living in a society that equated sexuality with reproduction, menopausal women were stereotyped as asexual, hard-to-live-with women who had endless hot flashes and were in need of tranquilizers or estrogen.

Although the words menopause and climacteric are often used interchangeably, by definition *menopause* means final cessation of menses. For women, *climacteric* is a broader term and refers to the transitional period between middle years and old age when reproductive function is diminished and eventually lost. In this chapter, the term "menopausal experience" will be used to denote the approx-

TABLE 6-1   *Nursing Intervention Process in Pre-Crisis: Pregnant and Postpartum Sexuality*

[ ] Refers to postpartum *only*

1. *Assessment* (nurse assesses or reviews records)
   a. Complete health history focusing on sexuality
   b. Physical exam and laboratory testing
   c. Client's perceptions:
      • Affective response to biophysical changes, adaptations in intimacy and lovemaking patterns, and problems [breastfeeding, labor and birth process, infant]
      • Influencing factors, such as attitudes about sex and intimacy during pregnancy and postpartum, health and comfort status, concerns about fetus/infant, support of others [type of delivery, complications]
      • Knowledge about normal pregnant and postpartal adaptations in sexual response patterns [sensuality and breastfeeding, involution and contraception]
      • Resources being utilized and needed
      • Anticipated effects of sexuality on partner, self, fetus
   d. Collaborative health teaching needs: as perceived by client and identified by nurse or others

2. *Planning* (a collaborative process to augment problem-solving)
   a. Explanation of biophysical changes and adaptations of sexual response cycle, contraceptive options, breastfeeding, techniques for preventing complications such as sore nipples
   b. Resources: community groups, referral to colleagues, and adjunct services (if needed)

3. *Intervention* (based on planning)
   a. Health teaching and counseling
   b. Liaison and support to significant other(s)

4. *Evaluation* of intervention and revisions needed for care, teaching, and follow-up

Adapted from Hunt. 1982. In *Crisis Theory—A Framework for Nursing Practice*, ed. M. S. Infante.

imately 10 to 15 years of normal maturational change that occurs in women. Some authorities describe the menopause experience as lasting only about five years. However, there is considerable variation. A woman often begins to experience some physiological changes in her early 40s and will stop menstruating by early to mid-50s. Some continue, however, to experience results of hormonal changes for many years. Therefore, it is difficult to establish specific parameters of this stage. This normal maturation period should not be confused with surgical menopause: the sudden interruption of reproductive integrity when the ovaries and uterus are removed.

Unfortunately, one of the most significant messages often conveyed is that the normal female menopause experience is something less than healthy. This is a misconception. While many women experience some discomfort associated with vasomotor instability, genital tissue change and/or feelings of anxiety, insomnia, depression, fatigue or emotional lability, others experience none of these. With the exception of the first two, these effects are not related solely to the menopause experience, but rather to mid-life developmental tasks and transitions. Other factors influencing the menopause include overall emotional and physical health, quality of diet, activity and exercise levels, and genetic aging patterns. Only about 10% of women require medical intervention to relieve severe problems.

Biophysical Reactions

Onset of the menopausal experience is brought about by an alteration in the relationship between the ovarian feedback system and the hypothalamic adenohypophyseal complex. Biophysically, the woman's equilibrium is disrupted during the normal physiologic process of aging. A gradual yet progressive decline in follicular ovum development and a decrease in corpus luteum activity occurs. These reductions produce decreasing levels of progesterones and estrogens, which, in turn, stimulate the anterior pituitary to overproduction of circulating FSH (follicle-stimulating hormone) and LH (luteinizing hormone) in an attempt to readjust the feedback mechanism. The ovaries become increasingly unable to synthesize estrogens and progesterones at previous optimum cyclical levels, even with the stimulation of high gonadotropin levels, and the hyperactivity eventually ends.

Consequences of these changes are increasing anovulatory cycles with eventual cessation of ovulation and resultant infertility and resultant changes in menstrual patterns. Considerable variation in individual menstrual cycles is typical. Some women experience irregular, infrequent, and scanty periods while others alternate between heavy flows and amenorrhea for several years prior to the end of menstrual periods.

Although progesterone production eventually ceases at some point, estrogen production does not. The gradual slowing of ovarian estradiol production, which began in the mid-20s, decreases more rapidly during these years of change. It is known, however, that the ovaries continue to produce diminished levels of steroids from converted theca-like cells in the ovarian stroma even after the cessation of menses. The body's fatty tissues are known to store and convert a biologically inactive male hormone — *androstenedione,* which is produced by the adrenals and ovaries — into

an endogenous estrogen known as *estrone.* Androstenedione is classified as an estrogen precursor. Women who are above average weight often experience fewer severe menopausal symptoms because of this phenomenon. During the menopause years, the higher estrogen levels and cyclical fluctuation that stimulates menstruation are gradually reduced, but somatic estrogen production is not entirely lost.

Although research is inconclusive, decreased estrogen levels appear to be responsible for many of the biophysical alterations characteristic of the menopausal experience. Vasomotor instability and genital atrophic changes are primary examples. Other alterations attributed to declining estrogen levels are osteoporosis, skin changes, joint and muscle pain, and urinary tract and cardiovascular disorders. It should be noted, however, that men experience these changes as well.

There seems to be agreement that hot flashes and flushes are linked to vasomotor instability. Approximately two-thirds of women experience these; approximately 10% of them seek intervention to alleviate their occurrence. A *hot flash* is perceived as a flash of heat throughout the body without related sweating or skin changes. These flashes are less commonly experienced than the *hot flush,* which causes rapid changes in blood vessels and produces sensations of heat (most often in the upper body and face), an increase in pulse and respiration, sweating, and chills. The duration and frequency of hot flashes and flushes vary; they are described as momentary to lasting for minutes, and occur infrequently to as often as five or six times a day. Symptoms of cold hands and feet, numbness and tingling, headaches, and palpitations have also been linked to vasomotor instability. Sources disagree on whether increased levels of FSH or erratic swings in hormones, especially estrogens, are primarily responsible for this phenomenon. The *"habituated cell theory"* has also been suggested as an explanation. This theory hypothesizes that groups of cells become addicted to certain levels of estrogen and when estrogen levels decline withdrawal symptoms are experienced.

Under the influence of lowered estrogen levels, the vagina gradually becomes less acidic and elastic, and the epithelium thins and loses its rugated texture. The introitus tends to narrow, the perineal epidermis thins, and supportive muscular and connective tissue to internal genitalia tend to relax. These gradual adaptations may cause postcoital discomfort, dyspareunia, spotting after coitus, and susceptibility to increased vaginal itching and infections and bladder infections.

Based on Masters and Johnson's clinical research and other self-report studies, both libido and sexual response patterns are characteristically altered, in part by the physiological changes that begin to appear in middle age. During the excitement phase, women often experience a one to three minute delay in lubrication and the amount produced is less. Although clitoral response is relatively unchanged, there is a decrease in labial swelling.

In the plateau phase, engorgement is less extensive, and there is reduced uterine elevation and less increase in the vaginal barrel. The number and duration of uterine contractions during the orgasmic phase is reduced. Additionally, this phase is somewhat shortened and some women experience painful contractions both during and following orgasm. The resolution phase is typified by rapid disengorgement.

Extragenital responses are also altered. There is a diminished increase in breast size, the sex flush occurs less frequently, is less pronounced and widely distributed, and myotonia reactions are lessened. These adaptations of the sexual response cycle are influenced to a great extent by lowered estrogen levels, but drugs and other nonphysiologic factors will also influence the cycle and libido.

The Male Climacteric

Increased attention has been evident in recent literature debating whether males have a mid-life experience analogous to menopause. Unlike women, men's mid-life sexuality has rarely been discussed, let alone written about. One of the first books written solely about men's middle years' sexual adaptations, *The Male Climacteric,* was not published until 1975.

Many of society's sex-negative images of female menopause have escaped men at middle age. To the contrary, middle-aged men in North American culture are often portrayed as virile, confident, and experienced. Sheehy comments, "In my experience, men will often dismiss any mention of the climacteric as a misery-loves-company idea cooked up by menopausal women" (1977, 317).

The language of men's adaptation to sexual mid-life is more ambiguous. The cliche "male menopause" is truly a misnomer because there is no monthly menstrual cycle and therefore no cessation of menses in men. Traditionally, it has been assumed that only women had monthly hormonal cycles. However, based on the few studies that have been done, there is some evidence that males experience more subtle biological and emotional cycles. "Climacteric," although not an ideal term, is more apt than "male menopause" in describing the maturational changes that variably affect middle-aged men. While the male maintains the potential for reproduction often into the eighth and ninth decade, there are both hormonal and biophysical adaptations to his sexuality.

Biophysical Reactions

Many men are seemingly unaware of these gradual changes; some do not perceive them as a threat to sexual integrity, while others are reluctant to admit to any sexual health disequilibrium. The latter attitude may be due, in large part, to cultural conditioning. However, approximately 15% of middle-aged men do experience profound physical and emotional changes that threaten their sexual self-esteem, body image, libido and/or sexual behavior.

A male's testosterone levels peak during his early 20s and then gradually decline until age 40 to 55, when the hormone levels decrease more rapidly. In addition, the size, firmness, and elasticity of the testes and scrotum begin to diminish. Hypertrophy of the prostate occurs in approximately 20% of late middle-aged men. Due at least in part to decreasing androgen output, men may experience a variety of mood changes, increased nervousness, irritability, depression, and insomnia. Some men report skin changes, fluid retention, urinary irregularities, headaches, hot flashes, and other reactions similar to those associated with female menopausal vasomotor instability.

Biophysical adaptations are also manifested in the sexual response cycle. During the excitement phase, erections may be less firm and full and take longer to achieve. Masters and Johnson report that erection takes two to three times longer after approximately age 50. Middle-aged men often report they need more stimulation to achieve and maintain an erection. During both the excitement and plateau phases, there is a decrease in testicular elevation. There is also difficulty in returning to full erection if it is partially lost. However, an erection can often be maintained without ejaculation for longer periods. The plateau phase is prolonged as a middle-aged man's ability to maintain an erection is increased.

During the orgasmic phase, ejaculation is somewhat less forceful, there may be a slight decrease in ejaculatory volume, and the sensual experience may be reduced. Resolution is gradually characterized by rapid detumescence and a longer refractory period. Decreased extragenital reactions are similar to those of the middle-aged female.

Testosterone replacement therapy is neither effective nor recommended unless plasma testosterone levels are significantly depressed, a relatively uncommon occurrence. Prostatic cancer may be stimulated by long-term testosterone therapy. The integrated mind-body changes characteristic of the male climacteric are regulated by the hypothalamus and autonomic nervous system and influenced by a mixture of intrinsic and extrinsic social, emotional, and biophysical factors. Biophysical changes can be (1) sudden or gradual in onset, (2) a reflection of an underlying organic problem or merely normal aging, and (3) perceived as a crisis or effectively coped with through realistic problem-solving.

Perceptions of the Problem: Men and Women

Perceived threats to mid-life sexual integrity may initially stimulate a rise in tension and mild anxiety. Perceptions of threats are influenced by multiple factors. The following are examples of issues the nurse may need to help the client clarify in order to identify needs and problems and facilitate realistic problem-solving:

- What importance does fertility have for the individual? For his/her significant others?
- What values and attitudes are held about pregnancy, sexual response, and the aging process?
- Has contraception, lovemaking, or menstruation been problematic?
- What kinds of menopausal/climacteric experiences have friends or family had?
- What is the reaction of the partner toward menopause/the climacteric?
- What are the cultural influences on the

individuals and their role in society/family?

- What emotional stressors is the individual experiencing with family, job, or the social environment?

Perceptions about the menopausal and male climacteric experiences are obviously as varied as the individual. Sheehy (1977) describes the anxiety of many men as they encounter the normal bio-psycho-social effects of middle age: [He] fears "losing his male powers as he has known them, that can so often make the first time he can't get an erection crippling. Even the slightest suggestion that his sexual prowess is diminishing can psych the mid-life man into a repeat of what too often seems to him to be a humiliating failure" (p. 304).

Others have described this vulnerability a self-fulfilling prophecy often resulting in erectile difficulties (impotence). A vicious cycle of performance anxiety and sexual failure can be triggered by only one incidence of failure to achieve or maintain an erection. As a man's anxiety increases, so too can vulnerability to crisis. The nature of crisis is unique to each individual; for some it may be loss of a relationship, to another depression or premature ejaculation.

The women's movement of the last decade has been a major factor in demystifying cultural attitudes about menopause. Increasingly, women are learning more about how to care for and about their bodies and maintain sexual health during middle age.

In a culture that places an enormous emphasis on sex, youth, and beauty, the middle-aged individual can perceive this time as a threat to sexual self-esteem and sexual identity. On the other hand, many individuals are beginning to view this time as a real challenge to re-define themselves as sexual people, to enjoy their sexuality without fear of pregnancy or worry about contraceptives, and to reconsider their sexual attitudes and values. With emphasis on health promotion and high-level wellness, the nurse is seen as a primary advocate for assisting the individual during middle years to achieve and maintain sexual health and integrity.

Suggested Nursing Interventions for Problem-Solving with Clients

1. *Estrogen replacement therapy* (ERT) is one of the most controversial health-care issues confronting the consumer today. Clients need to be aware that physicians' attitudes about prescribing this medication still vary widely. If female menopause is viewed as an estrogen deficiency disease, ERT may be indiscriminately given for virtually all menopausal manifestations. On the other hand, some physicians prescribe this therapy for only the most severe reactions. Most physicians now recommend that estrogen replacement be combined with progesterone, the latter being added during the last 10 days of the monthly regimen. Each woman needs to make an informed decision based on whether the benefits outweigh the risks. The decision should be made only after the client has had a complete history, physical examination, appropriate laboratory tests, and a discussion of both positive and negative, short- and long-term effects of this controversial therapy. Although research studies are as yet inconclusive, there is evidence that ERT with combined progesterone decreases the risk of endometrial and breast cancer. Estrogen therapy alone is linked with increased risk of endometrial and breast cancer and cardiovascular disorders. Contraindications to ERT use are given in Table 6-2.

TABLE 6-2   *Contraindications to ERT Use*

Absolute Contraindications (must not use ERT)

- Current or past blood-clotting disorders
- Stroke
- Cardiovascular disease
- Undiagnosed abnormal vaginal bleeding
- Cancer of the breast, reproductive organs, or skin
- Pregnancy

Strong Relative Contraindications (probably should not use ERT)

- Impaired liver function
- Hypertension (high blood pressure)
- Diabetes
- Fibrocystic disease or fibroadenoma of the breast
- Sickle cell disease
- High blood serum lipid levels
- Elective surgery planned in next four weeks

Relative Contraindications (must be followed very carefully)

- Fibroid tumor of the uterus
- Strong family history of diabetes
- Epilepsy
- Asthma
- Varicose veins

Adapted from Stewart, F., et al. 1979. *My body, my health.* New York: Wiley.

2. Clients should be skeptical of professionals who dismiss anxiety about menopausal/climacteric biophysical and emotional manifestations or concerns with a brief "this is to be expected at your age." Receiving answers and solutions through collaborative problem-solving is the right of the consumer. If the professional is unwilling, the client should seek another resource.

3. Clients should be instructed and encouraged to initiate or continue to do breast and testicular exams in order to recognize normal aging adaptations. This may be a problem for women who have been conditioned to avoid touching or looking at their sex organs or have relied solely on professionals at a yearly exam.

4. Women should be encouraged to continue to have periodic Pap smears and yearly pelvic exams. Many women erroneously consider these procedures unnecessary after menopause, whether natural or surgical. The American Cancer Society has suggested that non-high risk women up to age 65 who have had normal cell Pap tests two years in a row need this test only every three years. The American College of Obstetricians and Gynecologists states that every woman sexually active and/or over the age of 18 should have a Pap test annually. This is a highly controversial issue within the health-care delivery system.

5. As the middle-aged male's erection becomes less firm and angular it may be more pleasurable, may fit and feel better, for the woman whose vaginal tissues are thinner and less elastic. Does the client feel it necessary to have the penis in the vagina to have an orgasm or an intimate loving relationship?

6. Many studies indicate that the normal aging adaptations are accentuated in sexually inactive men and women. Maintenance of intercourse and/or masturbation stimulate muscle tone, cardiac and respiratory rates, adrenal glands, and sympathetic and parasympathetic nerves. Obviously, many factors will influence sexual ability: partner interest and availability, mental and physical health, diet, exercise, past and present lifestyles, cultural expectations and taboos, previous

sexual patterns, fatigue, and alcohol consumption, to name but a few.

7. Decreased vaginal lubrication can be a problem resulting from decreased estrogen levels. Lubrication can be enhanced by longer foreplay and the use of topical water-soluble jellies and creams applied in and around the introitus. Estrogen creams should be used sparingly and with caution after other methods have failed. Vaginal estrogen creams are systemically absorbed. Some women have found that vaginal insertion or topical application of *small* amounts of yogurt and vegetable oil (avoid olive oil) are very effective in increasing lubrication. Use of *small* amounts of vegetable oils alone may be helpful.

8. Nutrition and vitamin mineral supplements may counter the effects of mid-life hormonal imbalance as well as enhance nutritional status. Several of the most popular "natural treatments" for common menopausal effects follow:
    - *Vitamin E* is frequently labeled the menopause vitamin. Many women claim that vitamin E supplements relieve leg cramps, headaches, hot flashes/flushes, fatigue, and insomnia and at the same time promote general well-being. Food sources rich in vitamin E include vegetable oils, wheat germ, soybeans, peanuts, salmon, and spinach. Vitamin E supplements may be contraindicated in diabetes, hypertension, and rheumatic heart disease. Vitamin E is often recommended to smokers and those who have a high intake of processed food because they usually have a higher deficiency. The usual recommended dose is 100 to 1000 units of vitamin E per day, taken after a meal containing some fat. A woman should start with 100 units and gradually increase her intake as needed. Anyone taking digitalis should not take any vitamin E without a doctor's supervision. Effects of vitamin E are enhanced when it is taken with vitamin C. And vitamin E and ginseng taken together may give better results than vitamin E taken alone. The ginseng should be taken before meals and the vitamin E after. Women should not expect immediate relief; two to six weeks should be allowed. Note that there is an increase in FSH and LH in a vitamin E deficiency.
    - *Vitamin B complex and vitamin C*— Food sources rich in vitamin B complex (there are more than 15 B vitamins) include brewer's yeast, whole grains and seeds, yogurt, liver, milk, and wheat germ. Food sources rich in vitamin C include bell peppers, citrus fruits, rose hips, broccoli, and strawberries. The balanced combination of the B vitamins and vitamin C is described as a "stress formula." One or two tablets per day can be taken after meals (100–500 mg/day of vitamin B complex with extra B_6, and 1000 mg/day of vitamin C). Many women feel these help to relieve hot flashes, nervousness, and irritability, and promote the body's resistance to infection. B complex works to detoxify and eliminate FSH and LH through the liver.
    - *Calcium*— From 600 to 1000 mg can be taken daily along with 400 units/day of vitamin D. This combination is taken because many women suffer loss of bone density with aging (osteoporosis). Food sources of calcium are milk and milk products (yogurt, cheese, buttermilk), beets, chard, endive, kale, and mustard. Sunshine is the best natural source of vitamin D.
    - *Herbs*— Some plants are reputed to relieve hot flashes because of their natural

estrogen content. Among the more common of these are Dong quoi (female ginseng), angelica root, sassafras, ladyslipper, and passion flower. A tea is often brewed from these herbs as well as other herbs. Lack of research studies prevents giving much specific information about mechanism of action, side effects, and appropriate "dosages."

Reitz (1979) found that many women experienced fewer of the problems associated with menopause by limiting or avoiding their intake of salt, sugar, white flour, alcohol, coffee, nonherbal teas, chocolate, red meat, butter, and cream.

9. Some women have found that pure yogurt, used either in a warm water douche or inserted directly into the vagina, relieves symptoms of vaginitis or cystitis. These symptoms occur more readily in women who have experienced some loss of tissue integrity with decreasing hormone levels.

10. Contraception is recommended for one, and some suggest two, years following the last menstrual period. Ovulation and menstrual patterns are often irregular during the menopause and this may be problematic for couples. Contraceptive alternatives during this period are more limited. The birth control pill is not recommended for women over 35 and especially over 40. Diaphragms may be con-

---

TABLE 6-3 *Nursing Intervention Process in Pre-crisis: Clients Experiencing Menopause or the Climacteric*

1. *Assessment* (nurse assesses or reviews records)
   a. Complete health history with emphasis on menstrual, contraceptive, reproductive, and sexual patterns
   b. Physical exam including pelvic
   c. Appropriate screening and laboratory tests
   d. Client's perceptions:
      • Affective response to problems, concerns, needs of menopausal experience/climacteric
      • Influencing factors (age, cultural attitudes, support of significant others)
      • Knowledge about menopause/climacteric, adaptations of sexual responses at mid-life, biophysical mid-life changes, prevention techniques
      • Resources being utilized and needed
      • Anticipated effect of the problem, need, or concern on relationship, mental and physical health
   e. Collaborative health teaching needs: as perceived by client and identified by nurse or others

2. *Planning* (a collaborative process to augment client problem-solving)
   a. Explanation of biophysical changes and sexual response patterns, health-care needs, options, screenings, exams, prevention techniques
   b. Resources: dietary, referral to colleagues, adjunct services (if needed), community resources

3. *Intervention* (based on planning)
   a. Health teaching and counseling
   b. Liaison support to client's significant other(s)
   c. Referrals

4. *Evaluation* of intervention and revisions needed for care, teaching, and follow-up.

Adapted from Hunt. 1982. In *Crisis Theory—A Framework for Nursing Practice,* ed. M. S. Infante.

traindicated if a cystocele or rectocele is present. Natural family planning methods may be more difficult to use because of the irregularity of ovulation and menses. The use of condoms and spermicides may be one of the most appropriate methods. Sterilization for both men and women is an increasingly popular choice for permanent contraception. It is the most common method for couples over 30 (Hatcher et al. 1979).

11. Contrary to conventional medical assumptions, 30% to 50% of chronic male impotence is currently thought to be associated with an underlying organic cause. The etiology varies but is often associated with diabetic neuropathy, drugs and alcohol, circulatory impairment, and low testosterone levels. Thus, chronic erectile difficulties should be medically evaluated.

12. Many middle-aged and older women and men have been conditioned by a society that was often sexist and repressive in its approach to sex education and sexual health care. The health-care system, too, lacked both scientific knowledge and practitioners who were adequately prepared to include sexual health in holistic care. Discussing sex with clients was often avoided or discouraged. Thus, some clients will be unwilling to discuss their sexual health. The knowledgeable nurse will respect the client's needs but leave the door open with an invitation for future dialogue. The pre-crisis intervention process is outlined in Table 6-3.

13. Suggested readings for clients (see References and Bibliography for more sources):
    • *Total Sexual Fitness for Women* by Lance and Agardy
    • *Menopause—A Positive Approach* by Reitz

    • *Male Sexuality—A Guide to Sexual Fulfillment* by Zilbergeld
    • *The Passage through Menopause: Women's Lives in Transition* by Millette and Hawkins

The Nurse and the Client Experiencing Dysmenorrhea or Premenstrual Syndrome

Attitudes toward menstruation are changing. Vernacular terms such as "falling off the roof," "getting the curse" and routine monthly excuses from gym class are becoming obsolete. But myths linger and taboos about menstruation still exist in some places. Misconceptions are deeply rooted in the culture and often perpetuated by the family, the media, health professionals, and peers. Some of these myths insinuate that women cannot make good decisions during their periods or be depended on due to absenteeism. And, until recently, millions of women were told that the predictable monthly fluid retention, discomfort from GI symptoms, and debilitating effects of dysmenorrhea were primarily in their heads. Females have been traditionally "treated," all too often on the premise that they had emotional problems, were unstable, neurotic, or high-strung. Some were given talks designed to downplay their symptoms and help them cope with discomfort. Others were given prescriptions for tranquilizers, strong diuretics, narcotics, psychotropic drugs, and birth control pills. Psychological factors may, in fact, influence the perception of pain but, unfortunately, this idea was generalized to most women. Dysmenorrhea is perhaps the most common gynecological problem experienced by women of all ages. Budoff estimates that nearly half of the 75 million American women have some type of regular menstrual discomfort and that perhaps 3.5 million, or 10%, are "completely incapacitated for one or two days each month because of pain" (1981).

Dysmenorrhea

Dysmenorrhea is categorized as either *primary,* referring to menstrual pain of unknown etiology, or *secondary,* menstrual pain caused by an organic problem such as endometriosis, fibroids, an inappropriately placed IUD, or other gynecological pathology.

Primary dysmenorrha has been further delineated into two types: *congestive* and *spasmodic.* It should be noted that some women experience both types. Congestive dysmenorrhea is the perception of dull, aching, abdominal discomfort that occurs primarily before menstruation and is often relieved by the onset of the menses or after several days of flow. This discomfort is frequently accompanied by premenstrual tension and symptoms of nausea, bloating, weight gain, anorexia, back and headache, and breast tenderness. The discomfort may not lessen with age and, in fact, may increase. While congestive dysmenorrhea is often associated with symptoms of the *premenstrual syndrome* (PMS) and the terms are often used interchangeably, PMS should be distinguished from dysmenorrhea. PMS should not be considered an exaggerated form of dysmenorrhea.

The term spasmodic dysmenorrhea refers to more acute lower abdominal spasms, backache, and inner thigh pain, often accompanied by nausea, vomiting, and syncope. This type of pain begins primarily at the onset of menstruation and lasts several days; the most intense discomfort is felt on the first day. Episodes of spasmodic dysmenorrhea may lessen with age and are most commonly experienced in women between ages 14 and 25.

Historically, many theories have been advanced to explain the etiology of primary dysmenorrhea. Until recently, medical texts asserted that the pain was largely psychogenic. Other widely accepted, but now mostly outdated, theories cited cervical stenosis, endocrine imbalances, an "infantile" uterus, and poor posture as the cause of dysmenorrhea.

Traditional treatments, based on supposed cause and symptoms, varied widely: hysterectomies, presacral neurectomies and sympathectomies, cervical dilations, and more recently, oral contraceptives. Pregnancy was long recommended as the best "cure" for alleviating monthly dysmenorrhea. Dysmenorrhea often lessened or was completely alleviated following a pregnancy; however, this was not the case for many women. Dysmenorrhea is now primarily accepted as a biophysical response to ovulation and the growth and shedding of the endometrium under hormonal stimulus. This explanation accounts for absence of pain in anovulatory women and the relief often seen with oral contraceptives, pregnancy, and menopause.

Present documented evidence strongly suggests that primary dysmenorrhea is the result of biochemical imbalances caused by hormone-like substances called *prostaglandins.* Prostaglandins are synthesized from essential, unsaturated fatty acids and regulate smooth muscle control. They were first isolated from human semen in the 1930s. It was not until the late 1950s and early 1960s with the research of Pickles (1957) and others that the link between these lipids, extracted from menstrual blood, and dysmenorrhea was reported. Little further research focused on this link until the 1970s. To date, nine groups of prostaglandins have been identified; they are found in nearly every body cell. The two that are primarily implicated in dysmenorrhea are PGE_2, a myometrial relaxant, and PGF_2, a myometrial stimulant. Both are produced in the uterine endometrium. These prostaglandins are synthesized at their highest levels prior to and at the onset of menstruation. It is now thought that when there are excessive levels of PGF_2 or when PGF_2 levels exceed those of PGE_2 painful uterine contractions occur. Thus, it is not only the amount of prostaglandins synthesized but also the ratio between the two that is critical. Prostaglandin levels and balance can make the difference between mild cramping and the uterine ischemic reaction often likened to angina of the heart muscle. Systemic effects of dysmenorrhea are thought to result from excess prostaglandins escaping into the circulatory system where they stimulate the smooth muscle of the gut and blood vessels.

Based on this latest theory linking primary dysmenorrhea to prostaglandins, one of the most promising treatments is the use of antiprostaglandin drugs or prostaglandin inhibitors.

Premenstrual Syndrome

The precise etiology of a diversely complex number of symptoms known as premenstrual syndrome is still unknown. First reported in the literature 50 years ago, PMS has received little attention in the medical world until recently. Although very real to sufferers, it remains poorly understood, vaguely defined, wrongly diagnosed, and all too often inadequately treated.

The cause of PMS may be closely related to fluctuating hormone levels (estrogens, progesterones, and prolactin) during the menstrual cycle and the ratio of these hormones to prostaglandins and/or neurohormones. It has been estimated that 80% of women experience some effects of the premenstrual syndrome. Onset varies widely, frequently beginning three to six days prior to the menses. Many women experience some symptoms as early as 14 days before menstruation.

Common effects of this syndrome are tension, lethargy, irritability, depression, headache, nervousness, anxiety, hostility, fatigue, mood swings, crying, and dizziness. These effects can occur singly or in clusters, and can range from mildly annoying to severe. Often these effects are combined with one or more biophysical changes: diarrhea, edema, constipation, abdominal bloating and cramping, weight gain, breast tenderness, joint pain, facial acne, hypoglycemia, nausea and vomiting, to name a few.

Most women have some awareness when menstruation is imminent. Some experience little or no discomfort, many feel "witchy" or "not up to par," while others have serious bouts of physical illness and/or depression at this time.

Treatment has traditionally been directed at the symptoms since a specific cause has yet to be determined. No one remedy has proven to be universally effective. New research findings, especially in the areas of nutrition, may offer some promising relief from the effects of premenstrual syndrome.

Past and current therapies include progesterone, aldosterone antagonists, lithium, tranquilizers, oral contraceptives, vitamin B_6, prolactin inhibitors, diuretics, and antiprostaglandins. Some of these drugs have proven to be controversial or ineffective, while progesterone and others are under current research study. Natural progesterone has recently been identified by some women as an effective treatment. However, progesterone, a potent mineralocorticoid and known CNS depressant, can cause lethargy, depression, increased appetite, weight gain, fluid retention, and edema. Established in England as an accepted treatment for PMS, natural progesterone has not yet been approved by the FDA for large-scale manufacture in this country. Natural progesterone is ineffective in an oral tablet; currently, vaginal and rectal suppositories are the only effective routes of administration. In general, the effects of PMS therapies studied range from minimal to complete relief, *for some symptoms, for some women.* There is as yet, no "magic formula."

Suggested Nursing Interventions for Problem-Solving with Clients

1. Women with menstrual difficulties should avoid powerful diuretics, which often have potent side effects. If a diuretic is taken, it should be ingested with a glass of orange juice. Figs, bananas, tomatoes, leafy vegetables, melons, and carrots should be included in the diet to provide potassium, often lost when taking diuretics. Diuretics require close medical supervision.

2. Clients with PMS should reduce sodium intake seven to ten days prior to menstruation; this may decrease fluid retention symptoms. Avoid the following: adding salt to food; commercial salad dressings; canned/dried soups and boullion; ham, bacon, sausage, lox; soy and Worcestershire sauce; monosodium glutamate; potato and corn chips, pretzels, and nuts; sandwich meats and spreads; sauerkraut, pickles, olives; restaurant food (especially Mexican and Chinese); meat tenderizers, catsup, and chili sauce; most cheeses (except cottage); salted butter and margarine; frozen and instant dinners; canned foods (except fruits and juices); soft drinks and cocoa; canned tuna, salmon, and other seafood; peanut butter; salted meats, chipped or corned beef; regular bread, rolls, and buttermilk; and baking powder and soda.

3. Clients should avoid methylated xanthine-containing drinks. Xanthines are caffeine or caffeine-like chemicals found in tea, coffee, cola, or cocoa. These contribute to increased tension effects and may also increase heart rate and cause an irregular heart beat as well as systemic effects. The following list gives common sources and amounts of caffeine (Luke 1982):
   - instant decaffeinated coffee — 3 mg/5 oz serving
   - brewed coffee — 85 mg/5 oz serving
   - brewed black tea — 50 mg/5 oz serving
   - Coca-Cola — 65 mg/12 oz serving
   - TAB — 49 mg/12 oz serving
   - cocoa — 50 mg/6 oz serving

   One source suggests that 250 mg/day is excessive intake.

4. Symptoms of altered CHO metabolism and hypoglycemia such as fatigue and weakness may be relieved by small infrequent meals (+/− six times a day), and/or snacks of low-carbohydrate, high-protein, and low-fat foods. Cravings for chocolate and other sweets are common, but temptation should be avoided because these concentrated carbohydrates will cause the blood sugar level to skyrocket. This effect is short-lived, however, and the blood sugar level quickly plummets.

5. Vitamin B_6 supplements may help to counter fatigue and tension symptoms by increasing protein utilization and decreasing the effects of increased estrogen occurring at this time. Providers often suggest 100–200 mg/day on premenstrual days.

6. When antiprostaglandin therapy is prescribed, pills should be ingested with milk or food to avoid common GI side effects. Frequently prescribed antiprostaglandins are Motrin® (ibuprofen), Ponstel® (mefenamic acid), Anaprox® (naproxen sodium), Naprosyn (naproxen), Zomax® (zomepirac sodium — now unavailable), and Indocin® (indomethacin — more side effects). Antiprostaglandins are closely related to aspirin, which is also a prostaglandin inhibitor.

7. Avoid antiprostaglandin therapy if
   a. the individual suffers oxygen-induced asthma, hives, or nasal polyps.
   b. chronic GI tract inflammation exists.
   c. the individual is under age 12 to 14. Check specific drug literature.
   d. sensitivity occurs. Observe for rash and diarrhea.

8. Aspirin alone can provide relief for mild dysmenorrhea because it is a mild anti-prostaglandin. Aspirin is a potent drug and chronic, long-term use should be avoided. For *any* drug taken, suggested dosages and method of ingestion should be adhered to and drug combination avoided unless it has been discussed with health-care providers and the potential side effects are known.

9. Some women who take oral contraceptives may be deficient in vitamin B_6, a lack which can increase symptoms of depression. Supplementary B_6 (20 to 50 mg/day) may alleviate depression. Some may need higher dosages (see No. 5).

10. The use of an IUD for contraception may increase dysmenorrhea and should be avoided in these circumstances.

11. Some women experience increased sexual tension and libido prior to and during menstruation. Orgasm may relieve backache, feeling of pelvic fullness, and cramping.

12. Breast tenderness, which can fluctuate from month to month, may be helped by wearing a supportive bra continually when symptoms persist.

13. Stretch-relaxation exercises and other, more vigorous exercises, may decrease discomfort for the individual. She should avoid standing or walking on hard pavement.

14. Direct massage on the small of the back may relieve cramping and pressure sensa-tions. Effleurage (massaging the lower abdomen with the finger tips in a circular pattern), hot pads, tub baths, La Maze breathing techniques, yoga, and meditation may also be of help to some.

15. Suggested reading for clients:
    No More Menstrual Cramps and Other Good News by Budoff.

16. The nursing intervention process for dysmenorrhea and PMS is outlined in Table 6-4.

For more information about PMS write:

National Center for Premenstrual Syndrome and Menstrual Distress, Inc.
515 Third Avenue, Suite #1
New York, NY 10016
Telephone: 1-800-227-3800, extension 101

Reproductive Choice

While creating a human life can be magnificent, at the wrong time it can also be conceived as a depressing, unwanted, or catastrophic event. Decisions about whether, when, and under what circumstances to bear children touch most people at some time in their lives. Pregnancy, already considered a developmental hazardous event, can be compromised by the situation (age, genetic, health, or economic factors), and thus more readily result in crisis.

During the childbearing years there are multiple decisions for individuals to make. Today there are many choices involved in avoiding, spacing, and terminating pregnancies. This has not always been so. Reproductive freedom has historically been denied to most women. Numerous cultural, scientific, religious, biological, political, and socioeconomic factors have either denied or limited healthy, voluntary parenthood. While many

TABLE 6-4 *Nursing Intervention Process in Pre-Crisis: Clients Experiencing Dysmenorrhea and Premenstrual Syndrome*

1. *Assessment*
   a. Complete health history with emphasis on menstrual, reproductive patterns
   b. Physical exam including pelvic
   c. Appropriate screening measures and laboratory tests (if indicated)
   d. Client's perceptions:
      • Affective response to problem; pain, limitation of activity/functioning, etc.
      • Knowledge about menstruation and hormonal and menstrual cycle
      • Resources being utilized and needed
      • Anticipated effect of the problem
   e. Collaborative health teaching needs: as perceived by client and identified by nurse or others
2. *Planning* (a collaborative process to augment client problem-solving)
   a. Explanation of menstrual cycle and hormonal influence, medication, diet prevention techniques
   b. Resources: referral to colleagues and adjunct services (if needed) and community resources
3. *Intervention* (based on planning)
   a. Health teaching and counseling
   b. Liaison and support to client's significant other(s)
4. *Evaluation* of intervention and revisions needed for care, teaching, and follow-up.

Adapted from Hunt. 1982. In *Crisis Theory—A Framework for Nursing Practice,* ed. M. S. Infante.

barriers to self-determined parenting have been dismantled, other obstacles still exist. For example:

1. All currently available contraceptive methods have some degree of failure rate and many have dangerous side effects. Some have age, accessibility, and cost limitations.

2. Over 1 million adolescents become pregnant each year. There are limited alternatives for their childbearing and few support systems for child-rearing.

3. One-half of the adolescents (aged 15 to 19) are sexually active; 27% have never used birth control (*Teenage Pregnancy* 1981, 11).

4. Sexual health education (home, school, church) is often prohibited, inaccessible (through lack of consent or availability), or stigmatized.

5. Much of today's media bombards us with sexual emphasis, innuendo, and the "hard sell" about every product imaginable related to intimacy and body functioning. However, the National Association of Broadcasters' code does not permit information about contraception or birth control products to be aired.

For the client, the expansion of reproductive rights, methods, and information necessitates informed decision-making. For the nurse, this situation emphasizes the need for *practical* anticipatory guidance and health teaching and *collaborative* problem-solving.

The Nurse and the Client Who Chooses Contraception

One of the most significant yet controversial resources utilized to promote reproductive freedom is contraception. Most reliable methods used today had yet to be developed a mere 30 years ago. Withdrawal, abstinence, primitive barriers, and chemical methods have been used for centuries. Historically, however, family planning has been largely hit or miss, often religiously condemned, and services were prohibited by law. The "ideal" contraceptive does not exist, but if it did, it would meet the following criteria:

- low cost
- easy to use
- no side effects
- no religious barriers
- 100% effective
- widely available
- coitus-independent
- shared responsibility
- reversible when pregnancy desired
- comfortable

Although abstinence is obviously 100% effective, many people find this realistically unacceptable as a long-term solution. The nurse needs to acknowledge abstinence as a choice, however, and support those who see it as a viable option.

Perceptions of the Problem

Even if the ideal contraceptive existed and were widely available, it probably would not be utilized by all those hoping to avoid pregnancy. The use, nonuse, and misuse of birth control involves some risk-taking for everyone. The kind and amount of risk-taking is unique to each individual and is influenced by a number of factors: cultural and religious views and values, cost, availability of health-care and family planning services, sexual self-esteem, knowledge about sex and reproduction, and perceptions of partner or familial relationships.

While many realistically perceive and weigh the potential of pregnancy against contraceptive risks, others do not. Out of fear, ignorance, or ambivalence, high risk takers use ineffective methods, downplay, or deny the risk of unprotected intercourse, or avoid the issue altogether. One researcher links sex guilt with use of contraception; high sex guilt women are less likely to use contraception (Mosher 1973). Although many adolescents are high risk takers, this characteristic should neither be assumed nor negated by the health-care provider.

Problem-Solving

Augmenting client problem-solving and mobilizing contraception as a resource can more readily be accomplished

1. when the nurse recognizes and taps opportunities for teaching and counseling in a variety of settings with a variety of ages. A good deal of recent effort has been directed at adolescents in school and clinic settings. Little effort, for example, has been focused on the woman over the age of 40. She often faces 10 to 15 more years of potential fertility and contraceptive use, is highly vulnerable to the side effects of birth control pills, and may not be amenable to sterilization. Industrial and corporate settings have been largely overlooked for their potential in offering outreach health teaching and counseling to the individual of middle age.

2. if contraceptive services are more accessible and attractive, less authoritarian, and more flexible and comprehensive.

3. when professional providers are more "client"- rather than "problem"-oriented, encouraging a "couple" approach to contraceptive service and education.

All too often contraception is described or prescribed solely on the basis of what teacher/provider feels is appropriate. This tendency often results in inconsistent use or even non-use, especially if the client/consumer finds the method distasteful, difficult to use, prohibitively expensive, or fails to understand how it works to prevent pregnancy. It may also result in consumers who are unaware of the variety of methods available, their advantages and risks, the effectiveness of the methods, the side effects, and the costs involved. The best method for a woman/couple is not necessarily the one rated most statistically effective or selected by the provider. On the basis of collaborative problem-solving, the well-informed consumer makes a choice tailored to fit his/her unique needs, health status, and lifestyle.

Informed consent is of primary importance, not only to encourage a high level of sexual self-care awareness and responsibility but also for legal considerations. Many providers are now requiring written consent forms to be signed for contraception care. Hatcher (1980, 204) suggests all documenta-

---

TABLE 6-5 *Nursing Intervention Process in Pre-Crisis: The Client Who Chooses Contraception*

---

1. *Assessment*
   a. Complete health history with emphasis on menstrual, contraceptive, reproductive, and sexual activity patterns
   b. Physical exam including pelvic
   c. Appropriate laboratory testing (if indicated)
   d. Client's perceptions:
      • Affective response to need for/problem with contraception (use/misuse/nonuse)
      • Influencing factors (attributes about birth control, sexual activity, cultural and religious beliefs, relationships, sexual self-esteem)
      • Knowledge about birth control methods, reproduction, sexuality
      • Resources being utilized and needed
      • Anticipated effect of contraceptive use/misuse/nonuse on relationship with partner and significant others (peers, family)
   e. Collaborative health teaching needs: as perceived by client and identified by nurse or others

2. *Planning* (a collaborative process to augment client problem-solving)
   a. Explanation of various options and resources available
   b. Explanation of client's chosen method, examinations, and referral to colleagues and adjunct services (if needed)
   c. Obtain written informed consent using BRAIDED guidelines
   d. Referrals for surgical intervention (sterilization)

3. *Intervention* (based on planning)
   a. Prescribe chosen method (birth control pill) with physician collaboration
   b. Insert/fit method (diaphragm, IUD) or refer to qualified professional colleague for procedure
   c. Validate, review client records ("natural" family planning)
   d. Describe/demonstrate (using model) use of method (spermicides, condoms)
   e. Health teaching and counseling specific to method; arrange for follow-up
   f. Referrals

4. *Evaluation* of intervention and revisions needed for care, teaching, and follow-up.

Adapted from Hunt. 1982. In *Crisis Theory—A Framework for Nursing Practice,* ed. M. S. Infante.

tion be based on seven basic elements. Think BRAIDED:

Benefits of the method

Risks of the method (major/common, minor)

Alternatives (including abstinence or no method)

Inquiries about method are patient's right and responsibility

Decision to withdraw from using method OK

Explanation of method (what to expect and do)

Documentation of all of the above

Suggestions for nursing intervention with the client who chooses contraception are outlined in Table 6-5. Contraceptive methods — their operation, use, advantages, side effects or constraints, effectiveness, method and cost of acquisition, and health teachings offered by the nurse — are listed in Appendix A.

Ineffective Methods

Withdrawal (coitus interruptus) and douching are not described in Appendix A. Of all methods, withdrawal is the least effective, although it is probably one of the oldest known forms of birth control. Pregnancy may be caused by sperm present in preejaculate fluid drops. Vaginal penetration need not occur for some of this fluid to make its way into the vagina and uterus. It must also be said that it is extremely difficult for the man to time withdrawal before ejaculation (this is especially true of adolescents). Not only is this method unreliable, it can also be extremely frustrating to both partners (especially men in their teens) and can significantly decrease sexual pleasure. Withdrawal effectiveness: Theoretical, 9/100; actual use, 20–25/100 (Hatcher et al. 1980, 4).

Douching is really a "nonmethod." Even if douching could occur immediately, *some* sperm would have time to migrate through the cervical os into the uterus. Consider the fact that the average ejaculate (3 to 5 ml) contains 40 million to 200 million sperm (Stewart et al. 1979, 45). The force of the douching fluid (even gentle pressure) may force sperm into the uterus. Douching effectiveness: Theoretical, not known; actual use, 40/100 (Hatcher et al. 1980, 4). It is interesting to note the effectiveness of "chance" for a sexually active individual: Theoretical, 90/100; actual "use," 90/100 (Hatcher et al. 1980, 4).

Lactation is discussed under Postpartum Sexuality. Its effectiveness rate as a contraceptive method for 12 months: Theoretical, 15/100; actual use, 40/100 (Hatcher et al. 1980, 4).

The Nurse and the Client Who Chooses Abortion

As discussed in Chapter 4, induced abortion has been one of the most controversial healthcare issues of all time: socially, politically, ethically, and emotionally. A severe blow was leveled at those who seek to limit or deny reproductive freedom with the U.S. Supreme Court's January 22, 1973 landmark decision of two cases (*Roe v. Wade* and *Doe v. Bolton*). The political and legal aspects of this issue have intensified to the point that some describe abortion as the political battle of the 1980s ("Battle Over Abortion" 1981, 20). Although abortions, to date, remain legal under the guidelines of the 1973 Supreme Court decision, federal and state funding for pregnancy termination has become drastically restricted. Congress has eliminated abortion funding for armed forces personnel and their dependents, Peace Corps volunteers (National Women's Health Network 1980), and other federal government employees. Some states have eliminated coverage for abortions under health insurance plans. In 1982, various pieces of proposed "pro-life" legislation were introduced in the U.S. Congress. As noted in Chapter 4, these are attempts to make abortion once again illegal in this country.

Since 1973, the estimated number of elective abortions performed in the U.S. has risen to 1.5 million annually ("Battle over Abortion" 1981), a third of all pregnancies. According to the Centers for Disease Control Statistics (1977), at least 65% of women who electively terminate their pregnancies are less than 25 years old, white, and unmarried. No matter what the reasons for the choice, termination of pregnancy through an electively induced abortion is an outcome rarely arrived at without a great deal of emotional conflict.

Perceptions of the Problem

Undeniably, the legal and political environment have great implications for clouding or clarifying individual perceptions and influencing problem-solving. However, there are multiple factors that not only affect perceptions but often confuse and frustrate all those involved. Whether abortion is seen as an acceptable choice or an unacceptable solution or even considered at all will be influenced by a complex mix of variables: personal self-esteem, religious beliefs, financial status, interpersonal relationships, lifestyle, educational and career aspirations, family values, emotional and physical health status (fetal, parental and/or significant other[s]), and cultural expectations.

Parents, partners, and/or other significant individuals in a woman's life (her support system) can temper perceptions. They can be supportive and stabilizing forces. However, their influence can be coercive, destructive, or punitive. Many of these supportive others

may, in fact, be struggling with their own guilt, anger, or regret over the pregnancy.

The health-care delivery system itself can be a factor influencing perceptions and problem-solving. If a client's previous experiences with delivery of care have been positive, help may be more readily sought. If past experiences have been perceived as judgmental, ineffective, or unsuitable to needs, there may be reluctance to seek assistance. If services are not readily available—inaccessible or costly—client access will be compromised.

Problem-Solving

Individual problem-solving really begins once the possibility or probability of pregnancy is acknowledged. Pregnancy testing is realistically the next effective step. At this point, the client will most likely enter the health care delivery system. Unfortunately, denial, fear, ambivalence, lack of sexual and/or reproductive knowledge or awareness of appropriate community health care resources often delay the decision-making process. This can alter potential options and possible solutions. Delaying decision-making is especially characteristic of young, single, primigravidas (Lion 1982, 310).

Following positive confirmation of a perceived problem pregnancy, potential options, available resources, and the consequences, risks, and ramifications of possible solutions need to be explored with the woman and her supportive other(s). In order to reach an acceptable, realistic, and informed decision, alternatives should be considered:

1. Continuation of pregnancy and following birth
   a. Assumption of parenthood—shared or single
   b. Permanent relinquishing of the infant through adoption

TABLE 6-6 *Nursing Intervention Process in Pre-Crisis: Clients Experiencing an Induced Abortion*

1. *Assessment*
   a. Pregnancy testing
      Serum HCG radioimmunoassay: done as early as eight days following ovulation (or before first missed menstrual period)
      Urine HCG testing: Peak HCG levels occur 50–70 days after last menstrual period (LMP); sometimes accurate results 38–42 days post-LMP
   b. If positive pregnancy test and abortion chosen:
      1) Complete health history with emphasis on menstrual, contraceptive, reproductive patterns and pelvic pathology or surgery
      2) Physical exam including pelvic; possible chest x-ray
      3) Laboratory tests:
         Pap smears   Complete blood count (at least hemoglobin and hematocrit)
         GC culture   Blood type and Rh determination
         VDRL   Rho Gam eligibility screen (if Rh negative)
         Urinalysis
   c. Client's perceptions:
      • Affective response to problematic pregnancy (unplanned, genetic problems, threat to maternal health)
      • Influencing factors (personal attitudes about abortion and pregnancy, religious expectations, support of significant other[s], sexual self-esteem)
      • Knowledge about abortion methods, reproduction, contraception
      • Resources being utilized and needed
      • Anticipated effect of abortion on lifestyle, sexuality, family and partner relationships, further contraception
   d. Collaborative health teaching needs: as perceived by client and identified by nurse or others
2. *Planning* (a collaborative process to augment client problem-solving)
   a. Explanation of options available and resources available (clinic, hospital, private office) within limitations of gestational age
   b. Explanation of chosen method, tests, abortion procedure, examinations and referrals
   c. Obtaining written informed consent (in conjunction with agency guidelines)
   d. Discussion of plans for future contraception
3. *Intervention* (based on planning)
   Remain with client during procedure, providing physical and emotional support and concurrent explanations. Liaison and support to client's significant other(s). Provide pre- and post-abortion counseling, teaching and promote client/supportive other discussion. Make referrals and schedule follow-up appointment.
4. *Evaluation* of intervention and revisions needed for care, teaching, and follow-up.

Adapted from Hunt. 1982. In *Crisis Theory—A Framework for Nursing Practice,* ed. M. S. Infante.

c. Temporary relinquishing of the infant through formal or informal foster care

2. Termination of the pregnancy

Tapping the growth potential of the crisis model conceptual framework, the nurse initi-ates "prevention promotion" wherever and however opportunities present. In many health care settings the nurse is often the one to interpret pregnancy tests and relay the diagnosis. The client whose pregnancy test is negative may be overjoyed and is often dismissed with little or no additional comments other than test results. When this happens, the nurse fails to seize an excellent opportunity to focus on the original need for the pregnancy test. Contraceptive use, nonuse, or misuse, the client's plans for the future, sexual health and reproduction knowledge, as well as sexual self-concept perception are issues that may need to be explored by the nurse.

Although nurses can be primary resources when clients problem-solve about pregnancy and the abortion option, it is not always the case. Counseling about and direct intervention in induced abortion is described by some nurses as one of the most controversial and difficult areas of professional practice. The nurse may experience difficulty in communicating positive or nonjudgmental attitudes when there are conflicts between the nurse's and client's value systems or if the nurse has unresolved attitudes about sexuality or abortion. Nurses who have reservations or negative attitudes about abortion should not be expected to work with these clients. Many nurses who do choose this demanding role often describe pregnancy termination care as both challenging and emotionally draining.

The process of nursing intervention with clients choosing abortion is outlined in Table 6-6. Methods of abortion and suggested health teachings are described in Appendix B.

The Nurse and the Client Experiencing a Sexually Transmissible Disease

One of the most significant factors in the maintenance of sexual health and integrity is the extent to which one takes responsibility for his/her sexual behavior. Unfortunately, many people either ignore or are unaware of the potential implications sexual activity has on one's own health or that of a partner. More than 10 million Americans contract sexually transmissible diseases (STD) each year at a medical cost of about $1 billion. Of these, 85% are between the ages of 15 and 30 (Nass et al. 1981). An estimated 100,000 females are left sterile each year because of these infections.

Historically, the term *venereal disease* (VD) was used to describe the "classic" infections: gonorrhea, syphilis, chancroid, lymphogranuloma venereum, and granuloma inguinale. Biblical references dating to 1500 B.C. are found about gonorrhea. Literature dating to approximately A.D. 1495 refers to syphilis as the evil pox that was considered an acute systemic disease in earlier times.

STD is a broader, more inclusive term than VD and is used today in reference to infections/diseases that can be passed through sexual or intimate contact. These include vaginitis, urethritis, and parasite infection. Although not every occurrence of these conditions results from intimate or sexual transmission, all have that potential.

Certain STD are not often seen in the United States. For example, granuloma inguinale is considered endemic in the tropics but uncommon in this country. It is thought to be caused by a *Klebsiella* group bacteria formerly known as Donovan bodies. Chancroid, too, is common in tropical regions but not in the United States. It is caused by a bacteria; males are symptomatic while women are most often asymptomatic carriers. Lymphogranuloma venereum is seen worldwide, especially in developing countries, but is uncommon in this country. This disease, also bacteria caused, is one primarily affecting the lymphatic system. It is more common in men, but women tend to be carriers.

In general, sexually transmissible diseases

- can be transmitted through anilingus, during oral and/or genital intercourse, through intimate body contact, on occasion by self-inoculation, through contact with personal items such as towels, bedding or clothing, and congenitally.

- most commonly involve only the genitals and reproductive tract but may involve other body parts or produce systemic effects.
- can affect all ages, socioeconomic and cultural groups, males and females.
- can be annoying, painful, or incapacitating in acute phases but with no long-term effects.
- can be life-threatening or chronic in nature.
- can cause infertility, interfere with vaginal births, and/or threaten the well-being of the fetus and neonate.

Perceptions of the Problem

Substantial numbers of people are ambivalent about or ignorant of the signs, symptoms, and potentially serious and permanent consequences of STD. Many individuals have a tendency to deny or neglect any threat to sexual health and integrity. Others, suspecting an STD infection, often self-diagnose and treat in order to avoid embarrassment or possible negative judgments by partners, family, or health-care providers. Consumers may well be justified in these perceptions, especially in regard to professionals. Much of the ambivalence and the negative consumer attitude may stem from the rather traditional "fear approach" used by health-care providers in finding, treating, and educating about STD.

Prepared with an open nonjudgmental attitude, accurate information, and practical suggestions regarding prevention, treatment, and access to resources, the nurse not only facilitates effective collaborative client problem-solving but can stimulate the awareness of colleagues and the public at large.

Suggested Health Teaching for Primary Prevention

1. Males and females tend to get infections when their general health is compromised. Illness, fatigue, stress, and poor nutritional habits are among the many factors that will increase risk and vulnerability.

2. Use of spermicidal foam, cream, jellies with condoms, or condoms alone will decrease chances of infection. However, their effects extend only to those areas covered and do not guarantee protection.

3. Genital hygiene is a major factor in prevention.
   a. Wipe front to back after urinating or defecating.
   b. Avoid feminine hygiene sprays, strong soaps, scented and colored toilet paper, bubble baths, oils, lotions, and excessive powder use in the genital area. Powders can cake in moist genital areas and increase irritation. In addition to irritating the skin and mucous membranes (causing itching, swelling, redness, and tenderness), these products may also cause allergies from the dyes or perfumes they contain.
   c. Indiscriminate douching can alter the vaginal pH and decrease the protective organisms that help to maintain the vaginal environment. Douching can also be harmful if the pressure of the douche solution pushes an existing infection into the uterus. Douching should only be done for therapeutic use or, infrequently, to restore vaginal pH (adult pH is approximately 3.5 to 5.0). A more alkaline vaginal pH normally exists prepuberty and postmenopause, following intercourse (for about two hours) and with ovarian activity during the menstrual cycle.

Douche equipment should not be shared and should be thoroughly cleaned after each use; otherwise, it can be a medium for bacterial growth. Douching should be avoided during pregnancy, menstruation, and the early postpartum period. Due to increased vascularity at these times, air embolism or infection can potentially result. Douching, as well as use of vaginal spermicides, should be avoided for 48 to 72 hours prior to a pelvic exam when cultures are to be taken. Recent douching will alter vaginal and endocervical secretions and may distort test results.

d. Wear loose-fitting cotton underwear and avoid synthetic fabrics, pantyhose, tight jeans or slacks, jockey-type shorts, athletic supporters for long periods, and wearing underwear to bed. Cotton allows the genital area to "breathe" while synthetics tend to trap moisture and create a warm, dark, moist medium perfect for growth of organisms. A common fungus infection called "jock itch" occurs when there is poor genital hygiene or underwear is infrequently changed or washed. The synthetic-backed cotton crotch in panties made of man-made fibers does not allow for this "breathing" effect, although it may be advertised this way.

e. Washing hands before and after sex, washing genitals after sex, and emptying the bladder both before and after sex may give some protection.

f. Shower or bathe daily. Uncircumcised males should retract the foreskin and wash the glans to avoid the accumulation of smegma and urine, which provides another excellent medium for bacterial growth. This practice should be taught to young boys, emphasizing that the foreskin should be replaced after washing to prevent paraphimosis. Paraphimosis is edema of the glans, which can occur with decreased circulation when the retracted foreskin is not slipped back. Smegma can accumulate in women's labial folds and under the clitoral hood. Urine, vaginal mucus, menstrual discharge, and perspiration can also collect in the perineal area, producing bacterial growth and odor.

g. Avoid direct contact with public toilet seats or cover them with toilet paper before use. Some STD can be transmitted in this way: trichomonas, pubic lice, others.

h. Avoid the super-absorbent tampons. Alternate tampon use with pads during menstruation. Tampon use has been strongly linked to Toxic Shock Syndrome (see Chapter 7 for discussion). Tampons and pads should be changed at least four times a day.

i. Recognize characteristic patterns of vaginal discharge, which exist from puberty to menopause. They are often misinterpreted or misunderstood. They can serve as a baseline for self-assessment.
Following menstruation to before ovulation:
• white, cloudy, or slightly yellowish in color
• scanty in amount but increasing toward ovulation
• thick and sticky
Ovulation:
• thinner and slippery (like raw egg white)
• clear
Four days after ovulation to before menation:
• cloudy and milky in color
• thick and sticky
• becomes scanty again

j. Precoital inspection (see No. 2 under

Suggested Health Teaching to Reduce Hazardous Events, Prevent Recurrence, and Avoid Crisis, this chapter).

4. Some women find that eating pasteurized pure yogurt, inserting yogurt into the vagina, and douching with yogurt (2 tablespoons to 1 quart warm water) or buttermilk helps to maintain the vaginal environment with lactobacillus. Other women have found that eating citrus fruits, drinking cranberry juice, and taking vitamin C tablets can be helpful to increase the acidity of the vagina and urinary tract.

5. Inadequate lubrication during intercourse may cause irritation to vulval, penile, and vaginal tissues. Irritated and inflamed tissues are less resistant to microorganisms. Postmenopausal, postpartum, and anatomically and sexually immature women may be especially vulnerable. Longer foreplay and use of exogenous lubrication can be helpful. Use water-soluble (K-Y) jelly, coconut oil, cocoa butter, safflower oil, or contraceptive foam, cream, or jelly; petroleum-based products should be avoided. As indicated in Chapter 5, these lubricating agents may be beneficial to menopausal women and used instead of an estrogen vaginal cream. Estrogen creams should be used sparingly, if at all, as they are systemically absorbed. Altering coital positions may also decrease irritation and discomfort.

6. If STD exposure or infection is suspected, it should be checked with an exam and appropriate screening. If there is a wait for an appointment, use warm sitz baths to relieve irritating symptoms. Tampons (unscented and without deodorant) can be temporarily used to decrease discharge, odor, and itching while waiting. Tampons should be changed frequently.

7. Some women practice routine self-examination of the vulva and inspect the vagina with a speculum in order to familiarize themselves with the "normal" appearance of the genitals and cervix. Based on the same principles of breast self-exam, monitoring the normal characteristics will more readily enable detection of any abnormal change.

8. A pelvic exam, Pap smear, VDRL, and GC cultures should be part of routine physical examinations. Pap smears can detect early cervical epithelium cell changes which may be potentially cancerous. The smear can also provide information about cervical and vaginal infections. Further testing and examinations are needed if the Pap smear indicates atypical or abnormal results. These exams should be specifically requested; the client should not assume that they will be done. Yearly vaginal and periodic screening exams for sexually active young women, as well as all women over 18, are smart sexual health care. Men should have a VDRL, GC smears, and testicular and prostate exams with routine physicals.

9. If an increase in discharge or foul odor is noticed, the vagina should be checked. Diaphragms, cervical caps, condoms, tampons, or menstrual sponges may have inadvertently been left in the vagina. Young children often put foreign objects into the vagina.

10. It is essential that professional health teaching and counseling include appropriately integrated information about sexual anatomy and physiology.

11. Adolescents do not need parental permission for STD screening or treatment in any state. This fact needs to be stressed. Teenagers most often avoid the health-care system for fear parents will be told. Providers need to assess the client's knowledge and build on realistic understanding, but not assume client awareness or accuracy.

12. Questions and concerns about any sexually transmissible disease can be anonymously discussed by calling the toll-free V.D. Hotline — 7 days a week (1-800-227-8922).

13. Suggested readings for clients (see References and Bibliography for more sources):
    No More Menstrual Cramps and Other Good News by Budoff
    Our Bodies, Ourselves by Boston Women Health Book Collective
    Changing Bodies, Changing Lives by Bell et al. (especially for teenagers)
    Men's Bodies, Men's Selves by Julty

Suggested Health Teaching to Reduce the Hazardous Event, Prevent Recurrence, and Avoid Crisis

1. Avoid intercourse if symptomatic. Additional irritation to already inflamed tissues can spread organisms and slow down the healing process. Avoid using leftover medication or another's prescription even when symptoms are similar to a previous infection or to someone else's infection. Without an exam and screening measures, self-treatment can be ineffective and co-existing infections or underlying pathology remain unidentified.

2. Assuming that partners are unaffected because no symptoms exist is dangerous. Avoid intercourse with anyone who has symptoms; precoital inspection is one way to determine this. This is especially important when there is a new partner or multiple partners. Communicating about a real or potential problem can be the basis of a trusting relationship.

3. Follow prescribed treatments and medication directions carefully. Clients should
    a. know what the medication is, what effect it will have on the infection and general health, what its potential side effects are, and how to take medication. Drug allergies should be identified.
    b. take all the medication prescribed, at the times directed.
    c. lie down for at least 15 minutes to ensure drug absorption when using a vaginal cream or suppository. Avoid use of tampons to prevent leakage or staining, as tampons will decrease the localized effect by absorbing the medication. Mini-pads can be used.
    d. when using a diaphragm during treatment, soak it for 30 minutes with Betadyne® scrub (iodine) or 70% rubbing alcohol after two days of treatment and again when medication regimen is completed.
    e. have follow-up exams, cultures, smears, or tests as specified by the caregiver. This measure is extremely important. Disappearance of symptoms is not an indication that the infection has been eliminated, but clients often make this interpretation and fail to complete treatment or keep return appointments.
    f. be aware that laboratory tests may give inaccurate reports on the presence or absence of infection/disease: false-positive or false-negative readings. If symptoms persist or if there is doubt about test accuracy, more specific screening measures may be needed.
    g. have infections professionally diagnosed with reliable screening measures rather than relying on the "eyeball" approach to diagnosis. Clients should be encouraged to question this approach as well as request specific explanations about examination, diagnoses, prescribed treatments. Clients need not accept hasty dismissals and can be encouraged to ask for printed adjunct information.

TABLE 6-7   *Nursing Intervention Process in Pre-Crisis: Clients Experiencing a Sexually Transmissible Disease*

1. *Assessment*
   a. Complete health history with emphasis on infection problems, contraceptive and sexual activity patterns, and partner preferences
   b. Physical exam including pelvic
   c. Appropriate screening measures and laboratory tests
   d. Client's perceptions:
      • Affective response to the problem (hazardous event — insult to the body)
      • Influencing factors (attitudes about sexual health care, type and frequency of sexual activity, support of significant other[s])
      • Knowledge about STD, genital hygiene, prevention measures
      • Resources being utilized and needed
      • Anticipated effect of the problem on self, significant other(s)
   e. Collaborative health teaching needs: as perceived by client and identified by nurse or others

2. *Planning* (a collaborative process to augment client problem-solving)
   a. Explanation of screening, tests, and exams
   b. Resources: medications, treatments, and referral to colleagues and adjunct services (if needed)

3. *Intervention* (based on planning)
   a. Health teaching and counseling about infection process, prevention
   b. Exams, administration of medication, screening
   c. Liaison and support to client's significant other(s)
   d. Referrals

4. *Evaluation* of intervention and revisions needed for care, teaching, and follow-up

Adapted from Hunt. 1982. In *Crisis Theory — A Framework for Nursing Practice,* ed. M. S. Infante.

h. not use topical cortisone creams for more than three or four days as they are absorbed systemically and may potentiate adverse reactions.

i. do Kegel (pelvic floor) exercises because they increase circulation to the perineal area, promote tissue healing, and increase the tone of the pubococcygeus (PC) muscle.

Table 6-7 outlines the nursing intervention process for clients with STD; common STD and implications for practice are discussed in Appendix C. The format is designed for easy reference in clinical practice.

REFERENCES

Adams, M. M., G. P. Oakley, and J. S. Marks. 1982. Maternal age and births in the 1980s. *Journal of the American Medical Association* 247(4):493–494.

AIDS Update: Search for Agent X. 1983. *Science News* 123(16):245.

Allen, J., and G. Mellin. 1982. The new epidemic. *American Journal of Nursing* 82(110): 1718–1722.

Anderson, M. L. 1980. Talking about sex with less anxiety. *Journal of Psychiatric Nursing and Mental Health Services* 18:10–15.

The battle over abortion. 1981. *Time,* 117(4): 20–28.

Bell, R. 1980. *Changing bodies, changing lives.* New York: Random House.

Bettoli, E. J. 1982. Herpes: Facts and fallacies. *American Journal of Nursing* 82(6):924–929.

Bing, E., and L. Colman. 1977. Making love during pregnancy. New York: Bantam Books.

Bing, E., and L. Colman. 1980. *Having a baby after 30.* New York: Bantam Books.

Brewer, G. S., ed. 1978. *The pregnancy after 30 workbook.* Emmaus, Pa.: Rodale Press.

Budoff, P. W. 1981. *No more menstrual cramps and other good news.* New York: Penguin.

Campbell, C. E., and R. J. Herten. 1981. VD to STD: Redefining venereal disease. *American Journal of Nursing* 81(9):1629–1635.

Centers for Disease Control. 1983. Prevention of acquired immune deficiency syndrome (AIDS): Report of inter-agency recommendations. *Morbidity and Mortality Weekly Report* 32(8): 101–103.

Centers for Disease Control. 1977. Abortion surveillance, annual summary. Atlanta.

Dyer, R. A. 1979. Menopause—a closer look for nurses. In *Women in stress: A nursing perspective,* ed. D. K. Kjervik and I. M. Martinson. New York: Appleton-Century-Crofts.

Ellis, D. J. 1980. Sexual needs and concerns of expectant parents. *Journal of Obstetric, Gynecologic and Neonatal Nursing* 9(5):306–308.

Fogel, C. I., and N. J. Woods. 1981. *Health care of women.* St. Louis: C. V. Mosby.

Food and Drug Administration. 1983. Two dosage forms of acyclovir available. *FDA Drug Bulletin* 13(1):5.

Gordon, L. 1977. *Woman's body, woman's right.* New York: Penguin.

Guidelines. 1980. Storrs, Conn.: University of Connecticut Women's Health Clinic.

Hames, C. T. 1980. Sexual needs and interests of postpartum couples. *Journal of Obstetric, Gynecologic and Neonatal Nursing* 9(5):313–315.

Hatcher, R. A., G. K. Stewart, F. Stewart, F. Guest, D. Schwartz, and S. A. Jones. 1980. *Contraceptive technology 1980–1981.* 10th ed. New York: Irvington.

Hawkins, J. W., and L. P. Higgins, 1981. *Maternity and gynecological nursing—women's health care.* Philadelphia: Lippincott.

Infante, M. S., ed. 1982. *Crisis theory—a framework for nursing practice.* Reston, Va.: Reston Publishing.

Inglis, T. 1980. Postpartum sexuality. *Journal of Obstetric, Gynecologic and Neonatal Nursing* 9(5):298–300.

Kellum, M. D., and A. Loucke. 1982. Genital herpes infections: Diagnosis and management. *The Nurse Practitioner* 7(2):14–21.

Kitzinger, S. 1979. *Sex during pregnancy.* Seattle: The Penny Press.

Kyndely, K. 1978. The sexuality of women in pregnancy and the postpartum: A review. *Journal of Obstetric, Gynecologic and Neonatal Nursing* 7(1):28–32.

Lion, E., ed. 1982. *Human sexuality in nursing process.* New York: Wiley.

Luke, B. 1982. Does caffeine influence reproduction? *The American Journal of Maternal Child Nursing* 7(4):240–244.

Madaras, L., and J. Patterson. 1981. *Womancare.* New York: Avon.

Martin, L. L. 1978. *Health care of women.* Philadelphia: Lippincott.

Masters, W. H., and V. E. Johnson. 1966. *Human sexual response.* Boston: Little, Brown.

Mosher, D. L. 1973. Sex differences, sex experience; sex guilt and explicitly sexual films. *Journal of Social Issues* 29(3):95–112.

Naeye, R. L. 1979. Coitus and associated amniotic-fluid infections. *The New England Journal of Medicine* 301:1198–1200.

Nass, G., R. Libby, and M. P. Fisher. 1981. *Sexual choices.* Monterey, Calif. Wadsworth.

National Women's Health Network. 1980. *Abortion.* Washington, D.C.

Pearson, L. 1982. Climacteric. *American Journal of Nursing* 82(7):1098–1102.

Picconi, J. 1977. Human sexuality—a nursing challenge. *Nursing 77,* pp. 72D–72M.

Pickles, V. R. 1957. A plain-muscle stimulant in the menstrum. *Nature* 180(4596):1198–1199.

Reid, R., and S. S. C. Yen. 1981. Premenstrual syndrome. *American Journal of Obstetrics and Gynecology* 139(1):85–97.

Reitz, R. 1979. *Menopause: A positive approach.* New York: Penguin.

Ridenour, N. 1980. Chlamydia. *Nurse Practitioner* 5(5):45–48.

Riordan, J. M., and E. T. Rapp. 1980. Pleasure and

purpose: The sensuousness of breastfeeding. *Journal of Obstetric, Gynecologic and Neonatal Nursing* 9(2):109–112.

Ruebsaat, H. J., and R. Hull. 1975. *The male climacteric.* New York: Hawthorn Books.

Seaman, B., and G. Seaman. 1974. *Women and the crisis in sex hormones.* New York: Dutton.

Senator Bob Packwood's pro-choice report. 1982. Washington, D.C.

Sheehy, G. 1977. *Passages—predictable crises of adult life.* New York: Bantam Books.

Siemens, S., and R. C. Brandzel. 1982. *Sexuality— nursing assessment and intervention.* Philadelphia: Lippincott.

Sponge gets ok. 1983. *Science News* 123(17):261.

Stewart, F., F. Guest, G. Stewart, and R. Hatcher. 1979. *My body, my health.* New York: Wiley.

Swanson, J. 1980. The marital sexual relationship during pregnancy. *Journal of Obstetric, Gynecologic and Neonatal Nursing* 9(5):267–270.

Teenage pregnancy: The problem that hasn't gone away. 1981. New York: Guttmacher Institute.

Weaver, P. 1980. *Strategies for the second half of life.* New York: Signet Books.

Weinberg, J. S. 1982. *Sexuality: Human needs and nursing practice.* Philadelphia: Saunders.

Yarber, W. L. 1978. Preventing venereal disease infection: Approaches for the sexually active. *Health Values: Achieving High Level Wellness* 2(2).

BIBLIOGRAPHY

Canavan, P. A., and C. A. Lewis. 1981. The cervical cap: An alternative contraceptive. *Journal of Obstetric, Gynecologic and Neonatal Nursing* 10(4):271–273.

Cervical cap use studied in U.S. 1983. *NAACOG Newsletter* 10(6):1, 7.

Fairbanks, B., and B. Scharfman. 1980. The cervical cap: Past and current experience. *Women & Health* 5(3):61–80.

Fasano, N. F. 1979. The psychological aspects of contraception. *Issues in Health Care of Women* 1(5):17–27.

Frey, K. A. 1981. Middle-aged women's experiences and perceptions of menopause. *Women & Health* 6(1):25–36.

Glass, R. 1982. *Women's choice: A guide to contraception, fertility, abortion and menopause.* New York: Basic Books.

Gunn, T., and M. Stenzel-Poore. 1981. *The herpes handbook.* Portland, Ore.: VD Action Council.

Hawkins, J. W., and L. P. Higgins. 1982. *Health care of women: Gynecological assessment.* Monterey, Calif.: Wadsworth.

Himell, K. 1981. Genital herpes: The need for counseling. *Journal of Obstetric, Gynecologic and Neonatal Nursing* 10(6):446–450.

Kambic, R., M. Kambic, A. M. Brixius, and S. Miller. 1981. A thirty-month clinical experience in natural family planning. *American Journal of Public Health* 71(11):1255–1258.

Levinson, D. J. 1978. *Seasons of a man's life.* New York: Knopf.

Lopez, M. C., J. Costtow, E. Adams, P. Romero, J. Gladfelter, and M. Morrison. 1980. *Menopause, a self care manual.* Santa Fe, N. Mex.: Santa Fe Health Education Project.

Magenheimer, E. A. 1979. An alternative contraceptive method: Fertility awareness. *Issues in Health Care of Women* 1(6):39–50.

The menopausal woman. 1978. *Issues in Health Care of Women* 1(2).

Millette, B., and J. W. Hawkins, with M. Kurien and R. Schiffman. 1983. *The passage through menopause: Women's lives in transition.* Reston, Va.: Reston Publishing.

National Institutes of Health. 1980. *Q and A about genital herpes.* Bethesda, Md.

National Women's Health Network. 1980. *Menopause.* Washington, D.C.

Nixon, S. A. 1979. Some very friendly diseases— watch out. *Issues in Health Care of Women* 1(5):39–43.

Page, J. 1977. *The awkward age menopause.* Berkeley, Calif.: Ten Speed Press.

Rafferty, E. G. 1981. Chlamydial infections in women. *Journal of Obstetric, Gynecologic and Neonatal Nursing* 10(4):299–301.

Robinson, B. H. 1978. Nutritional effects of oral contraceptives. *Issues in Health Care of Women* 1(1):37–60.

Rothman, L., and L. Punnett. 1978. *Menstrual extraction.* Hollywood: Feminist Women's Health Center.

Santa Cruz Women's Health Center. 1978. *Herpes.* Santa Cruz, Calif.

Santa Cruz Women's Health Center. 1979. *Menopause self-help resources and bibliography.* Santa Cruz, Calif.

Santa Cruz Women's Health Center. 1978. *P.I.D.* Santa Cruz, Calif.

Scarf, M. 1980. *Unfinished business: Pressure points in the lives of women.* New York: Doubleday.

Stone, M. T. 1979. Female sterilization: The nurse's role. *Issues in Health Care of Women* 1(5):45–60.

Wade, R. C. 1980. *For men about birth control.* Boulder, Colo.: Roger C. Wade.

Wade, R. C. 1978. *For men about abortion.* Boulder, Colo.: Roger C. Wade.

Weideger, P. 1976. *Menstruation and menopause the physiology and psychology, the myth and the reality.* New York: Knopf.

Westoff, L. A. 1980. *Breaking out of the middle-age trap.* New York: Signet Books.

Wirth, V. 1979. Condoms and foam: Traditional forms of contraception still going strong. *Issues in Health Care of Women* 1(5):29–36.

Introduction

Sexual Assault and Exploitation

Incest and Sexual Abuse of Children
Incest patterns
Non-familial sexual abuse
Effects on the child
Assessment of the sexually abused child
Interventions
Child Pornography
Sexual Assault of Adolescents and Adults
Legal aspects
Reactions of the victim
Interventions
Legal and emotional counseling
Attitudes of health-care providers
Rape crisis centers
Education and prevention
The assailant
Prostitution, Stripping, and Sexual Slavery
Interventions
Battering
Interventions
Sexual Harrassment
Interventions

Loss of Reproductive Integrity

Infertility and Involuntary Sterility
Causes of infertility
Sterility
Reactions to inability to conceive
Interventions
Support for infertile couples
Voluntary Sterilization
Parenting of a Child with Ambiguous or Anomalous Genitalia
Hysterectomy
Castration
DES Exposure

Toxic Shock Syndrome

Loss of Sexual Function

Impotence
Premature or Retarded Ejaculation
Lack of Orgasm or Sexual Responsiveness in the Female
Vaginismus
Lack of Desire
Dyspareunia

Summary of Implications for Nursing Practice

Human Sexuality and Nursing Interventions: Crisis

Joellen W. Hawkins

Introduction

Loss or impairment of sexual function can be devastating to the individual who values expression of sexuality. The potential for crisis for the individual is present, whether actual loss occurs or only the threat of loss. Crisis may be biophysical and/or psychosocial. The individual who has sustained a biophysical insult such as castration or sexual assault may experience a psychosocial crisis as well in facing an altered body image, lifestyle, or change in relationships. Loss of reproductive integrity through sterilization, infertility, hysterectomy, or having a child with ambiguous genitalia can affect one's sense of worth as a sexual being. Even inability to perform sexually can constitute a crisis for the individual.

In this chapter, we will look at events that occur outside the realm of developmental phenomena. These are the unforeseen and unexpected events that can precipitate a crisis for the individual, family, and/or community that have implications for sexuality. The presentation will focus on the impact of the event on the expression of sexuality or upon identity as a sexually intact being, and on interventions by health-care providers.

Sexual Assault and Exploitation

Sexual assault, abuse, or exploitation of one human being by another poses a threat to the sexual integrity of the victim. The victim's family and community may also be affected. Sexual molestation of a child will raise the ire of a community to its maximum. Sexual assault of an adult woman generates mixed responses, from anguish and anger to casual acceptance and derogatory remarks about the morality of the victim. Sexual assault and exploitation generate controversy in most communities; responses are heavily influenced by emotions. Victims may, therefore, look to health-care providers for special support in coping with the crisis of assault.

Sexual assault, abuse, and exploitation take several forms in our society. From a life-span perspective, abuse can begin at home with small children as its victims, and extend all the way through assault of the elderly.

Incest and Sexual Abuse of Children

Incest is the most common form of sexual abuse and exploitation of children. It is generally defined as sexual acts that constitute deviant behavior occurring between related persons, including stepparents and stepchildren. No nationwide studies on incest have been done, so statistics must be pieced together from case reports and estimates by those who have expertise in working with victims and their families. Estimates range from 100,000 to over 300,000 cases a year. Three-quarters of these constitute sexual abuse by a family member. One girl in every four in this country will be sexually abused in some way before the age of 18 (Weber 1977, 64). The average age of victims is 11 years, but victims as young as 8 months have been identified. Abuse knows no socioeconomic or ethnic boundaries and ranges from "fondling" to vaginal intercourse (Weber 1977, 64).

Interestingly, nearly every society in the history of humankind has made some attempt to regulate or legislate against incestuous acts (Bluglass 1979; Fox 1980, 9). In 37 states

sexual abuse is a reportable crime and in 21 states suspected abuse must be reported. All 50 states have laws governing the reporting of child abuse (Lean 1978, 642–644). However, there are many obstacles to reporting, particularly in cases of incest, and few convictions ever occur. Emotional and personal factors color interactions between health-care professionals and families and may mask the possibility of incest when emergencies occur. The victim is often very young and/or does not understand what is occurring (Luther and Price 1980, 161–162).

Incest Patterns

Incest may be divided into five dyads: father-daughter, mother-son, brother-sister, father-son, and mother-daughter.

Father-daughter incest is most frequently reported and has received the most attention from health-care providers. There is conflict in the professional literature over descriptions of the type of father who engages in sexual acts with his daughter or stepdaughter. Some clinicians describe the father as passive, introverted, and socially isolated (Peters 1976; Kempe 1978; Poznanski and Bloss 1975, 57), whereas others describe the father as strong, authoritarian, and domineering (Nakashima and Zakus 1977; Kempe 1978; Finkelhor 1978). The common denominator between the two types is a high degree of alcoholism; figures as high as 30% to 50% have been cited (Finkelhor 1978, 440).

The potential for incest extends beyond the personality traits of the father, however. Until recently, the myth that incestuous fathers were usually rural or blue collar was largely unchallenged, but unsatisfactorily substantiated. Recent surveys have uncovered substantial evidence of incest both in urban settings and in middle-class families (Finkelhor 1978, 42–43). Disorganization in family life and other forms of overt and socially questionable sexual activity such as pimping and prostitution also contribute to the incidence of incest (Sagarin 1977, 130; Finkelhor 1978, 47).

Families with a history of or the threat of abandonment seem prone to incest. The incestuous relationship may occur after desertion by the father (Finkelhor 1978, 46). This observation may also, in part, offer one explanation for the occurrence of incest between a stepfather and his stepdaughter. Having experienced the loss of her father, the girl may compensate through compliance with the stepfather in order to avoid another loss.

The mothers are generally active nonparticipants in the incestuous relationship. That is, the mothers are usually aware of the relationship, but do not intervene in any way. A poor relationship between mother and daughter is almost a given when incest occurs. Sexual attention from the father, then, represents some attention for the child (Poznanski and Blos 1975, 57). The literature is replete with case examples of mothers who overtly "set up" the relationship by encouraging father and daughter to sleep together or arranging for them to be home alone (Kempe 1978; Peters 1976; Luther and Price 1980, 163; Gutheil and Avery 1977; Finkelhor 1978). At the same time, the mother denies that the relationship exists. When confronted, she may accuse her daughter of being a whore or seducing the father (Poznanski and Blos 1975, 57). The role the daughter plays in the incestuous relationship may relieve the mother of unwanted duties to her husband (Luther and Price 1980, 163).

Victims have been exploited as early as a few months of age, but the average is between 6 and 11 years. Although an "innocent victim," the child is usually passive and sometimes even cooperative or actively seductive (Poznanski and Blos 1975, 59). Children lack the experience or stage of moral development to sort out right from wrong in such a com-

plex situation (Luther and Price 1980, 163). As the child grows older, incest represents attention. Groth and Burgess point out that "good" children, those who acquiesce readily to adult authority, make easy victims for abuse (1977). The victim is often the oldest daughter (Kempe 1978). Although most victims are of normal intelligence, some have a special problem such as retardation or seizure disorders (Weitzel et al. 1978). Emotionally, the girls are immature, dependent, lonely, and frightened (Poznanski and Blos 1975, 62).

Father-daughter incestuous relationships generally begin with caressing and fondling and then move to genital contact, particularly in postpubertal girls. They vary from rape experiences in that they are generally ongoing in duration and do not usually involve physical force and violence (Finkelhor 1978, 42).

Sexual activity between siblings is probably a very common occurrence, due to the awakening sexual drives of puberty and the proximity of siblings for experimentation (Finkelhor 1980, 171–172; Poznanski and Blos 1975, 69). Activities may range from mutual exploration and experimentation to overt victimization of a younger sibling by an older one (Burgess et al. 1978). A recent survey of undergraduates in New England colleges revealed that 15% of female and 10% of male participants had had sexual experience involving a sibling. Some researchers believe that brother-sister incest is the most common, but probably least frequently reported form of incest, as it is usually transient and has few long-term emotional effects (Nakashima and Zakus 1977).

Mother-son relationships occur rarely according to the literature (Poznanski and Blos 1975, 67–68). Inhibitions seem to be stronger. Also, mother-son separation is less common than father-daughter and the age differential acts as a deterrent (Sagarin 1977, 131–132).

Father-son incest is documented in the literature in case presentations (Dixon, Arnold, and Calestro 1978). Interestingly, family patterns mimic those of father-daughter incest, with violent behavior and alcoholism characterizing the father and knowledgeable compliance characterizing the mother (Dixon et al. 1978, 837).

Mother-daughter relationships, although generally believed to occur, are rarely reported. Emotional repercussions do not surface frequently in counseling. However, this possibility should not be ignored as a risk for children and adolescents.

Nonfamilial Sexual Abuse

Although nonfamilial-sexual abuse constitutes a small proportion of all child sexual abuse (Peters 1976), ranging in estimates from 3% to 30%, it represents a risk health-care providers must consider. Most of the victims are girls and most of the abusers are male (DeFrancis 1969). Activities range from exposure of genitals, manipulation, fondling, and kissing, to intercourse, although the latter is rare (Peters 1976). Usually the abuse is not physically violent and the coercion takes the form of rewards such as candy, money, toys, or affection (Groth and Burgess 1977). Sometimes there seems to be an almost tacit cultural permission for such activities (Rush 1980).

Child sex rings have received the attention of health-care providers over the last few years. Burgess and McCausland (1979a) believe these represent a precursor to prostitution of young persons (pp. 45–46). Their investigations and those of colleagues uncovered six such rings, involving 36 children ranging in age from 6 to 14. Both boys and girls were involved, and rings were both heterosexual and homosexual (pp. 46–47). They define a sex ring as "a group of peer-aged children under 14 years, who are controlled by an adult for self-serving motives and sexual activities that are against the law" (p. 48). Rings were of three types: random, organized youth sex rings, and syndicated sex rings. The latter exploit the children through films and/or photographs used for advertising purposes to entice a customer to order a child (Burgess and Birnbaum 1982, 48).

Effects on the Child

Risks to the child who is the victim of incest or nonfamilial sexual abuse are many. The biophysical risks include bruises and other physical trauma, damage to the genitals such as tearing of the hymen, vaginal lacerations, and injury to penis or scrotum, sexually transmitted diseases, oral or anal lacerations, and pregnancy. Cases of gonorrhea have been reported in children as young as a few months of age, and pregnancy has occurred in 9-year-old girls.

Aside from the biophysical risks, the psychosocial ramifications may be tremendous. Symptoms such as insomnia, anxiety, recurrent bad dreams, and antisocial behaviors such as school failure, truancy, and running away can reflect the turmoil the child is experiencing (Luther and Price 1980, 164). Hysterical seizures have been reported in adolescents who have experienced incestuous relationships (Goodwin, Simms, and Bergman 1979; Gross 1979). Adolescents often have poor self-image and exhibit this through running away, drug abuse, and prostitution (Luther and Price 1980, 164). After the incestuous relationship has ended, girls have been found to exhibit difficulties in the area of sexuality. These include sexualizing all relationships, moving toward overt homosexuality or extreme promiscuity, frigidity, or marrying early (Poznanski and Blos 1975, 62).

Assessment of the Sexually Abused Child

Sexual abuse of children comes to the attention of health-care providers in a number of ways. For example, a young girl with vaginal itching and discharge may have contracted gonorrhea. A school-age child may exhibit behavior disturbances that come to the attention of the school nurse or may have bruises or signs of pregnancy. An adolescent may present with a sexually transmitted disease or pregnancy. If pregnancy occurs in an incestuous consanguineous relationship, the pregnancy is at greater risk for stillbirth, mental retardation, and congenital anomalies (Poznanski and Blos 1975, 76). Thus, the relationship may first come to light if the child resulting from the union is anomalous and genetic evaluation is undertaken.

When sexual abuse is suspected, careful assessment of the child for injury in addition to presenting symptoms is indicated. Parents need honest information about findings and they should be questioned about the circumstances leading to the child's injuries or behavioral manifestations. A young child cannot be relied on to be an accurate historian, but an older child can usually recount enough detail to identify the extent of sexual exploitation and any untoward results. The technique of identifying body parts by playing has been used to elicit details from young children. Having the child draw pictures or act out in play what he or she is thinking or feeling can also help to provide clues to the child's experience and reactions (Thomas 1980, 27–28; Gorline and Ray 1979, 111).

Conferring with parents will help to clarify their perceptions of what has happened to the child and confirm any role they have played. The caregiver should be prepared for anger, frustration, and/or denial. Support for the parents' perspective is essential if the child is to be helped and the trauma minimized (Thomas 1980, 28).

Physical examination may be traumatic for the child. Recognizing this, the approach of health-care providers needs to be particularly sensitive, nonthreatening, and supportive. The small child should have a parent or support person present during the exam and an older child should be given the choice. Offering explanations ahead of time, demonstrating equipment, and allowing the child to handle it can be reassuring.

If the child is brought in immediately after assault, exposing the child's clothing to a Wood's lamp will cause semen to fluoresce dark green. The child should be allowed to remove his or her own clothes or be assisted by parents. Secretions can be present on hair, skin, and buttocks and can be collected as evidence, as can hairs or fingernail scrapings (Thomas 1980, 28). Most emergency rooms or clinics have protocols and specimen containers for evidence. Whether assault has occurred in close proximity to the time of examination or has occurred over time, the child should be examined for lacerations, bruises, and evidence of old injuries such as scars. The provider should check for penile bleeding, hematuria, hematoma of glans or vulva, injuries to shaft, frenulum, and scrotum, rectal and vaginal erythema, abrasions, fissures, or lacerations. The caregiver should also look for evidence of crab lice and of sexually transmitted diseases such as gonorrhea, syphilis, herpes 2, condyloma, and trichomonas. If there is no evidence of vaginal entry and/or the hymenal ring is intact, a vaginal examination may be omitted. If vaginal penetration has occurred in a young child, sedation analgesia or anesthesia may be necessary for a speculum examination to be done.

Screening for trauma should proceed, as with other exams, from the less threatening areas (head, trunk, and extremities) to the genital area. The young child may be examined on a parent's lap. The older child may be examined on the examination table. Allowing the child to assist in the examination to the extent of his or her ability and interest can help to minimize the trauma. The child, for example, can spread the labia so the caregiver can inspect the hymen, or help by lifting his penis or retracting the foreskin. The status of the hymen has legal significance but does not prove or disprove penetration. It may be intact, free of signs of trauma or old scarring, or be recently ruptured or absent. The hymen may allow penetration without rupture or be ruptured by activities or accidents unrelated to sexual abuse (Gorline and Ray 1979, 112–113).

The female who is ovulating can be impregnated without penetration. If semen has been deposited on her perineum, it is possible for sperm to enter the vagina and travel through the uterus to the site of fertilization in the fallopian tube. Thus, it is important to rule out pregnancy. A urine pregnancy test and bimanual or ultrasound examination can be done.

Interventions

Biophysical interventions are based on findings. In some settings, penicillin prophylaxis is advocated to treat possible gonorrhea exposure. Tetanus immunization should be brought up-to-date. Sitz baths can help to heal perineal trauma and decrease pain.

Referral may be necessary for the child and, in most cases, the family when sexual exploitation or assault occurs. The safety of the child must be assured. This may mean referral to social service or child-protection agencies (Gorline and Ray 1979, 113).

If the abuser is a member of the household or a child-care person, reporting the incident to police and child-protection authorities is required in every state (Thomas 1980, 29). Prosecutions for incest are rare; other statutes such as rape and child abuse are usually reverted to (Poznanski and Blos 1975, 76). This situation in no way diminishes the importance of reporting cases of consanguineous abuse.

Comprehensive programs designed to meet the needs of both victims and offenders are being established based on a model developed in California (Weber 1977, 66–67).

Rape crisis centers, child-abuse hotlines, and sexual assault services in hospitals reflect the concern of society for the victims of incest and sexual abuse (Weber 1977, 67).

In the state of Washington a network of centers works with families and individuals who are victims of sexual assault in various forms, including incest. Their booklet on prevention of incest is a model for communication between parents and children (He Told Me Not to Tell 1979). Recognizing the needs of families in which incest occurs and providing services through special centers, programs, and lay literature reflect the concern of health-care providers for the victims, the offenders, and family members.

Prevention programs are aimed at educating children about sexual exploitation and abuse before they become victims. The idea of the child's right to his or her own body is emphasized in such programs. Children are also informed about sources of help if exploitation is threatened or occurs (Herman 1981a, 63–64; Herman 1981b) (see Box).

Child-rearing courses and prenatal classes can also be used as vehicles to discuss the sexual development and needs of children and situations that lead to abuse (Luther and Price 1980, 164–165).

Child Pornography

Pornography that exploits children has been receiving more attention as women speak out against the exploitation of their own bodies and those of their children.

Pornography has been defined as representations of sexual behavior, whether verbal or pictorial, that are explicit and portray, as a distinguishing characteristic, the degradation of human beings, usually women, in such a manner as to endorse the degradation (Longino 1980). Child pornography, which is about 5% of the business, exploits both boys

Personal Safety Advice for Children
(Parents/Guardians Too!)

Dear Children,

Personal safety is more than learning how to cross the street, ride a bicycle or swim.

Public restrooms should be used with caution. If you must use such facilities, it is best to have someone accompany you. Don't loiter in or around the restroom area. Don't speak to strangers—leave immediately.

Every child should know his/her full name, address, telephone number, school, and the name, address, and telephone number of a relative or friend who can be contacted in case of emergency. You should be instructed in the proper use of the telephone to get help in emergency situations.

Report to your parents, school authorities, or a police officer—anyone who exposes "private parts" or attempts to expose your "private parts." Don't go over to strangers in automobiles who may ask you for directions or pretend to have something for you—such as a message, gift, money, or candy.

Stay with your group. On an outing don't wander off alone. If you should get separated, have a prearranged meeting area to wait for your group, preferably a location where someone in authority would be present. For example, in a movie—the manager's office; or in open areas where a security office is not available—choose a location where there are many people, so that you are not alone until your friends find you.

Only parent/guardian, doctor, nurse should be allowed to touch your body in a personal manner. If a stranger, relative, or friend wants to touch your "private parts" or have you do the same to her/him—state that you are not allowed—and get away as fast as you can. Never keep it "secret"; tell your parent or guardian.

Never hitchhike—or accept an offer of a ride from a stranger. Learn to use the public transportation that is available to you. If for some reason you can't, then have your parent/guardian or another responsible person take you to or from your destination. Hitchhiking is equally as dangerous for boys as it is for girls.

Always tell your parent/guardian where you are going, with whom you will be, and when you will return. If you will be late in getting home, call and let someone know you have been detained and where you are.

Lock doors and windows and never indicate to strangers that you are home alone. If someone telephones asking for your parents/guardians—state that they can't come to the phone. Take a message, or have them call back. Don't open the door to strangers—if your parents are home let them answer the door. If you are alone, don't let strangers know there is no one at home with you.

Shortcuts through deserted areas, alleyways, vacant lots or abandoned buildings can be dangerous. Walk or play out in the open where you can see or be seen by other people. Don't stay in the schoolyard when the rest of your playmates have left. Walk to and from school with a friend or group of friends, if possible.

Always discuss with your parent/guardian any incident which has disturbed or confused you. Confide in them freely even when you feel embarrassed or ashamed about the situation. Any questions about sex should be directed to them and not to your friends, who may not know as much as you.

Familiarize yourself with your neighborhood. Remember the places you can go to if you should need immediate help: stores, gas stations, a friend's house nearby, the local police and fire stations. Always let your parent/guardian or school authorities know about anyone who tries to touch you or convince you to go along. Try to remember what the person looked like and what was said.

Every parent should exercise care in the selection of baby-sitters. Young people who baby-sit should also know something about the families for whom they sit. Make arrangements to be brought to and from the location—especially if it involves coming home late at night, or travelling in an area with which you are not familiar.

To be alert is important—alert to the fact that

there are those who might try to take advantage of you (will try to win you over by offering you money, candy, or a gift of some kind for favors of a very personal nature). The requests might embarrass you or make you feel uncomfortable. This person, whether a total stranger or known to you or your family, should be reported to your parent/guardian.

Your personal safety is important—don't be embarrassed at being afraid. Discuss things openly with your parents/guardians. Don't be misled by promises or offers that may seem good at the moment. Your parents/guardians, school authorities, and police want to help you; confide in them. BEING AWARE IS A GOOD HABIT. Tell your friends about personal safety, too!

SOURCE: Reprinted with permission from the Police Department, City of New York Detective Bureau, 1981.

and girls in sexual behavior ranging from undressing and fondling to genital penetration (Steinem 1977, 44). This pornography, known as "chicken porn," centers on magazines and films; the latter is more explicit and exploitive. "Models" range in age from as young as 3 to teenagers. Publications bear titles such as *Lollitots* and *Moppets.* They command grossly inflated prices, suggesting exploitation that is not only biophysical and psychosocial, but economic as well. The average customer is a white, middle-class, middle-aged, married male (Dudar 1977, 46).

Although parental involvement may occur, it is rare. Most "models" are victims of child molesters and many are runaways who pose for survival (Dudar 1977, 80).

During the mid-1970s, sexual exploitation of children through pornography began to draw national attention. Congress passed several laws to curb the use of children and restrict interstate travel for sexual purposes. According to federal investigators, the bulk of child pornography available in this country today is of the homemade variety (Press 1982a, 5).

Child pornography materials are sometimes seized by law enforcement officers, but legislative attempts to curb exploitation are tempered with concern over the First Amendment. Prosecution thus is aimed at the producers and recruiters and not at the peddlers, who are much easier to identify. Information on those who produce child pornography is difficult to obtain. Although much of the material originates in large cities (Dudar 1977, 47), in recent years a large enterprise was uncovered in a small, rural community in northeast Connecticut.

Cognizance of the existence of this form of child sexual abuse on the part of health-care providers can assist authorities in the prosecution process. The child who has been sexually exploited should be viewed as a potential victim of this form of abuse as well, particularly the unaccompanied older child or adolescent who presents for care unaccompanied. Exploitation can precipitate a crisis, either at the time of "modeling" or later in life. Education programs need to address this form of exploitation to alert children to their potential as victims.

As parents and as those who work with parents, nurses can encourage listening to children, communicating about what may happen, and observing for changes in children's behavior (Press 1982c, 4). As concerned professionals and as citizens, we can support legislation that separates this form of pornography from others, categorizes it as child abuse, and makes it a federal crime to transport both boys and girls under 18 (Mann Act) across state lines for immoral purposes (Steinem 1977, 44).

Sexual Assault of Adolescents and Adults

Sexual assault, often referred to as rape, is a considerable risk for adolescents and adults, particularly women.

Rape is, in essence, forced sexual intimacy. It is a crime primarily against women, a deadly insult to the personhood of the victim, and "deprivation of sexual self-determination" (Medea and Thompson 1974, 11). Only the boundaries of human imagination limit the insult and humiliation the victim of rape may endure (Hawkins and Higgins 1981, 99). Rape is a crime of violence, power, and mastery and not, as many believe, a crime of sex (Hawkins and Higgins 1981, 9).

According to federal estimates, over 276,000 women are probably raped each year in the United States (NARAL 1981). Disturbingly, there seems to be a trend in this country toward the acceptance of forced sex and the use of sexual force. The myth that the victim was being "seductive" or "asking for it" is corroborated by findings from a study; 54% of male respondents indicated that under some circumstances it is all right to force a woman and that what happens is the result of her actions (Fingler 1981, 23). These findings coincide with statistics indicating tht more than 50% of attackers are known to their victims (Medea and Thompson 1974, 29).

Burgess and Holmstrom found that victims of rape or sexual assault fell into three main categories: rape-sex without consent, accessory-to-sex (inability of the victim to consent — as with a younger victim), and sex-stress (sex with initial consent — as in a date rape) (Burgess and Holmstrom 1974, 19). Women who are raped are either the victims of blitz rape (the sudden attack) or of confidence rape (the assailant gains trust and then betrays it) (Burgess and Holmstrom 1974, 20).

Males are the victims of sexual assault as well (Burgess and Holmstrom 1974, 257).

Although most male victims are children, adolescents and adults may also be exploited and assaulted, sometimes with deadly intent and consequences. However, this material will focus on female victims, simply because most victims are females.

One out of every three women in the United States will be raped at least once in her lifetime: 96% of rapes occur between people of the same race and 75% of rapes are planned. Rapes occur anytime, anyplace, and to anyone. Over 50% of rapists are married men with seemingly normal sex lives (Fox 1981, 1). Although nearly half of rapes occur in large cities, the incidence in suburbia has increased (Ledray et al. 1979, 197).

There appears to be a high correlation between alcoholism or heavy drinking and rape, at least among convicted rapists (Rada 1975, 444). This information, although not consistently reported in all studies, suggests a compounding variable in carefinding, prevention, and interventions for health professionals.

Health-care providers are not immune from being rapists or perpetrators of sexual assault. Physicians have been convicted of sexual assault on their clients. Nurses who witness such assaults may be indicted if they fail to report the crimes (Horsley 1980, 71–72).

Rape on campuses is a particular threat to adolescents and young adults. Statistics are hard to find since most university health services are not required to report rapes to law enforcement authorities. The campus offers particular advantages to rapists: concentrations of victims in low security areas, multiple sites for rape to occur, predictable mobility patterns of women, empty buildings, and often poorly lit areas (Project on the Status and Education of Women, no date, 2-3).

Married women may be victims of undesired sexual assaults by their husbands. Forty states offer protection to women from sexual assault by their legal husbands. Ten states, at this writing, continue to grant absolute immunity to spouses from prosecution for sexual assault (Parisky 1981, 33).

Myths about rape perpetuate the expectations of society that men are aggressors and possessors of women's bodies. Viewed in this way, rape is, in effect, a crime against a man because it violates his possession. Women continue to be viewed as responsible for sexual dynamics. Therefore, they are seen as responsible for seduction of the male, which leads to rape. As noted earlier, actual rape is not often associated with sex and is the expression of aggression and power (Hawkins and Higgins 1981, 100). Rape fantasies are not uncommon among women, but they emphasize control by the woman over the circumstances, an imagined position that differs markedly from the reality of sexual assault. The view of rape as a crime has come to the attention of the public only in recent years, with the help of the women's movement in debunking the myths that had long masked the criminal nature of sexual assault.

Legal Aspects

The prosecution rate for rape continues at a slow pace, while the rate of rapes rises. Fewer than 1% of cases are ever tried out of the less than 10% that are even reported (Sredl et al. 1979, 38–39). The ideologies associated with rape change slowly and influence criminal prosecution. The first is that women report their assailants out of spite or revenge. The second is that women ask to be raped by the clothes they wear, by their seductive behavior, or by going out of their homes. The third is that true rape is limited to virgins. The fourth is that women are property owned by their fathers, lovers, or husbands (Ross 1973).

The choices a victim has in prosecuting are to bring criminal charges or civil charges against the rapist or to file civil charges against a third party who might be held responsible (Project on the Status and Education of Women, no date, 3–4). What constitutes rape changes in meaning depending upon the perception, whether it be that of the rapist, the victim, the attorney, the police, or the jury (Hawkins and Higgins 1981, 101).

According to law, conviction of rape requires evidence beyond a reasonable doubt and testimony by the victim. Her assailant is not required to testify (Sredl et al. 1979, 41). Evidence sufficient to prove guilt beyond a reasonable doubt includes the initial police report, examination of the rape scene, results of the physical examination, photographs of the victim, and polygraph evidence from the victim (Sredl et al. 1979, 40). Most states now have legislation requiring hospitals to render emergency service to rape victims who request it and, in some cases, to require the state to reimburse costs. Any legislation does not guarantee a maximum rate of conviction, however (Sredl et al. 1979, 39).

Reactions of the Victim

Rape and sexual assault represent a crisis for the victim and often for the family, significant others, and the community as well. They pose a direct threat to the reproductive integrity of the victim, as well as to her psychosocial well-being. The reactions of the victim depend on the person's previous coping skills and internal and external resources.

Burgess and Holmstrom (1976) found that victims used a variety of coping strategies when confronted with danger; only one-third were unable to act (p. 415). Strategies used included cognitive assessment and attempts to find alternatives, verbal tactics (talk one's way out), and physical action to prevent the attack. A number of victims tried more than one strategy (Burgess and Holmstrom 1976, 414–415).

In coping with the actual rape attack, women focused on survival. They used cognitive strategies, focusing on a specific thought to block out the reality, to survive, and to remain calm. Some memorized details of the event or used coping strategies drawn from previous traumas. Verbal strategies included yelling, screaming, talking to and trying to calm the assailant and dissuade him from further abuse or to gain control. Some women fought and struggled. Victims also utilized psychological defenses: denial, dissociation, suppression, rationalization, and resignation. Involuntary physiological responses included choking, gagging, nausea, pain, urination, hyperventilation, loss of consciousness, and seizure activity (Burgess and Holmstrom 1976, 415–416).

After the attack, victims tried to alert others to get help, bargained for freedom, or had to physically free themselves (Burgess and Holmstrom 1976, 416–417).

The initial reactions following the assault are usually shock, anxiety, and agitation. The victim may be hysterical or may appear to be calm and in control (Medea and Thompson 1974, 101). Burgess and Holmstrom identified two emotional styles among victims, each of which is exaggerated under stress. In *expressed* style, victims emote feelings of fear, anger, and anxiety either verbally or by their behavior. In *controlled* style, victims mask or hide feelings and reactions under a facade of calm and composure. The primary reaction of almost all women, regardless of emotional styles, however, was fear (Burgess and Holmstrom 1973, 1743).

Interventions

When victims present for help from healthcare providers, some clear implications should emerge from the victims' responses to the crisis and their reported needs. Burgess and Holmstrom point out the need for health-care providers to recognize rape as a situational crisis, to view the victim as a consumer of emergency health-care services, and to provide crisis intervention in the form of primary prevention (1973, 1744). The victim should be extended privacy and given priority as an emergency. She should be allowed to call a support person and/or be offered the services of a rape crisis counselor, when available. A thorough history, taking into account the emotional style of the victim, will elicit data about the event that may be used later as court evidence. It will also give the woman an opportunity to share her perception of the attack.

Preparation for physical examination includes procurement of the necessary specimen receptacles. This will assure collection of data important to the prosecution, should the victim choose to pursue legal recourse against the assailant. Clothing should be carefully handled and evidence such as hairs removed from it and labeled. All signs of trauma should be carefully assessed and carefully documented. X-ray and laboratory studies will confirm or rule out fractures and internal injuries to organs. It is sometimes appropriate, with permission of the victim, to take photographs for court evidence. The pelvic examination must be done carefully, with great sensitivity and care. Any data should be collected scrupulously because of their relation to the assault. The perineum is checked for lacerations and bruising and observed with a Wood's lamp. Specimens of secretions and any loose hairs are collected. A urine specimen is obtained after the victim has been cautioned not to wipe away any seminal fluid. After vaginal insertion of the speculum, swabs are obtained of cervix, vagina, and vulva, as well as gonorrhea cultures. Samples of the victim's pubic hairs are taken to compare with any that may belong to the assailant (Sredl et al. 1979, 39–40).

Treatment includes interventions for any lacerations, bruises, or fractures, penicillin prophylaxis, and tetanus toxoid. Sometimes pregnancy prophylaxis is offered in the form of diethylstilbestrol (DES), a dilatation and curettage, or vacuum suction of the uterus (Stredl et al. 1979, 42).

Adequacy and completeness of records is essential to court evidence in the event of arrest and prosecution. Burgess and Laszlo stress the need for precise recording of signs and symptoms of trauma, both biophysical and psychosocial (1977, 64). The information included in the record can help to corroborate the testimony of the victim. Include the victim's statements about the physical assault and the assailant's threats of harm (Burgess and Laszlo 1977, 66–67).

After completion of the examination, the caregiver's attention should focus on the biophysical needs of the victim. She may need tissues, something to eat and/or drink, safety pins or needle and thread to repair her clothing, and a private place to wash with warm water, soap, and mouthwash. She should be offered the opportunity to call someone to take her home or to a safe place and to bring her something to wear (Burgess 1978, 15; LeFort 1977, 43–45).

Legal and Emotional Counseling

Victims also need assistance in decision-making concerning police involvement. The decision to call police should rest with the victim, if she is capable of making that decision. If she does decide to report the crime, the police will want to question her and obtain a description of the assailant. There is disagreement as to whether a female police officer or a sensitive male officer is of more benefit to the victim (Burgess and Holmstrom 1974). The rate of reported rape increases when victims have access to an anonymous telephone counseling service. In order to increase arrests and convictions from reported rapes, the victim must have legal protection, long-term supportive counseling services, and knowledge of successful prosecutions reported in the media (Kaufman et al. 1974). Burgess and Holm-

strom describe the court processes a victim will experience if she chooses to prosecute (1974).

Emotional support for the victim is critical, both during the crisis and in post-crisis follow-up. Long-term effects following the initial shock include paranoia, inability to concentrate, distrust of males, and a distortion in sense of self (Sredl et al. 1979, 42).

Identification of coping strategies used by the victim can be useful in follow-up therapy. First, the clinician can provide the victim with information about coping behavior and positive adaptation to a crisis. This helps alleviate any guilt experienced by the victim in feeling she did not do enough to prevent the assault. It also reinforces positive feelings for the victim about her abilities to restore herself to wellness post-crisis. Such identification also helps to ascertain further crisis and post-crisis interventions (Burgess and Holmstrom 1976, 417; Burgess and Holmstrom 1979a).

Victims need assistance in reaching phase two — a seemingly satisfactory adjustment post-crisis — and to move successfully on to phase three. Phase three is characterized by reliving of the episode and is the time during which the victim has to resolve her feelings about her world, her life, and the assailant (Medea and Thompson 1974, 103). She must work through any negative feelings about herself, reestablish a sense of security, resolve any guilt she may feel, and work through feelings about the person who assaulted her (Medea and Thompson 1974, 103–106).

Another problem victims must be helped to deal with is if and how to tell their families. Burgess and Holmstrom found in their study of disclosure to parental family members (1979b) that the majority of victims told selective parental family members, one-third told all the family, and a full one-quarter told no family member. In most cases in which family members were told, the victim was the one to tell them (p. 258). Four components of the process were identified: deciding whether to tell, deciding how to tell, timing the news, and dealing with the initial responses of the persons told (p. 259). Burgess and Holmstrom feel that disclosure is a component of the crisis counseling process. Victims need help in predicting family responses to the news; deciding whether or not to tell should be based on the advantages and disadvantages. After the news has been disclosed, follow-up support should be provided for the victim (pp. 266–267).

Those who counsel rape and assault victims should also be cognizant of long-term effects once the immediate crisis has passed. Victims report difficulties in sexual expression that persist for months or years. Most victims report a return to normal activity within four to six months, but a small number experience ongoing problems (Ellis et al. 1980, 47).

Follow-up counseling sessions after the crisis may be conducted by telephone or in person. A follow-up call made within 48 hours after the rape or assault is useful in assessing the coping abilities of the victim (Burgess and Holmstrom 1974). The needs of each client should be considered and plans for time and frequency of contact in the post-crisis period made accordingly. Referrals to other health-care professionals may be made if warranted. For example, social workers may provide counseling and also help the victim to identify resources in the community (Abarbanel 1976, 481).

The victim who chooses to prosecute will need special help and support through the court processes, which can last months and even years. In fact, the health-care professional could be subpoenaed as a court witness. The victim may need follow-up after the case is over, too, to help her put her life together and take up the tasks of living once more. Thus, crisis intervention during the period immediately following the sexual assault is but one part of the process of helping those who are victims.

Attitudes of Health-care Providers

Attitudes of health-care providers toward victims of sexual assault will, of course, affect the efficacy of interventions. A recurrent theme in cases of rape and sexual assault is blaming the victim. Interestingly, one study of attitudes found that nonwhite police officers blamed victims more than white officers. Nurses who viewed themselves as potential victims were more likely to blame victims than those who did not see themselves as potential victims. In general, though, most nurses and police officers do not blame victims and are similar in their assignments of blame. Attitudinal and personality variables of these two groups seem particularly influential in assignment of blame (Alexander 1980, 76–77). Another study showed that perceived carelessness on the part of the victim is a factor affecting attitudes of student nurses toward the victim (Damrosch 1981, 168–170). The victim needs recognition of her role by others. If staff members exhibit attitudes that suggest that "nothing happened" or blame the victim, then the victim's needs are not being met (Burgess and Holmstrom 1973, 1745).

Rape Crisis Centers

Rape crisis centers have evolved over the past years in response to the needs of victims. Such centers may exist as independent entities offering 24-hour counseling and support services or as integral parts of hospital emergency wards. The programs are aimed at supporting victims through the crisis and then providing follow-up or referral for the post-crisis period. One such center offers follow-up, in-service education for staff, consultation for police, courts, schools, and other agencies that work with victims, public education, and clinical research (Rape Crisis Intervention 1978). The Sexual Assault Resource Program is a nurse-designed and nurse-directed research/demonstration project. It serves as a model for assisting victims to return to a prerape level of functioning (Ledray 1982). For rape crisis centers to be effective, evaluation would seem to be an integral and ongoing component, designed to improve services to clients and to increase the sensitivity and response to victims of other components of society: police, hospitals, and the entire legal system. One center has instituted an extensive evaluation program based on objectives for the services of the center. Information generated has led to changes in program design, goals, and objectives (Bushnell et al. 1980, 61–80). Problems identified by another center included the hospital setting, an overbalance of emphasis on medical and legal aspects of intervention, the length of police interrogations prior to crisis intervention at the center, and the maze of the legal system (Ruch and Chandler 1980, 60–62).

Education and Prevention

One aspect of care for victims that is often overlooked is that of education and prevention. Education programs should include not only victims and potential victims, but also all of those who work with victims: police, lawyers, courts, and health-care providers. Prevention programs can be aimed at high risk target areas such as college and university campuses. Raising public awareness, instituting better security measures (escort and transport services, good lighting, patrolling, locking dormitory doors), and providing self-defense courses are all strategies to prevent assault (Project on the Status and Education of Women, no date, 4–5). Providing women with personal safety tips is also a strategy for prevention (Medea and Thompson 1974, 59–96; Brownmiller 1975, 347, Abarbanel and Rebello 1981; National Institute of Mental Health 1981) (see Box). Older women are not immune and deserve special consideration as potential victims when preventive strategies are planned.

The Assailant

What of the rapist, the perpetrator of the crime of sexual assault? Specific programs have been started in some areas to treat sexual offenders (Bush 1975). These programs are

---

Safeguards Against Sexual Assault

Sex crimes are not crimes of passion. Sex crimes are crimes of violence. Far from being impulsive behavior, most sexual assault is planned. This crime could happen to you, no matter your age, color, wealth or marital status. . . . BE AWARE . . . TAKE PRECAUTIONS.

At Home

1. If you live alone you should list ONLY your initials and last name in the phone directory and on a mailbox.

2. Be sure to lock your doors, even if you are at home, and even if you only leave for a few minutes (to walk the dog, get the mail, put out the garbage, hang out the laundry, etc.).

3. Shades or blinds should be on every window.

4. If you live in a basement or first floor apartment, bars should be put on the windows by the landlord.

5. NEVER open the door automatically. Require the caller to identify himself/herself satisfactorily (repairpersons, delivery persons, police

officers, public servants, etc.). Utilize chain bolt when checking identification.

6. If a stranger asks to use your phone, DO NOT permit him/her to enter. Offer to summon emergency assistance or make the call for that person.

7. Inside and outside lights give you a good deal of protection. Leave lights on at night, even when away from home. Change the location of inside lighting from time to time.

8. Leave light on over door you will be using when you return home after dark. Use timers. Have key READY so that door can be opened immediately.

9. If a window or door has been forced or broken while you were absent, DO NOT ENTER OR CALL OUT. Use a neighbor's phone IMMEDIATELY to call police and wait outside until they arrive.

In Elevators

If you live in an apartment building in which you know the other residents and find yourself in the lobby with a stranger, let that person take the elevator and wait for it to return for you. . . . If you are on the elevator and someone gets on whose presence makes you uneasy, get off at the next floor. ALWAYS STAND NEAR THE CONTROL PANEL. If threatened, hit the alarm button and press as many of the other buttons as you can reach with your arm, elbow, etc., enabling the door to open at any of several floors.

Walking

1. Whenever possible, AVOID WALKING ALONE AT NIGHT.

2. After getting off a bus or leaving a subway station, LOOK AROUND to see whether you are being followed.

3. If someone suspicious is behind you or ahead of you, cross the street. If necessary, crisscross from one side to another, back and forth. DON'T BE AFRAID TO *RUN*. (One of the criminal's greatest assets is his ability to surprise you, to attack when you least expect it. Should you continue to be followed, be prepared to SCREAM AND RUN. . . .)

4. BE EXTRA *AWARE* OF WHAT'S AROUND YOU. Walk closer to the curb to avoid passing too close to shrubbery, dark doorways, and other places of concealment. Shun shortcuts, especially through backyards, parking lots, and alleyways.

5. If a car approaches you and you are threatened, SCREAM AND RUN in the direction opposite that of the car. (The driver will have to turn around to pursue you.)

6. Dress for mobility. Many styles are nice but make moving harder on you.

7. Try not to overload yourself with packages, books, large purses, etc.

8. Never hitchhike or accept a ride from a stranger.

9. When arriving home by taxi or private auto, request the driver to wait until you are inside.

10. Have your key ready in hand, so your house door can be opened immediately.

Driving

1. When practicable, travel on well lighted, more populated streets and thoroughfares. Keep windows closed and doors locked.

2. Keep your car in gear while halted at traffic lights and signs. If your safety is threatened, hold down on the horn and drive away as soon as possible.

3. Check your rear view mirror. If you believe you are being followed by another car, do not drive into your driveway or park in a deserted area. Pull over to the curb at a spot where there are people, and let the car pass you. If the car continues to follow, drive to the nearest place where you can get help (gas station, police station, fire house, etc.).

4. If you should be followed into your driveway, stay in your car with the doors locked until you can identify the occupants or know the driver's intent. Sound horn to get the attention of neighbors or as an effort to scare the other driver off.

5. When parking at night select a place that will be lighted when you return. Check for loiterers before leaving the car.

6. Never leave car keys in the ignition, even if you are only parked for a short time. Take them with you, and make sure that the car is locked.

7. Never pick up a hitchhiker or offer a ride to a stranger. Offer to summon emergency assistance or make a phone call for someone whose auto is apparently disabled. (Stay inside your locked auto when making offer.)

8. Be conscious of your own auto maintenance. If a breakdown occurs, tie a white cloth to the door handle or antenna, wait for police assistance inside your locked auto. If a "good samaritan" offers help (mechanical or otherwise) pass money for an appropriate phone call via your slightly opened window.

9. Don't let your auto's fuel gauge go below "half" before filling the gas tank FOR SAFETY'S SAKE. . . .

Checklist for Victims of Sexual Assault

Report CRIME IMMEDIATELY to the POLICE DEPARTMENT. . ."DIAL 911."

1. Do not wash or douche.

2. Do not touch, move, or destroy any article that may be evidence.

3. Have medical exam and internal gynecological exam at the nearest hospital emergency room, as soon as possible.

a) Inform doctor of exact acts committed upon you. He should note any medical evidence of them.

b) Semen smears must be taken by doctor.

c) Doctor will note any bruises or injuries (bleeding, lacerations, etc.), external or internal.

d) Doctor should test for venereal diseases and pregnancy later (if relevant).

4. Inform police department investigator of ALL details of attack, however intimate, and of anything unusual you may have noted about the attacker. Remember what he said and how he said it. It could lead to his arrest.

5. Show police any external bruises or injuries, however minor, resulting from the attack. Also show injuries to a friend or relative who might be available as a corroborative witness at the trial.

6. Give any clothing that was stained or torn (including undergarments) during the commission of the crime to the police for analysis.

7. WHEN CALM . . . make note of events of attack. This includes unusual details, direction in which you last saw him running, description (height, weight, clothing, type of build, color of skin, hair, facial oddities, scars, jewelry, etc.).

THE VICTIM IS *NOT* TO BLAME, THE VICTIMIZER IS.

source: Reprinted with permission from the Police Department, City of New York Detective Bureau, 1981.

generally predicated on several premises: deviant behavior is learned and therefore can be modified; sex offenders, with guidance, can help each other; the treatment environment and process of learning acceptable behavior must be reality oriented (Bush 1975, 38). Castration, once heralded as a treatment for sex offenders, has no scientific or ethical basis (Heim and Hursch 1979).

Clinical research being conducted on the rapist identifies four patterns: rape with an aggressive aim, rape with a sexual aim, rape with sex-aggression defusion, and the impulse rape (Burgess and Holmstrom 1974, 21–34).

These descriptions closely match those of victims as they describe the circumstances of the assault and behavior of the rapist.

Men who commit crimes of sexual assault are not necessarily sexually deviant persons. Often they are known to their victims. They may be participants in normal social roles as fathers, husbands, and productive members of the work force. What, then, in the nature of our society perpetuates the myths about rape which, in a sense, allow men to abdicate responsibility for their own sexual actions? Why is it that the victim must suffer guilt, accusation, and insinuations about her morality (Medea and Thompson 1974, 45)? The rapist/victim dyad reflects the social positions of men and women. Until those change, women will continue to be victims of a crime that society continues to condemn legally, but perpetuates by its values and myths. As discussed in Chapter 4, some critics feel that violent pornography encourages violence against women; others note that it reflects the deeper issue of the power imbalance between men and women in our culture.

Prostitution, Stripping, and Sexual Slavery

Prostitution, stripping, and sexual slavery pose risks not only to adolescents and adults, but to children as well. Individuals who as children experienced sexual advances by adults and then experience rape seem to develop an abusive sexual self-identity. This in turn seems to lead some of these persons to choose prostitution as a way of life (James and Meyerding 1977, 40–41). Those persons who choose prostitution run the gamut from "in-house" jobs, to walking the streets and soliciting, to housewives and drug addicts who do not view prostitution as their profession, but rather as a means to other ends. All of these groups sometimes exhibit psychopathology (Exner et al.

1977, 484–485). Some interesting books on the lives of prostitutes have been published recently (Shulman 1981; Jaget 1981).

Teenage prostitution is often a desperate bid for survival by runaways and is rampant in large cities. Unable to get other employment, these teenagers turn to prostitution as a last resort. They are easy prey for those who make their living off the prostitution of others. An estimated 75% of teen prostitutes come from poor households, and they are easily lured by a pimp who promises them money and glamour (Ritter and Weinstein 1979, 20–21).

The dynamics between pimp and prostitute may not be altogether exploitive (James 1973). Usually the pimp is male and the prostitute female, although this stereotype does not always hold. The pimp offers male protection and assistance in the business details of the occupation.

It is unlikely that prostitution will go away. Some attempts to deal with it include legislation to outlaw it and vigorous campaigns to bring about prosecutions and convictions. A second way to deal with it is to legalize and regulate it as an occupation (Bullough and Bullough 1978, 292–294). Bullough and Bullough also suggest "decriminalization of sexual activities between consenting adults," regardless of exchange of money (pp. 294–295). Law enforcement officials could then focus on protection of minors under statutory rape and age of consent legislation (p. 295).

Stripping for a living sometimes represents another form of sexual exploitation. Studies of decision-making indicate that women choose stripping because it means more money than other occupations open to them, and because it offers glamour and the chance to be in show business (Boles and Garbin 1974, 119–121). The occupational opportunities open to women with limited education, besides exploiting them through wage discrimination, may make alternatives such as stripping seem attractive. However, strippers run the risk of being injured by customers or may use violence themselves to repel undesired approaches. Interactions with customers outside the work setting may include sexual intercourse; some houses expect their "girls" to engage in prostitution (Boles and Garbin 1974).

Sexual slavery, known in the 19th century as "white slavery," is now more accurately called female sexual slavery. It may involve the capture and exploitation of young women ranging in age from teens to 30. These women are kept in brothels in various countries throughout the world, and may be transported from city to city or out of their own countries to others. Coercion and violence are used to keep the women captive (Barry 1979a).

Barry, in her exhaustive study of female sexual slavery, contends that it is carried out by individuals, privately within families, and by international gangs. It ". . . is present in *all* situations where women or girls cannot change the immediate conditions of their existence, where regardless of how they got into those conditions they cannot get out, and where they are subject to sexual violence and exploitation" (Barry 1979b, 33).

Josephine Butler, an English woman, was the first person to speak out against forced prostitution in the 19th century. She challenged the Contagious Diseases Acts in England as attempts to formalize and legalize sexual enslavement of women and campaigned for their repeal. Those who supported her protests included Florence Nightingale (Barry 1979b, 12–13). At last, in 1886, the Acts were repealed, but by that time international trafficking in women was well established (Barry 1979b, 25).

The exploitation of women through sexual slavery at present is thought to be widespread, although little official documentation is available through agencies such as INTERPOL. It is suspected that much of the traffic in women is disguised (Barry 1979b, 250–252).

Interventions

As health-care professionals, we have responsibilities to our clients to provide care, regardless of their lifestyle or occupation. During the care-giving process, evidence may present itself suggesting a case of sexual abuse or exploitation. When the client is an adult, issues of the right of self-determination may arise. At the same time, when taking the history of a client, evidence may emerge to indicate infringement of the client's rights by another person. It is then the responsibility of the professional to offer support, help to identify resources, and provide for follow-up.

Adults who are sexually exploited are vulnerable to sexually transmitted diseases, pelvic inflammatory disease, pregnancy, injury to the perineum and genitals, and psychosocial and sexual sequelae. Assessments, therefore, are based on risks and acceptable interventions based on the data collected. Strategies for prevention such as contraception should also be included when appropriate.

Health-care providers need to be alert to the occurrence of teenage prostitution and be active in finding youngsters caught in this lifestyle. Public clinics and emergency rooms are sites where victims may present for care. Particular risks include sexually transmitted diseases, pregnancy, and genital trauma. When prostitution is suspected, a social service referral may be useful for counseling, identifying resources, and helping the young person choose an alternative lifestyle or return home. Shelters such as Covenant House in New York City offer not only a place to stay, but an opportunity to talk with volunteers about their lives (Ritter and Weinstein 1979, 20).

Battering

Battering may be related to sexual exploitation and abuse. Children who are victims of incest or sexual abuse by unrelated persons may also suffer physical abuse to elicit compliance, prevent disclosure, or as part of the sexual activity. Adults who suffer sexual abuse or exploitation may also be battered. The woman who presents with possible pregnancy or exposure to a sexually transmitted disease as the result of undesired sexual activity should be assessed carefully for signs of physical injury. If the woman has bruises, it is important to determine their origin. The woman may need reassurance and offers of protection before she will admit to being a victim. Abuse of women, mostly by their husbands, occurs more frequently than rape (Gingold 1976, 51). Some of the myths about rape also pertain to battering. The woman is supposed to have provoked the man into beating her, and she has to prove that she is a victim. Like rape, battering is a crime that knows no sociocultural or economic boundaries (Gingold 1976, 52). Men, too, can be battered (Brehm, no date).

Persons who have been beaten will suffer injuries ranging from bruises, lacerations, and fractures to concussions and miscarriages. In addition, they suffer the psychological effects of terror, degradation, guilt, and fear from living in a milieu of violence. However, economic pressures and the effects of socialization are constraints against leaving a violent situation. In addition, although battering is a crime, prosecutions are not frequent; victims earn retaliation for reporting their assailants, especially if they are spouses (Gingold 1976, 52). The importance of emotional attachments to the batterer must not be overlooked (Dutton and Painter 1981).

Interventions

In addition to care for the physical insults the victim has sustained, he or she will need assistance in dealing with violence in the family and/or the relationship. It is important to elicit the victim's perception of violence as a problem. Then the caregiver must ascertain whether or not the victim is ready to act on the situation (Valenti 1979, 192–193). Identification of community resources such as shelters, legal services, and financial assistance are critical (Valenti 1979, 187). Many resources are available to women and their children to help them escape from a violent situation (Kashimer 1976, 97–98). Health-care professionals can be knowledgeable about those resources in their communities.

Sexual Harassment

Sexual harassment is also a threat to the sexual integrity of the individual. Most victims are women, and the harassment most often occurs at the place of employment, although it may also occur in public places. One survey reported that 88% of respondents had experienced unwanted sexual advances in the workplace (Project on the Status and Education of Women 1978, 1). Another, a study of nurses, reported that over 60% of the sample of 89 had experienced harassment at work. Typical harassers were physicians or supervisors (Duldt 1982, 336–337). Often the victim is in a subordinate position and may, therefore, be intimidated or coerced into submitting to continued harassment. The victim of harassment may be subjected to verbal abuse, pressure for sexual activity, sexist remarks about her body, clothing, or sexuality, unwanted physical advances, leering, demands for sexual favors accompanied by threats concerning job, grades, and so on, and/or physical assault (Project on the Status and Education of Women 1978, 1–2).

Interventions

Consciousness-raising is a first step in curtailing sexual harassment. Women need to know they do not have to submit to unwanted sexual abuse and harassment. Several lower court rulings have confirmed harassment as a violation of Title VII of the Civil Rights Act. Test cases have elicited rulings that employers must investigate complaints of harassment and deal with offenders. "Sexual harassment of students may constitute a violation of Title IX" (Project on the Status and Education of Women 1978, 4).

We as health-care professionals can help to educate those members of our own professions as well as the public at large. In addition, we can offer support and identify resources for victims of harassment (Lindsey 1977; Lefkowitz 1977; Alliance 1981).

Loss of Reproductive Integrity

Reproductive integrity means being able to parent as many or as few children as one desires, when one desires, without significant biophysical or psychosocial insult to any member of the triad (woman, man, and fetus). Threats to reproductive integrity include any developmental or situational hazardous events that interrupt the normal cycle from fertility and fertilization through the puerperium and neonatal periods. Interruptions in or anomalies in biophysical development of reproductive organs may result in infertility and/or sterility. Loss of reproductive integrity includes sterility, hysterectomy, and production of an anomalous child. Even when sterility is voluntary, the potential for crisis exists and should be recognized.

Infertility and Involuntary Sterility

Reproduction is still the expectation of many persons who marry or choose a long-term relationship while in their teens, 20s, and 30s. The birth rate is, indeed, dropping and individuals may expect to have fewer children. Nonetheless, many men and women view parenting as an expected developmental event. Echoing this expectation, Greenbaum believes that ". . . both men and women have a need to rear children in order to enhance their own self-realization and to achieve fulfillment of some of their emotional, mental, and social aspirations" (1973, 1264). This kind of statement, of course, does not support those who do not want children. But the sentiment has a strong emotional impact on those who do want to bear children but cannot. It has been estimated that 3.5 million couples in this country are involuntarily childless, comprising about 15% of married couples (Green 1977, 356).

Causes of Infertility

Infertility is defined as lack of conception after one year or more of unprotected intercourse (Friedman 1981, 2041). Some sources attribute cause equally to men and women. According to one source, 35% of cases are due to each partner and the remaining 30% to the couple together (Menning 1975, 1).

Male factors in infertility include "either faulty sperm production (spermatogenesis) or faulty delivery of sperm" (Taymor 1978, 17). Impaired spermatogenesis can be due to problems with necessary hormones, endocrine disorders, and genetic anomalies. Excessive heat to the scrotal area, presence of a varicocele, generalized illness, physical and chemical agents, and infections in the testicles can disrupt spermatogenesis. Sperm transport is disrupted by blockage of the epididymis or vas deferens as a result of infection, injury, congenital anomaly, nerve injury, or impotence (Taymor 1978, 17–21). Occasionally retrograde ejaculation or hypospadias (misplaced urethral opening) is the problem (NAACOG 1982).

Causes of infertility in women are more numerous. Obstruction of the vagina, vaginitis, and/or anatomical aberration may prevent coitus or conception. Cervical mucus may be hostile or impenetrable to sperm or congenital anomalies may be present. The uterus may be anatomically anomalous, tumors may be present, or there may be adhesions from surgery or infection. A common cause of infertility is occlusion of the fallopian tubes. Salpingitis is usually the result of gonorrhea, but may be due to other pathogens. The tube may be dislocated by adhesions, so that the tube and ovary are not adjacent. Endometriosis is another cause.

Ovarian cysts, tumors, or congenital anomalies may cause infertility, but the major ovarian cause is disruption in the normal ovulatory cycle. Irradiation and mumps may damage the ovaries (Taymor 1978, 23–26).

The increasing incidence of sexually transmitted diseases may also affect fertility. The age at which a woman tries to conceive may be an additional factor in success. Choosing to delay conception until after 30 will mask any fertility problems that may exist and delay treatment.

The role of emotions should not be overlooked; physical effects of emotional state are well demonstrated. Emotional factors must be considered in assessing causes of infertility (Taymor 1978, 27–31).

The couple's sexual technique may also affect conception. The couple may not be having vaginal intercourse. Pain or lack of knowledge may prohibit vaginal penetration. On the other hand, in some cases frequency of intercourse can actually reduce the chance of conception.

Sterility

Sterility means that an individual cannot procreate. A distinction is made between primary and secondary sterility in women: primary sterility means the woman has never been pregnant and secondary sterility is sterility that occurs after one or more pregnancies (Leridon 1977, 96). Involuntary sterility is due to immaturity, anomaly, or absence of reproductive organs, exposure to excessive amounts of radiation, and/or surgical trauma.

Reactions to Inability to Conceive

The individual or couple grappling with threat to or loss of reproductive integrity may exhibit a variety of responses. If he or she had experienced ambiguity toward parenting, a sense of relief may ensue when pregnancy does not occur. On the other hand, inability to conceive may be perceived as a blow to masculinity or femininity and/or loss of a desired experience. The person may feel sexually inadequate or the news of infertility or sterility may cause alterations in sexual expression. Perceptions of blame for the inability to conceive can cause resentment and accusations. Feelings of guilt and of being sexually less than adequate may arise. The partners may blame each other. At a time when they most need each other's support, that support may be lacking.

For the woman who has a career, infertility or sterility may exaggerate any feelings of guilt about trying to combine career and traditional roles. Conversely, for the woman who expects to assume a traditional role as wife and mother, threats to reproductive integrity may distort or destroy her self-image. A man may perceive his lack of ability to father a child as a severe blow to his image as a man and as a sexual being. This threat may pervade not only his personal and sexual life, but his social and professional life as well (Hawkins 1982).

A couple experiencing infertility may seek a variety of medical evaluations and procedures, ever hopeful that pregnancy may result. Some couples decide to pursue adoption or become foster parents as an alternative. Others may decide not to parent and to invest their energies in other activities together and/or as individuals.

TABLE 7-1 *Infertility Workup*

Woman	Both	Man
Menstrual history	Complete medical history— diet, habits, exercise, sleep	Semen analysis
Cervical mucus test		Urologic evaluation
Basal body temperature graph (several months)	Sexual history	Testicular biopsy
Huhner test	Fertility history	Seminal fructose level
Tubal insufflation (Rubin)	Physical examination	Seminal volume
Hysterosalpingogram	Postcoital test	Scrotal thermography and venography
Hydrotubation	Lab studies for infection of genital tract	
Laparoscopy	Sperm antibody studies	
	Hormonal assays	

SOURCE: Data from: Friedman, B. M. 1981. Infertility Workup. *American Journal of Nursing* 81(11):2041–2046 and Taymor, M. L. 1978. *Infertility.* New York: Grune & Stratton.

Interventions

Assessment is the first step for couples who experience infertility. The workup begins with a comprehensive interview and history to elicit data about menstrual cycles, sexual history, fertility indices, and habits of daily living such as diet, smoking, and exercise. Health-care professionals must be careful not to convey a message to the couple that they are "doing something wrong." The health history, physical examination, and laboratory assays help to rule out anomalies and systemic disease. The workup for both the man and the woman is complex and time-consuming (Friedman 1981) (see Table 7-1). It should proceed from least to most intrusive procedures.

Obtaining a *semen sample* yields information about the presence or absence, number, and motility of sperm. A *Huhner test* is done to view the motility of sperm in cervical fluid. It is usual for the woman to keep a *basal body temperature record,* which helps to determine occurrence and timing of ovulation. (Keeping this chart can "control" people's lives, so care-

givers must be sensitive to client's reactions). The *tubal insufflation test* (Rubin), *hysterosalpingogram* (dye outlining uterus and tubes), and *hydrotubation* (saline in tubes to demonstrate patency), are means by which assessment of tubal patency and anatomic normalcy of reproductive organs are determined. An *endometrial biopsy* is done to ascertain characteristics of the endometrial lining and provide data concerning its readiness for implantation. A *laparoscopy* is done to visualize the uterus, tubes, and ovaries.

Therapeutic interventions for infertility include counseling, treatment for any specific problems identified, and support for the couple through the process of assessment, planning, and active interventions. Couples struggling with infertility need a great deal of support. They may feel the problem "runs their lives," and that they must have sex "on demand." They may be deluged with advice from friends and family and they may not be ready for alternatives until the whole grieving process has occurred; that is, grieving for loss of reproductive abilities. Only then will they be ready to hear about new techniques.

The health-care community continues to develop new interventions to assist infertile couples achieve parenthood. The process of assessment and treatment is slow and years may pass before successful conception occurs (Kolata 1979, 85). The assessment process may be threatening. Both men and women may feel inadequate when confronted. As Kolata reports, "Some men feel so threatened that they will not have a sperm test" (1979, 85).

Microsurgery offers new hope to women with blocked fallopian tubes. Success rates are considerably better than those claimed for traditional tuboplasty techniques.

If the vas deferens is occluded by voluntary sterilization or by anomaly or disease, reconstruction may be attempted. Microsurgery can be used for this procedure (Decker 1978, 258–259).

Failure to ovulate can be treated with clomiphene citrate. This compound is a weak estrogen and competes with estrogen for binding sites in the hypothalamus. Thus, administration causes FSH (follicle-stimulating hormone) and LH (lutenizing hormone) to rise and production of estrogen in the ovary to increase. This latter effect triggers LH release, causing ovulation to occur (Taymor 1978, 182–183). Those women who do not produce sufficient gonadotropins to induce ovulation may be treated with menotropins (human menopausal gonadotropins) (Oelsner et al. 1978). When excessive amounts of prolactin are being produced, bromocriptine mesylate can be used to reduce its secretion (Kolata 1978, 86–87).

Work on extrauterine fertilization techniques has reached the point of clinical application. In 1981 the first "test-tube" babies were born (First 'Test-Tube' Baby 1981, 38; Strickland 1981). The technique involves using a laparoscope to visualize an egg cell about to rupture, suctioning the egg cell out of the ovary, removing the egg from the cell and placing it in a culture dish with sperm and certain chemicals. The egg, once fertilized and developing as a blastocyst, is then inserted into the woman's uterus through her cervix where, hopefully, implantation and normal development will occur (First 'Test-Tube' Baby 1981, 311).

Artificial insemination is a technique used to help certain infertile couples. If the partner's sperm count is low, several ejaculations can be collected, concentrated, and insemination attempted during the woman's fertile period. Sometimes clomiphene citrate is used to induce ovulation in the woman in combination with artificial insemination. Other reasons for homologous insemination are disturbances in sexual function, structural anomalies of the cervix or vagina, epispadias and hypospadias, and hostile cervical mucus (Gilbert 1976, 259).

When the male partner is sterile, has a severe hereditary defect, or if there is an ABO or rhesus incompatibility, heterologous insemination may be chosen. Unlike partner donors, however, heterologous donation has legal implications. A few states have statutes that legitimize donor insemination (Taymor 1978, 206). In others, the legal status is ambiguous and some suits have occurred in the lower courts. The psychological effects of artificial insemination with donor sperm can be profound; the couple should be carefully counseled prior to choosing this procedure.

When sperm antibodies are present, use of a condom for some time prior to conception (if the woman has antibodies) or methylprednisolone therapy (if the male has antibodies), may allow conception to occur (Friedman 1981, 2046).

Other alternatives available to the couple experiencing infertility include surrogate mothering and adoption. *Surrogate mothering* is an alternative when the woman is sterile, has an anatomic anomaly that precludes pregnancy such as congenital absence of the uterus or ovaries, or has undergone hysterectomy prior to childbearing. In surrogate mothering, the host mother is artificially inseminated with sperm from the male member of the couple desiring a child. When the baby is born, the couple become the legal parents. In 1983, several legal cases resulted from the practice of surrogate mothering. In one case, the biological mother wanted to keep the child. In another, the father refused to take the child, due to the presence of a congenital anomaly. The practice of surrogate mothering is very controversial and is surrounded by some serious legal and ethical questions.

Adoption has become more difficult within the past decade or two as the result of several changes in our society. The availability of safe legal abortion has given women an alternative to bearing an unwanted child and then releasing that child for adoption. In addition, a large number of women who bear a child and are not involved in a committed relationship now choose to keep their children. Thus, the children most readily available for adoption are those who are past infancy, those with congenital anomalies, those of mixed racial origins, and those from foreign countries. The process of adoption is a very long and tedious one, usually requiring a wait of a year or more after approval for the placement of a child.

Support for Infertile Couples

Couples who are faced with loss of reproductive integrity need a great deal of support from health-care professionals through the long processes of assessment and intervention. The process may seem endless and the results are not guaranteed. Since sexuality is an integral part of self, threats to or loss of reproductive integrity affect self-image. As a result of the stresses infertility imposes, in 1973 a support group—RESOLVE—was formed to assist couples (Menning 1976, 258–259). It began as a small, free telephone counseling service and has grown to be an important source of information and support for involuntarily childless couples.

Individuals who experience infertility invariably go through periods of crisis during the processes of diagnosis and treatment. The nurse, therefore, should be constantly alert to signs of crisis and intervene by encouraging communication between the partners, by enhancing communication with other family members, by explaining all procedures and discussing alternatives in the diagnostic and therapeutic regimens, and by referring the couple for professional counseling if necessary. Loss of self-esteem and threats to masculinity and femininity are common among couples. Acknowledging that these feelings are common and normal and discussing them can be very helpful (NAACOG 1982, 5).

Couples who experience prolonged infertility will often experience the same stages of grieving that would occur with the loss of a loved one. The first response is usually denial, followed by anger, guilt, rage, and depression. Nurses are in key positions to help couples resolve their grieving (NAACOG 1982, 5).

Nurses working with couples experiencing fertility problems can also help in other ways. The nurse can help to interpret and describe the various steps in a fertility workup and can perform some of the tests. She/he can discuss with the couple the need for and value of various procedures and help them make informed decisions regarding the steps they wish to take in diagnosing and treating the problem. She/he can be a sounding board for feelings and frustrations and a source of support and counseling. Most of all, she/he is a resource person for the couple to help alleviate the emotional stress that inevitably accompanies infertility (NAACOG 1982, 6).

Voluntary Sterilization

Control of fertility probably predates written history. Voluntary sterilization has now superseded the use of oral contraceptives as a means of fertility control in the United States (Kash 1984, 17). Most people are sterilized by choice and are happy with that choice. However, since sterilization represents loss of an important and intimate function, it is understandable that some men and women will perceive loss of reproductive integrity through sterilization as a threat to self-image and sexuality at a time subsequent to the procedure (Stone, 1979).

Clients are informed that sterilization must be considered a permanent and irreversible procedure (Association for Voluntary Sterilization 1979). Some, however, seek reversal because of changes in life situations and the desire to become a parent. As the demand for sterilization has increased, so has the demand for reversal. Health-care professionals need to be cognizant of the crisis voluntary sterilization may subsequently produce if reversal is desired. Desire for more children and infant deaths are major reasons for reversal requests (Gomel 1978, 41). The latter crisis, then, compounds the crisis of sterility. If a change in marital status precipitates the decision, that, too, may represent crisis for the individual (Harrison and deBoer 1977, 95). The increase for requests for reversal in recent years underlines the need for careful counseling and informed consent prior to sterilization. Exploration of perceived effects on sexuality will help to prevent crises precipitated by sterility, whether or not reversal is ultimately sought.

Parenting of a Child with Ambiguous or Anomalous Genitalia

The first question parents usually ask when a baby is born concerns its sex. When a child is born with ambiguous genitalia, one or both parents may perceive a threat to or loss of their reproductive integrity and, possibly, an assault on their sexuality. After the initial assessment confirms the observation of external genitalia, in-depth assessment should be done promptly so that sex assignment and treatment can be undertaken (Hill 1977, 810). If delay occurs, parents will assign a sex. If they are incorrect, later relinquishing a son or daughter can be a painful experience. Support for parents transfers to a healthy shaping of gender role for the child (Hill 1977, 813).

Demythologizing sexual ambiguity for parents is important to their relationship with their child, as well as to their feelings about themselves as sexual human beings. Correct use of vocabulary terms for genital structures and for the anatomical parts present or absent in their child will help the parents communicate with family and friends (Hill 1977, 813).

Children with ambiguous genitalia may experience a crisis in sexual identity as well. They will need not only the love and support of parents, but also that of health-care professionals. As they mature, they need honest answers about their own sexual development and reproductive potential. Surgery may be necessary or desired to ensure the most normal psychosexual development possible. Sex change may also be requested to grant psychosexual compatibility (Hill 1977, 814).

Health-care providers must be aware of the potential for crisis and the needs of parents who produce a child with ambiguous genitalia and those of the child at each developmental stage. Sensitive interventions can help to avert crisis and/or assist the individuals to an optimal level of wellness post-crisis (see Chapter 1).

Hysterectomy

Hysterectomy is the most frequently performed major surgical procedure in the United States (see Figure 7-1). It is estimated that between 750,000 and 800,000 hysterectomies are performed each year (Krauss 1979, 289). For the woman whose identity and femininity are defined by the ability to bear children, a hysterectomy may represent a crisis. The woman may respond to loss of her reproductive integrity with a decrease in sexual desire, depression, and perceived loss of femininity. Her husband, too, may view hysterectomy as synonymous with loss of sexuality (Wolf 1970). In one study, the majority of women did not appear to experience major changes in sexuality after hysterectomy (Humphries 1980, 12). However, a significant number indicated some problems appropriate for preoperative/postoperative counseling regarding sexuality (Humphries 1980, 10–13). In another study, some unrealistic beliefs about sexual sequelae were identified (Cosper et al. 1978, 11), but most women reported positive feelings about sexuality (p. 10).

Burchell points out that the uterus has three possible functions: reproductive, menstrual, and sexual (1977). It follows, then, that a woman's response to hysterectomy will be related to how she views and values these functions. One woman may feel relief when she no longer has to cope with menstruation or fear of pregnancy, whereas another woman may feel empty or stripped of her femininity. The reason for the surgery will, of course, affect the woman's response. If it is for cancer, sexual issues will be overshadowed by issues of death.

Masters and Johnson (1966) found in their research that the uterus is involved in all four stages of sexual arousal. It would seem probable, then, that a woman would experience some changes in sexual response after a hysterectomy. Pressure on the vaginal cuff during penile thrusting can cause pain for the woman who has had a hysterectomy. The optimal position for the cuff is on the superior wall of the vagina (Morgan 1978, 5). The vagina may be shortened after surgery. Resuming intercourse as soon as it is comfortable to do so will

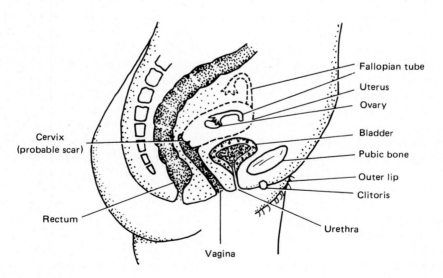

FIGURE 7-1
Hysterectomy.

SOURCE: Adapted from Boston Women's Health Collective, 1976. *Our bodies, ourselves.* 2nd ed. New York: Simon & Schuster.

help the vagina expand to accommodate penetration. Trauma to the bladder during surgery can mean pain during sex. Excess flatus beyond the immediate postoperative period can impede sexual feelings (Morgan 1978, 5). Preparing the woman for the effects of complications, if they occur, will help her cope with temporary effects on her sexuality.

If the ovaries have been removed, the resulting decrease in estrogen can cause vaginal atrophy and dryness. Lubrication is scanty and occurs more slowly. Supplementary lubrication with water-soluble jelly, saliva, coconut oil, cocoa butter, safflower oil, or other vegetable oils can be helpful, as well as counseling the woman and her partner to allow more time for arousal and lubrication to occur. Estrogen replacement therapy will resolve the problem, but the dangers mediate against its routine use (Morgan 1978, 6), as discussed in Chapter 6. Topical estrogen creams are absorbed systemically and bypass the liver, so the danger may be even greater than that for oral forms. Less vasocongestion occurs, so the feeling of arousal may be less intense (Morgan 1978, 6). Women need to know about these possible changes in order to realize they are normal and cope with them appropriately. Coming as a surprise, they may reinforce some women's feelings of sexual inadequacy or the perception that their lives as sexual beings have ended.

The responses of the woman's partner to the procedure will affect her coping. Some men taunt their partners with being "neutered" or "half a woman" or refuse to have sex. These men are rare, but the lesson they teach us is to be sensitive to the needs of the partner for support and accurate information (Morgan 1980, 26).

Implications for nursing include teaching women about biophysical changes they can expect after surgery that may affect sexual expression, emphasizing positive influences on sexuality (freedom from fear of pregnancy and from menses, relief of symptoms), and dispelling myths. Women need to know that hysterectomy does not mean an end to sexuality or femininity (Williams 1976, 439). The influence of cultural patterns should be considered when assessing a woman's response to her hysterectomy. The common experience of depression should be recognized, especially for its effects on sexual desire and expression.

Castration

Although castration (removal of the testicles) is a rare surgical procedure for a male, it usually, if not always, precipitates or occurs in conjunction with crisis. Castration is generally done only as a treatment measure for carcinoma or in the case of devastating and irreparable trauma. The reactions of the individual and society are far different when a man is castrated than when a woman has her ovaries removed. Since a man's genitals are mostly external, his sexual identity is closely tied to the reassurance he receives from touching or viewing them. The biophysical changes are notably more profound when testicles are removed than when an oophorectomy (removal of one or both ovaries) is done: erection problems, weight changes, fat deposits, breast growth, flabby skin, hair loss, hot flashes, brain pressure, dizziness, and heart disorders (Nass, Libby, and Fisher 1981, 401–402). The psychosocial consequences are, therefore, also greater.

Since the operation is so rarely performed, most men have no peer group for support. A man who has undergone this operation may, therefore, be almost completely dependent on health-care professionals for information and support through the crisis. His family and significant others, too, will need support, correct information, and help in reaching out and caring. The crisis in the client's sexuality will need to be dealt with sensitively and openly if he is to make the necessary adjustments to achieve an optimum possible level of biophysical and psychosexual wellness after the surgery.

DES Exposure

Those persons who were exposed in utero to diethylstilbestrol (DES) have sustained a unique threat to their sexual and reproductive integrity. As indicated in Chapter 4, during the decades between 1940 and 1970 DES was prescribed to pregnant women at risk for pregnancy loss under the belief that it would help to prevent loss. In 1971 a link was found between DES exposure in utero and a rare form of vaginal or cervical cancer called clear-cell adenocarcinoma (National Institutes of Health [NIH] 1977, 2–3). Although this form of cancer is rarely found, other benign conditions have been associated with DES exposure. These included extra tissue around the cervix ("hooded" cervix) or vagina (adenosis) and cell changes in the vaginal and mucosa and cervical epithelium (ectropion) (NIH 1980). Ridges in the vagina have been noticed in some women (O'Brien et al. 1979, 300). Although development of clear-cell adenocarcinoma is rare after initial negative exams, cases are beginning to appear in the literature (Anderson et al. 1979). The carcinogenic effects seem to have latent phases of 10 to 20 years. Malignancies occur in women between 14 and the mid-20s, peaking at age 19 (Anderson et al. 1979, 297). Women who have been exposed in utero also have a more frequent incidence of miscarriage and stillbirths (NIH 1980).

Significant differences in pregnancy outcome have been demonstrated in DES daughters. Infertility rates are higher than for unexposed women. A high rate of premature births seems to occur. Some women exhibit T-shaped or hypoplastic uteri and incompetent cervix. Those women who have cervico-vaginal ridges seem to have more pregnancy failures (Herbst et al. 1980, 67–68; Barnes et al. 1980; Kaufman et al. 1981).

Effects have also been detected in male offspring exposed in utero. Noncancerous changes in the testicles and penis have been found such as undescended testicles, cysts, and lowered sperm counts (DES Action 1978; DES 1976, 99).

Women who took DES during their pregnancies may be at greater risk for cancers of the breast and reproductive organs. Data are less conclusive than for their daughters and further study is underway (NIH 1980).

Women and men exposed to DES need to have complete history and physical examinations done. The daughters need, in addition, to have a Schiller's test and a colposcopy. Pap smears should be done, but will detect only cervical changes unless four quadrant vaginal scrapings are done (Reagan and Olaizola 1980, 101). These must be accompanied by palpation and biopsy of suspicious tissue (Anderson et al. 1979, 298).

When carcinoma does occur, radical surgery is often done. Vaginectomy and hysterectomy followed by vaginoplasty may be the treatment of choice. Some women have also had an oophorectomy and cystectomy done. Several young women have died as a result of metastatic cancer originating as clear-cell adenocarcinoma secondary to DES exposure in utero (Stilbestrol 1973, 15).

Mutilating vaginal surgery can have profound effects on the women who are its victims. Both biophysical and psychosexual crises are common when young women, at the threshold of their adult sexuality, experience the most devastating effects of DES exposure. Men who have abnormalities of their genitals are also at risk for crisis in relation to their reproductive and psychosexual integrity. Even when carcinoma is not present, those who have been exposed must live with this threat to their sexual integrity. Support and help groups for victims of DES exposure have been formed (Rockwood 1977, 18; National Women's Health Network 1980). A number of class-action suits have been filed against drug companies asking that funds be set up to assist victims with special examinations and treatment (Worthington 1977, 17).

Toxic Shock Syndrome

Toxic shock syndrome was first described as a distinct entity in 1978. In 1980, the Centers for Disease Control in Atlanta confirmed several hundred cases, some of which were fatal (1980). The syndrome has come to be associated with the use of vaginal tampons, although nonmenstruating women, men, and children can also be affected. The organism responsible for the syndrome is *Staphylococcus aureus,* a normal inhabitant of the vaginas of some women (Helgerson 1981, 99).

In its acute form, toxic shock syndrome is characterized by sudden onset of a very high fever, vomiting, and diarrhea, and, if not recognized and treated, proceeds rapidly to hypotension and shock. Accompanying symptoms include an erythematous macular sunburn-like rash that after ten days or so desquamates and is particularly marked on the palms of the hands and the soles of the feet. Other organ systems can be involved including gastro-intestinal, renal, muscular, mucous membranes, hepatic, hematologic, and the central nervous system (Wroblewski 1981, 82–83; Pope 1981, 31–32).

Approximately two-thirds of the cases have occurred in women between 15 and 24 years of age who are menstruating and using tampons. As of July 1, 1982, 95% of all reported cases have occurred in women and 90% occurred during a menstrual period; almost all of the latter group were using tampons (Tampons and Toxic Shock 1982, 2). The mecha-

nism of the relationship with tampons is unknown at present (Toxic Shock 1982; Oram and Beck 1981).

The most important implications for health-care professionals include education of clients in tampon use, the early recognition of signs and symptoms, and prompt reporting and treatment. Recommendations on tampon use include avoidance of superabsorbent brands, alternating use of tampons with pads, avoiding prolonged use, and using tampons only when flow is heavy to avoid damage to the mucosa on insertion and removal (Wroblewski 1981, 85).

Loss of Sexual Function

The loss of one's ability to function as a sexual being can constitute a crisis. We all have criteria for our sexual "performance" and when we are unable to meet those criteria, we experience loss of a very important function. How each individual views his or her sexuality will, of course, affect the perception of crisis. A person can be said to be sexually dysfunctional, at least in a relative way, if he is impotant or has disturbances of ejaculation, or if she does not experience orgasm, has vaginismus, or if either partner experiences sexual aversion or dyspareunia (Bransfield 1979). Or put another way, "sexual dysfunction is a physiologic alteration in the sexual response cycle, specifically in the excitement, plateau, orgasm, or resolution phase" (Elmassian and Wilson 1982, 14). Some authors distinguish between sexual performance and psychological-perceptual dysfunctions (Kaplan 1974; Lief 1977).

General approaches to therapy for sexual dysfunctions are described in Table 7-2. The following sections discuss specific dysfunctions, their causes, and possible self-help or

TABLE 7-2   *Therapies for Loss of Sexual Function*

Therapists	Techniques
Masters and Johnson	Behavior modification strategies Couple counseling Male and female therapist teams Sexual "tasks" (such as spending a minimum specified time on foreplay) Specific techniques for problems identified
Kaplan	Combines Masters and Johnson with in-depth psychoanalysis Generally one therapist Unravel sources of problems, fears Develop insight into sexual dysfunction
Hartman and Fithian and others	Based on high-level wellness sexology exam to measure sexual response Help individual understand his/her own response Hypnosis used sometimes
Heiman, LoPiccolo, LoPiccolo	Work with singles and couples Become familiar with one's own genitals and attitudes toward sex Explore own body Learn self-stimulation to climax Share with partner

SOURCE: Data from: Nass, G. D., R. W. Libby, and M. P. Fisher. 1981. *Sexual choices.* Monterey, Calif.: Wadsworth; Masters, W. H., and V. E. Johnson. 1970. *Human sexual inadequacy.* Boston: Little, Brown; Kaplan, H. S. 1974. *The new sex therapy.* New York: Brunner/Mazel; Kaplan, H. S. 1979. *Disorders of sexual desire.* New York: Simon & Schuster; Hartman, W. E., and M. A. Fithian. 1972. *Treatment of sexual dysfunction.* Long Beach, Calif.: Center for Marital and Sexual Studies; Heiman, J., L. LoPiccolo, and J. LoPiccolo. 1976. *Becoming orgasmic: A sexual growth program for women.* Englewood Cliffs, N.J.: Prentice-Hall.

professional measures for overcoming these difficulties.

Impotence

Inability to attain or maintain an erection to have intercourse is known as *impotence.* A small percentage of men experience difficulties with erection due to biophysical causes; the rest are due to psychosexual origins. Biophysical causes are many: anomalies in anatomy; cardiorespiratory, genitourinary, hematologic, endocrine, vascular or neurologic problems; drug use; infection; and miscellaneous, such as obesity (Kolodny et al. 1979, 376–377; Cooper 1972). Heavy drinking has been implicated as a cause of impotence (Lemere and Smith 1973). Psychosexual reasons include developmental, affective, interpersonal, and cognitive factors (Kolodny et al. 1979, 378).

The first step in helping men with problems of erection is a careful history and physical examination to ascertain the cause or causes. Sometimes there is more than one cause such as the presence of a chronic disease and fear of death or serious risk if orgasm occurs. Or the man may fear for the safety of his partner if she has a chronic or terminal disease or is recovering from an illness or surgery. The partner may be included in the assessment process, when desired and appropriate, as the cause may rest with both persons.

Interventions focus on minimizing the effects of biophysical factors, whenever possible, and on providing appropriate counseling or therapy for the individual and/or the couple (Finkle and Thompson 1972; Holdsworth and Daines 1978; Kolodny et al. 1979, 386–389). Special training as a sex therapist or counselor is usually necessary to intervene, especially when psychosexual causes are identified.

A relatively new form of therapy for organic impotence is the penile implant. Two types are available, one of which is inflatable. Nurses are involved in the hospital care of men undergoing implant (Wood and Rose 1978). Being well informed about the type of implant, the surgical procedure, and any complications—as well as the organic reasons creating the need for implant—will help the nurse respond professionally and empathically. A new inflatable penile prosthesis is described in the literature (Googe and Mook 1983).

Premature or Retarded Ejaculation

In the male, disturbances of orgasm involve either premature or retarded ejaculation. Definitions vary as to what time span constitutes premature ejaculation. It is generally agreed that premature ejaculation is present when the man can exert little or no control over the timing of ejaculation or when the man cannot delay ejaculation to allow his partner to reach orgasm more than 50% of the time (Elmassian and Wilson 1982, 19).

Causes of premature ejaculation are rarely physical. The only physical factors usually identified include chemical irritation of the glans (making it inordinately sensitive) and infection of the prostate or urethra. Because ejaculation and orgasm can come under voluntary control, the man who ejaculates prematurely may not have learned to recognize the signs of impending orgasm and learned to control the sensations. The anxiety surrounding first hurried sexual encounters may mediate for hasty ejaculation in order to avoid interruption or "being caught." Petting to the point of orgasm while fully clothed can also condition the man to associate orgasm with body pressure and rubbing instead of vaginal penetration (McCary and McCary 1982, 513). One should also not dismiss the man's perceptions of women and their sexual needs. Achieving orgasm too quickly can deprive the woman of sexual release and perpetuate the man's control and lack of concern for her needs.

Various techniques are suggested to delay ejaculation (Harrison and deBoer 1977, 87–89; Kolodny et al. 1979, 391–394). The squeeze technique prescribed by Masters and Johnson (1970) involves pressure to the penile glans when the man feels that he is about to reach orgasm. The pressure needs to be strong, short of the point of causing pain, and sustained until erection is nearly lost and the pressure of impending orgasm has passed. Semans suggests a similar start-stop sequence in which the partner stimulates the man to the point of imminent ejaculation and then ceases all stimulation. Semans (1956) suggests using several of these stimulation-stop sequences and then allowing the man to ejaculate. Once the man can sustain erection without orgasm for 15 to 20 minutes, the couple then proceed to intercourse, using the same technique of thrusting to the point just short of orgasm and repeating the sequence several times before going on to ejaculation. Siemens (1982) describes a similar technique.

Failure to ejaculate (ejaculatory incompetence or retarded ejaculation) is usually related to organic or drug-related causes or long-standing use of coitus interruptus (Harrison and deBoer 1977, 88). It has been estimated that 15% of the most-used prescription drugs can cause sexual problems (Sperm Count 1982). Ejaculatory problems may also be related to psychosexual factors such as a traumatic experience, dislike of the partner, or interruption of privacy.

The treatment for retarded ejaculation depends, of course, on the cause. If drugs are implicated, then perhaps dosage can be altered or the timing of ingestion changed to accommodate sexual habits. If the cause is related to sexual habits and activity, then attention should be focused on these. Assurance of privacy, a partner of the man's choosing and liking, and adequate stimulation are prerequisites to orgasm. The man may need extravaginal stimulation from his partner using oral or manual techniques. A cream or lotion that simulates the consistency of vaginal secretions may be helpful (McCary and McCary 1982, 516–517). If the origins of the problem lie in a deep sexual trauma, then the individual may need therapy with a professional in order to work through his feelings. If the man can ejaculate only through self-stimulation, then he needs a period of desensitization, progressing from masturbating alone, to doing so in the presence of his partner, and then to allowing the partner to stimulate his penis to orgasm (McCary and McCary 1982, 517).

Lack of Orgasm or Sexual Responsiveness in the Female

Women, too, may experience lack of orgasm; this is much more common than in men. They may have never achieved orgasm or may not be orgasmic at present. Organic causes account for only a small percentage of cases. These include hormonal imbalance, injuries or anomalies in anatomy, infections or lesions on the genitals, nerve impairment, aging, and abuse of drugs or alcohol. The rest are related to psychosocial cultural factors.

Relational disorders — that is, disruption of the relationship between partners — may suggest that the partner, too, is suffering from a sexual dysfunction. Lack of desirability in the partner, lack of privacy, and perception of the partner as the "wrong person" can disrupt intimacy. Shame, fear, and guilt are the most common causes of sexual dysfunction in women. These have their origins in religious and cultural upbringing, in lack of knowledge about the anatomy and physiology of the reproductive tract, in a whole series of myths about female sexuality and sexual responsiveness, and in fear of pregnancy. As with a man, careful assessment for biophysical and psychosocial factors is essential prior to institution of any interventions.

There are several forms that a woman's sexual dysfunction can take. The first of these is lack of responsiveness, ranging from feeling completely devoid of desire to inability to achieve orgasm. McCary and McCary (1982, 520) make the following suggestions for the woman who has little or no desire for sex: choosing an optimal time when the woman is free from distractions and well rested; choosing a time when the relationship is as free from disharmony as possible; kindness, consideration, caring, and multiple expressions of love by the partner, who should be intimately familiar with the woman's body including communicating with her about what she likes and doesn't like in stimulation; prolongation of foreplay and use of stimulants if desired; use of fantasy by the woman, and a combination of stroking, verbal endearments, body pressure, and rhythm.

Inability to reach orgasm is a problem many women experience. Those women with primary orgasmic dysfunction have never achieved orgasm; those women in the situational category experience disturbance in orgasmic response secondary to once having achieved orgasm. Causes are essentially the same as with sexual unresponsiveness (McCary and McCary 1982, 521).

Manual self-stimulation is usually useful in helping the woman experience the levels of sexual excitation leading to orgasm. If masturbation is unacceptable, however, preparation for such activity or alternate means of stimulation must be sought. Use of a vibrator or stimulation by the partner may be acceptable to the woman. She may also need to communicate her needs more clearly — where and when she wishes to be touched, and how. Combining vaginal penetration and thrusting with direct clitoral stimulation may be helpful.

Vaginismus

Vaginismus is involuntary spasm or constriction of the distal third of the vaginal musculature and around the introitus. These spasms may either prevent penetration or trap the penis. Organic causes can sometimes be identified or contribute to occurrence as in the case of a painful episiotomy or anterior-posterior repair. In most cases, the cause is psychosocial in origin. Some common psychosocial causes are rape trauma, fear of pain in penetration, or a partner's repeated impotence.

Intervention is based on careful history and assessment for cause(s). Inclusion of the partner may be helpful in resolving the problem. Sometimes fingers or graduated dilators are used to reprogram muscles (Kolodny et al. 1979, 405–408). Application of local anesthetic agents to the vagina and vaginal introitus can help reduce the pain. Many of the techniques for increasing responsiveness are also useful with vaginismus.

Lack of Desire

"Sexual aversion" is an inexact term for disturbances in sexual desire (Watts 1979, 1570). It may be exhibited either as a long-term phenomenon or secondary to a particular sexual experience or life crisis.

Social and cultural factors are influential in shaping one's attitudes toward sexuality and sexual expression. Experiences beginning with the identification of body parts as a very young child affect perceptions of the genitals and their functions. Parental reactions to masturbation give the child cues to sexual behavior. So does the information (or lack of it) concerning sexuality that parents feel they can share with their children.

Exposure to pornography can affect the individual's feelings about his or her body or that of the partner. A crisis experience focused on sexuality — such as sexual assault, incest, mutilating genital surgery, or undesired sterility — can change the individual's interest in sex.

Fear of pregnancy can inhibit responsiveness. So can the relationship drawn between sex and sin. The cultural milieu of the United States still has unwritten mores concerning sexuality outside of legal marriage. Sexuality is supposed to be suppressed until the wedding night. While this is often far from the case, such "rules" can serve to affect sexual desire or responses.

The importance or priority sexuality is given by an individual will affect his or her responses to sexual overtures and degree of sexual desire.

Role definitions affect our sexual desires. Men are supposed to have insatiable sexual appetites, whereas women are supposed to be disinterested and passive. Outdated and false as these mythical roles are, they live on.

The obsession of our society with cleanliness, with euphemisms for urinating and defecation, and our discomfort with body issues carry mixed messages. It is difficult for some persons to disassociate sex and genitals from processes of elimination (Nass, Libby, and Fisher 1981, 147).

Clinical depression, certain pharmacologic agents, and interpersonal conflicts can also account for a decrease or absence of sexual desire (Watts 1979, 1571).

When the level of sexual desire is significantly diminished for a period of time, the individual may be motivated to seek help. Assessment of the history of desire and sexual experiences is a first step to identifying causes. Often complex factors are involved. Referral for sex therapy or other professional counseling may be appropriate. Nurses can participate in many levels of care depending upon their experience, preparation, and rapport with the client. Some self-help materials are also available (Heiman et al. 1976; Nowinski 1980).

Dyspareunia

When an individual experiences pain during intercourse (*dyspareunia*), it can precipitate a crisis for that individual and/or the partner. Pain other than that associated with vaginismus or psychogenic causes during sex can be due to organic causes. Some causes of pain include infection (vaginitis, sexually transmitted diseases), pelvic pathology (pelvic inflammatory disease), local irritation of vulva, vagina, clitoris, penis, or scrotum, inadequate lubrication, and bumping of the cervix or tension of the uterine ligaments, especially during deep thrusting (Boston Women's Health Collective 1976, 58). Pain can also be due to congenital misplacement of the urethral meatus at the edge of the vaginal opening. This condition can be corrected surgically by creating a space between the introitus and the meatus to relieve the chronic irritation and dyspareunia (Hensel 1982, 67). Tension and preoccupation or attempts at penetration prior to sufficient arousal can cause vaginal pain during intercourse.

When professional help is sought, the first step is a careful history and physical examination to identify a reason for the pain. Most of the organic causes have straightforward medical and nursing interventions. For the woman experiencing ligament or cervical pain, altering position, depth, and angle of penetration may relieve the symptoms. Individuals need support and help through any threat or crisis involving sexual performance or response and reassurance that the problems are often experienced by others and can be resolved.

Summary of Implications for Nursing Practice

A crisis or threat to sexual integrity can affect all aspects of the life of the individual. Sexuality is an integral part of self and sexual health can be an important index of well-being for an individual. Nurses play a critical role in assessing and intervening in crisis and helping the individual achieve the optimal level of wellness post-crisis. In issues of sexuality, they may be the primary intervenors or work collaboratively with other members of the team. Cognizance of the variety of hazardous events an individual can experience that may precipitate crisis will help the nurse in planning preventive strategies, as well as recognizing the event responsible for crisis when it does occur.

REFERENCES

Abarbanel, G. 1976. Helping victims of rape. *Social Work* 21(11):478–482.

Abarbanel, G., and S. Rebello. 1981. *Being Safe.* Santa Monica, Calif.: Rape Treatment Center.

Alexander, C. S. 1980. Blaming the victim: A comparison of police and nurses' perceptions of victims of rape. *Women & Health* 5(1):65–79.

Alliance Against Sexual Coercion. 1981. *Fighting sexual harassment.* Boston: Alyson and Alliance Against Sexual Coercion.

Anderson, B., W. G. Watring, D. D. Edinger, E. D. Small, A. T. Netland, and H. Safaii. 1979. Development of DES-associated clear-cell carcinoma: The importance of regular screening. *Obstetrics & Gynecology* 53(3):293–299.

Association for Voluntary Sterilization. 1979. *Voluntary sterilization.* New York: Association for Voluntary Sterilization.

Barnes, A. B., T. Cotton, J. Gundersen, I. L. Noller, B. C. Tilley, T. Strama, D. E. Townsend, P. Hatab, and P. C. O'Brien. 1980. Fertility and outcome of pregnancy in women exposed in utero to diethylstilbestrol. *The New England Journal of Medicine* 302(11):609–613.

Barry, K. 1979b. *Female sexual slavery.* Englewood Cliffs, N.J.: Prentice-Hall.

Barry, K. 1979a. Terror and coercion, the female sexual slave trade. *Ms.,* 8(5).

Berger, A. S., W. Simon, and J. H. Gagnon. 1973. Youth and pornography in social context. *Archives of Sexual Behavior* 2(4):279–308.

Blitman, N., and R. Green. 1975. Inez Garcia on trial. *Ms.,* 3(11).

Bluglass, R. 1979. Incest. *British Journal of Hospital Medicine* 22(2):152–157.

Boles, J. M., and A. P. Garbin. 1974. The choice of stripping for a living. *Sociology of Work and Occupations* 1(1):111–123.

Boles, J. M., and A. P. Garbin. 1974. The strip club and stripper-customer patterns of interaction. *Sociology and Social Research* 58(2):136–144.

Boston Women's Health Collective. 1976. *Our bodies, ourselves.* 2d ed. New York: Simon & Schuster.

Bransfield, D. D. 1979. Female sexual dysfunction definitions. Paper presented at conference, Human Sexuality for the Health Practitioner, 1 December, at the University of Connecticut Health Center, Farmington.

Brehm, A. K. no date. *Defining the problem of battering questions and answers.* Luverne, Minn.: Southwestern Mental Health Center.

Brown, C., J. Anderson, L. Burggrat, and N. Thompson. 1978. Community standards, conservatism, and judgments of pornography. *The Journal of Sex Research* 14(2):81–95.

Brownmiller, S. 1975. *Against our will.* New York: Simon & Schuster.

Bullough, V., and B. Bullough. 1978. *Prostitution: An illustrated social history.* New York: Crown Publishers.

Burchell, R. C. 1977. Hysterectomy: Functional versus anatomic considerations. *Cancer* 27:241–242.

Burgess, A. W. 1978. The rape victim: Nursing implications. *The Journal of Practical Nursing* 28(11):14–15.

Burgess, A. W., and H. J. Birnbaum. 1982. Youth Prostitution. *American Journal of Nursing* 82(5):832–834.

Burgess, A. W., A. N. Groth, L. L. Holmstrom, and S. M. Sgroi. 1978. *Sexual assault of children and adolescents.* Lexington, Mass.: Lexington Books.

Burgess, A. W., and L. L. Holmstrom. 1979a. *Rape Crisis and Recovery.* Bowie, Md.: Robert J. Brady.

Burgess, A. W., and L. L. Holmstrom. 1974. *Rape: Victims of crisis.* Bowie, Md.: Robert J. Brady.

Burgess, A. W., and L. L. Holmstrom. 1973. The rape victim in the emergency ward. *American Journal of Nursing* 73(10):1741–1745.

Burgess, A. W., and L. L. Holmstrom. 1979b. Rape: Disclosure to parental family members. *Women & Health* 4(3):255–268.

Burgess, A. W., and A. T. Laszlo. 1977. Courtroom use of hospital records in sexual assault cases. *American Journal of Nursing* 77(1):64–68.

Burgess, A. W., and M. P. McCausland. 1979a. Sexual exploitation of children through sex rings. In *Clinical and scientific sessions.* Kansas City, Mo.: American Nurses' Association.

Bush, M. 1975. Sex offenders are people! *Journal of Psychiatric and Mental Health Services* 13(4):38–40.

Bushnell, J. L., M. J. Burke, M. Arnsdorf, and P. D. Steele. 1980. Evaluation of a sexual assault treatment center. *Nursing Administration Quarterly* 4(3):61–80.

Centers for Disease Control. 1980. Toxic-shock syndrome—United States. *Morbidity and Mortality Weekly Report* 29:229–230.

Cooper, A. J. 1972. Diagnosis and management of "endocrine impotence." *British Medical Journal* 2:34–36.

Cosper, B., S. S. Fuller, and G. J. Robinson. 1978. Characteristics of post-hospitalization recovery following hysterectomy. *Journal of Obstetric, Gynecologic, and Neonatal Nursing* 7(3):7–11.

Damrosch, S. P. 1981. How nursing students' reactions to rape victims are affected by a perceived act of carelessness. *Nursing Research* 30(3):168–170.

Decker, A. 1978. *Why can't we have a baby?* New York: Warner Books.

DeFrancis, V. 1969. *Protecting the child victim of sex crimes committed by adults.* Denver: American Human Association.

DES Action. 1978. *If you were born after 1940, you may be a DES daughter.* San Francisco: Coalition for the Medical Rights of Women.

DES: Potential risk for men, too? 1976. *Medical World News,* 26 Jan, 99–100.

Dixon, K. N., L. E. Arnold, and K. Calestro. 1978. Father-son incest: Underreported psychiatric problem? *American Journal of Psychiatry* 135(7):835–838.

Dudar, H. 1977. America discovers child pornography. *Ms.,* 6(2).

Duldt, B. W. 1982. Sexual harassment in nursing. *Nursing Outlook* 30(6):336–343.

Dutton, D., and S. L. Painter. 1981. Traumatic bonding: The development of emotional attachments in battered women and other relationships of intermittent abuse. *Victimology: an International Journal* 6(1–4):139–155.

Dworkin, A. 1981. *Pornography: Men possessing women.* New York: Putnam/Perigee.

Ellis, E. M., K. S. Calhoun, and B. M. Alkeson.

1980. Sexual dysfunction in victims of rape. *Women & Health* 5(4):39–47.

Elmassian, B. J., and R. W. Wilson. 1982. Assessment and diagnosis of sexual problems. *The Nurse Practitioner* 1(6):13–15,19,22.

Exner, J. E., J. Wylie, A. Leura, and T. Parrill. 1977. Some psychological characteristics of prostitutes. *Journal of Personality Assessment* 41(5):474–485.

Fingler, L. 1981. Teenagers in survey condone forced sex. *Ms.,* 9(8):23.

Finkle, A. L., and R. Thompson. 1972. Urologic counseling in male sexual impotence. *Geriatrics* 27(12):67–72.

Finkelhor, D. 1980. Sex among siblings: A survey on prevalence, variety, and effects. *Archives of Sexual Behavior* 9(3):171–194.

Finkelhor, D. 1978. Psychological, cultural and family factors in incest and family sexual abuse. *Journal of Marriage and Family Counseling* 4(4):41–49.

First 'test-tube' baby. 1981. *Science News* 119(20):311.

Fox, L. 1981. Rape: A violent crime that affects us all. *Nursing Pulse* 1(2):1–2.

Fox, R. 1980. *The red lamp of incest.* London: Hutchinson.

Friedman, B. M. 1981. Infertility workup. *American Journal of Nursing* 81(11):2041–2046.

Gilbert, S. 1976. Artificial insemination. *American Journal of Nursing* 76(2):259.

Gingold, J. 1976. One of these days—pow, right in the kisser. *Ms.,* 5(2):51–54.

Goodwin, J., M. Simms, and R. Bergman. 1979. Hysterical seizures: A sequel to incest. *American Journal of Orthopsychiatry* 49(4):698–703.

Gorline, L. L., and M. M. Ray. 1979. Examining and caring for the child who has been sexually assaulted. *The American Journal of Maternal Child Nursing* 4(2):110–114.

Gomel, V. 1978. Profile of women requesting reversal of sterilization. *Fertility and Sterility* 30(1):39–41.

Googe, M. C. S., and T. M. Mook. 1983. The inflatable penile prosthesis: New developments. *American Journal of Nursing* 83 (7): 1044–1047.

Green, T. H. 1977. *Gynecology essentials of clinical practice.* Boston: Little, Brown.

Greenbaum, H. 1973. Marriage, family, and parenthood. *American Journal of Psychiatry* 130:1261–1265.

Griffin, S. 1981. *Pornography and silence: Culture's revenge against nature.* New York: Harper & Row.

Gross, M. 1979. Incestuous rape: A cause for hysterical seizures in four adolescent girls. *American Journal of Orthopsychiatry* 49(4):704–708.

Groth, A. N., and A. W. Burgess. 1977. Motivational intent in the sexual assault of children. *Criminal Justice Behavior* 4(3):253–264.

Gutheil, T. G., and N. C. Avery. 1977. Multiple overt incest as family defense against loss. *Family Process* 16(1):105–116.

Harrison, R. G., and C. H. deBoer. 1977. *Sex and infertility.* New York: Academic Press.

Hartman, W. E., and M. A. Fithian. 1972. *Treatment of sexual dysfunction.* Long Beach, Calif.: Center for Marital and Sexual Studies.

Hawkins, J. W. 1982. Loss of reproductive integrity. In *Crisis theory: A framework for nursing practice,* ed. M. S. Infante. Reston, Va.: Reston Publishing.

Hawkins, J. W., and L. P. Higgins. 1981. *Maternity & gynecological nursing: Women's health care.* Philadelphia: Lippincott.

Heiman, J., L. LoPiccolo, and J. LoPiccolo. 1976. *Becoming orgasmic: A sexual growth program for women.* Englewood Cliffs, N.J.: Prentice-Hall.

Heim, N., and C. J. Hursch. 1979. Castration for sex offenders: Treatment or punishment? A review and critique of recent European literature. *Archives of Sexual Behavior* 8(3):281–304.

Helgerson, S. D. 1981. Toxic shock syndrome. Tampons, toxins, and time: The evolution of understanding an illness. *Women & Health* 6(3/4):93–104.

Hensel, H. A. 1982. Surgical relief of dyspareunia. *The Female Patient* 1(67–69).

Herbst, A. L., M. M. Hubby, R. R. Blough, and F. Azizi. 1980. A comparison of pregnancy experience in DES-exposed and DES-unexposed daughters. *The Journal of Reproductive Medicine* 24(2):62–69.

Herman, J. L. 1981a. Incest: Prevention is the only cure. *Ms.,* 10(5):63–64.

Herman, J. L. 1981b. *Father-daughter incest.* Cambridge, Mass.: Harvard University Press.

He told me not to tell. 1979. Renton, Wash.: King Co. Rape Relief.

Hill, S. 1977. The child with ambiguous genitalia. *American Journal of Nursing* 77(5):810–814.

Holdsworth, A. V., and B. Daines. 1978. Sex problems in marrige. *Nursing Mirror* 147:23–25.

Horsley, J. 1980. MD rape: Why you can be indicted. *RN* 43(9):71–72.

Humphries, P. T. 1980. Sexual adjustment after a hysterectomy. *Issues in Health Care of Women* 2(2):1–14.

Jaget, C., ed. 1981. *Prostitutes: Our life.* Falling Wall Press.

James, J. 1973. Prostitute-pimp relationships. *Medical Aspects of Human Sexuality* 7(11):147–160.

James, J., and J. Meyerding. 1977. Early sexual experience as a factor in prostitution. *Archives of Sexual Behavior* 7(1):31–42.

Jury finds for nurse plaintiff in rape trial, convicts MD's. 1981. *Nursing Pulse* 1(23):1.

Kaplan, H. S. 1974. *The new sex therapy.* New York: Brunner/Mazel.

Kaplan, H. S. 1979. *Disorders of sexual desire.* New York: Simon & Schuster.

Kaplan, H. S. 1974. *The new sex therapy: Active treatment of sexual dysfunction.* New York: Brunner/Mazel.

Kash, S. 1984. Birth-control survey: Sterilization tops list in U.S. *Ms.,* 12 (7):17.

Kashimer, M. 1976. Where to get help. *Ms.,* 5(2):97–98.

Kaufman, A., P. DiVasto, R. Jackson, J. Vandermeer, D. Pathak, and W. Odegard. 1977. Impact of a community approach to rape. *American Journal of Public Health* 67:365–367.

Kaufman, R. H., E. Adam, G. L. Binder, and E. Gerthoffer. 1981. Upper genital tract changes and pregnancy outcome in offspring exposed in utero to diethylstilbestrol. *Obstetrical and Gynecological Survey* 36(3):137–140.

Keaveny, M. E., L. Hader, M. Massoni, and G. A. Wade. 1973. Hysterectomy: Helping patients adjust. *Nursing 73* 3:9.

Kempe, C. H. 1978. Sexual abuse, another hidden pediatric problem: The 1977 C. Anderson Aldrich lecture. *Pediatrics* 62(3):382–389.

Kolata, G. B. 1979. Early warnings and latest cures for infertility. *Ms.,* 7(12):85–87.

Kolodny, R. C., W. H. Masters, V. E. Johnson, and

M. A. Biggs. 1979. *Textbook of human sexuality for nurses.* Boston: Little, Brown.

Krauss, R. H. 1979. Review of *Hysterectomy,* by S. Morgan. Women & Health 4(3):289–291.

Ledray, L. E. 1982. A nursing developed model for the treatment of rape victims. In *From accomodation to self-determination. Nursing's role in the development of health care policy.* Kansas City: American Academy of Nursing.

Ledray, L. E., S. H. Lund, and T. J. Kiresuk. 1979. Impact of rape on victims and families, treatment and research considerations. In *Women in stress: A nursing perspective,* ed. D. K. Kjervik, and I. M. Martinson, 197–217. New York: Appleton-Century-Crofts.

Lefkowitz, R. 1977. Help for the sexually harassed. *Ms.,* 6(5):49.

LeFort, S. 1977. Care of the rape victim in emergency. *Canadian Nurse* 73:42–45.

Lemere, F., and J. W. Smith. 1973. Alcohol-induced sexual impotence. *American Journal of Psychiatry* 130(2):212–213.

Leon, D. B. 1978. Sexual abuse of children. *ARON Journal* 27(4):642–644.

Leridon, H. 1977. *Human fertility.* Chicago: University of Chicago Press.

Lief, H. 1977. Inhibited sexual desire. *Medical Aspects of Human Sexuality* 11:94–95.

Lindsey, K. 1977. Sexual harassment on the job and how to stop it. *Ms.,* 6(5).

Longino, H. 1980. Pornography, oppression and freedom: A closer look. In *Take back the right: Women on pornography,* ed. L. Lederer. New York: Morrow Quill.

Luther, S. L., and J. H. Price. 1980. Child sexual abuse: A review. *The Journal of School Health* 50(3):161–165.

Malamuth, N. M., N. Heim, and S. Feshbach. 1980. Sexual responsiveness of college students to rape depictions. *Journal of Perspectives in Social Psychology* 38(3):399–408.

Malamuth, N. M., and B. Spinner. 1980. A longitudinal content analysis of sexual violence in the best-selling erotic magazines. *Journal of Sex Research* 16(3):226–237.

Masters, W. H., and V. E. Johnson. 1970. *Human sexual inadequacy.* Boston: Little, Brown.

Masters, W. H., and V. E. Johnson. 1966. *Human sexual response.* Boston: Little, Brown.

McCary, J. L., and S. P. McCary. 1982. *McCary's human sexuality.* 4th ed. Monterey, Calif.: Wadsworth.

Medea, A., and K. Thompson. 1974. *Against rape.* New York: Farrar, Straus, & Giroux.

Menning, B. E. 1975. *Infertility: Facts and feelings.* Belmont, Mass.: Resolve.

Menning, B. E. 1976. RESOLVE, a support group for infertile couples. *American Journal of Nursing* 76(2):258–259.

Morgan, R. 1978. How to run the pornographers out of town (and preserve the First Amendment). *Ms.,* 7(5).

Morgan, S. 1978. Sexuality after hysterectomy and castration. *Women & Health* 3(1):5–10.

Morgan, S. 1980. Hysterectomy. In *Hysterectomy.* Washington, D.C.: National Women's Health Network.

NAACOG. 1982. *Infertility: An overview.* Washington, D.C.: Nurses Association of the American College of Obstetricians and Gynecologists.

Nakashima, I. I., and G. E. Zakus. 1977. Incest: Review and clinical experience. *Pediatrics* 60(5):696–701.

NARAL. *The facts about rape and incest.* Washington, D.C.: National Abortion Rights Action League, 1981.

Nass, G. D., R. W. Libby, and M. P. Fisher. 1981. *Sexual choices.* Monterey, Calif.: Wadsworth.

National Institute of Mental Health. 1981. *National directory: Rape prevention and treatment resources.* Rockville, Md.: U.S. Dept. of Health and Human Services.

National Institutes of Health. 1980. DES-exposed daughters. *NIH, the search for health.* Bethesda, Md.: National Institutes of Health.

National Institutes of Health. 1977. *Questions and answers about DES exposure before birth.* Bethesda, Md.: U.S. Department of Health, Education, and Welfare.

National Women's Health Network. 1980. *DES.* Washington, D.C.: National Women's Health Network.

Nowinski, J. 1980. *Becoming satisfied.* Englewood Cliffs, N.J.: Prentice-Hall.

Now it's test-tube twins. 1981. *Science News,* 119(3):38.

O'Brien, P. C., K. L. Noller, S. J. Robboy, A. B. Barnes, R. H. Kaufman, B. C. Tilley, and D. E.

Townsend. 1979. Vaginal epithelial changes in young women enrolled in the National Cooperative Diethylstilbestrol Adenosis (DESAD) Project. *Obstetrics & Gynecology* 53(3).

Oelsner, G., D. M. Serr, S. Mashiach, J. Blankstein, M. Synder, and B. Lunenfeld. 1978. The study of induction of ovulation with menotropins: Analysis of results of 1897 treatment cycles. *Fertility and Sterility* 30(5):538–544.

Oram, C., and J. Beck. 1981. The tampon: Investigated and challenged. *Women & Health* 6(3/4):105–122.

Palmer, C. E. 1979. Pornographic comics: A content analysis. *The Journal of Sex Research* 15(4):285–298.

Parisky, F. B. 1981. The 'right' of sexual assault. *Hartford Courant* 144(74):B3.

Peters, J. J. 1976. Children who are victims of sexual assault—the psychology of offenders. *American Journal of Psychotherapy* 30(3):398–421.

Pope, T. L. 1981. Toxic shock syndrome. *The Nurse Practitioner* 6(5):31–32.

Poznanski, E., and P. Blos. 1975. Incest. *Medical Aspects of Human Sexuality* 9(10):46–76.

Press, R. M. 1982a. The continuing battle to halt child pornography in the U.S. *Christian Science Monitor* 74(126):5.

Press, R. M. 1982b. Secrecy in child pornography thwarts law enforcement. *Christian Science Monitor* 74(127):9.

Press, R. M. 1982c. How parents can aid fight against child pornography. *Christian Science Monitor* 74(128):4.

Project on the Status and Education of Women. no date. *The problem of rape on campus.* Washington, D.C.: Association of American Colleges.

Project on the Status and Education of Women. 1978. *Sexual harassment: A hidden issue.* Washington, D.C.: Association of American Colleges.

Rada, R. T. 1975. Alcoholism and forcible rape. *American Journal of Psychiatry* 132(4):444–446.

Rape crisis intervention. 1978. *The Journal of Practical Nursing* 28(11):17–19.

Reagan, J. W., and M. Y. Olaizola. 1980. Using cytology to study DES daughters. *Contemporary OB/GYN* 15:95–110.

Ritter, B., with B. Weinstein. 1979. The tragedy of teenage prostitution. *Senior Scholastic* 3(2):20–21.

Rockwood, M. 1977. Help for DES victims. *Ms.,* 5(9):18.

Ross, S. C. 1973. *The rights of women: The basic ACLU guide to a woman's rights.* New York: Avon.

Ruch, L. O., and S. M. Chandler. 1980. An evaluation of a center for sexual assault victims: Issues and problem areas. *Women & Health* 5(1):45–63.

Rush, F. 1980. *The best kept secret.* Englewood Cliffs, N.J.: Prentice-Hall.

Sagarin, E. 1977. Incest: Problems of definition and frequency. *The Journal of Sex Research* 13(2):126–135.

Semans, J. H. 1956. Premature ejaculation: A new approach. *Southern Medical Journal* 49:353–358.

Shulman, A. K. 1981. *On the stroll.* New York: Knopf.

Siemens, S. 1982. *Making sexual decisions.* Monterey, Calif.: Wadsworth.

Sperm count. 1982. *Women's Occupational Health Resource Center* 4(3):1.

Sredl, D. R., C. Klenke, and M. Rojkind. 1979. *Nursing 79* 9(7):38–43.

Steinem, G. 1978. Erotica and pornography, a clear and present difference. *Ms.,* 7(5).

Steinem, G. 1977. Is child pornography about sex? *Ms.,* 6(2):43–44.

Stilbestrol. 1973. *Science for the People* 5(1):14–16.

Stone, M. T. 1979. Female sterilization: The nurse's role. *Issues in Health Care of Women* 1(5):47–60.

Strickland, O. L. 1981. In vitro fertilization: Dilemma or opportunity? *Advances in Nursing Science* 3(2):41–51.

Tampons and toxic shock syndrome. 1982. Washington, D.C.: National Women's Health Network.

Task Force on Pornography at the University of Connecticut. 1981. Pornography and violence against women, issues and answers. Storrs, Conn.: University of Connecticut. mimeo.

Taymor, M. L. 1978. *Infertility.* New York: Grune & Stratton.

Thomas, J. N. 1980. Yes, you can help a sexually abused child. *RN* 43(8):23–29.

Toxic shock syndrome. 1982. Washington, D.C.: National Academy Press.

Van Gelder, L. 1980. When women confront street porn. *Ms.,* 8(8).

Valenti, C. 1979. Working with the physically abused woman. In *Women in stress: A nursing perspective,* ed. D. K. Kjervik, and I. M. Martinson, 187–196. New York: Appleton-Century-Crofts.

Walker, A. 1980. When women confront porn at home. *Ms.,* 8(8).

Watts, R. J. 1979. Dimensions of sexual health. *American Journal of Nursing* 79(9):1568–1572.

Weitzel, W. D., B. J. Powell, and E. C. Penick. 1978. Clinical management of father-daughter incest. *American Journal of Diseases of Children* 132(2):127–130.

Williams, M. A. 1976. Easier convalescence from hysterectomy. *American Journal of Nursing* 76(3):438–440.

Weber, E. 1977. Sexual abuse begins at home. *Ms.,* 5(10):64–67.

Wolf, S. R. 1970. Emotional reactions to hysterectomy. *Postgraduate Medicine* 47:165–168.

Wood, R. Y., and K. Rose. 1978. Penile implants for impotence. *American Journal of Nursing* 78(2):234–238.

Worthington, J. 1977. The cancer time bomb: Did your mother take DES? *Ms.,* 5(9):16–18.

Wroblewski, S. S. 1981. Toxic shock syndrome. *American Journal of Nursing* 81(1):82–85.

Introduction

Sexuality and Hospitalization

Sexuality after Surgery

    Mastectomy
        Assessment and treatments
        Effects on sexuality
        Adjustment: opportunities for caring support
    Sexual Reassignment: Working with Clients
    Genital Mutilation
        Interventions
    Pelvic Procedures: Alterations in Body Image
        Ileostomy and colostomy
        Cystectomy
        Pelvic exenteration

Risks for Adolescents

    Scoliosis
    Seizure Disorders
    Cerebral Palsy
    Chronic Illness

Sexuality and Disability

    Sexuality during Institutionalization
    Sexuality and Multiple Sclerosis
    Sexuality and Parkinson's Disease
    Sex with Arthritis
    Sex and Limb Amputation
    Spinal Cord Injury
        Nursing implications
    Sexuality and the Individual with a Learning Disability

Living with Chronic Conditions: Issues in Sexuality

    Obesity
    Chronic Kidney Disorders
    Sexuality and Diabetes
    Sexuality and Cardiac Conditions
    Sexuality and Respiratory Compromise
    Sexuality and Stroke
    Sexuality and Hypertension

Sexuality, Death, and Dying

Summary of Implications for Nursing Practice

CHAPTER **8**

Human Sexuality and Nursing Interventions: Post-Crisis

Joellen W. Hawkins

Introduction

Numerous hazardous events have implications for sexuality in the post-crisis or rehabilitation phase. Although an event such as a coronary or kidney failure represents an immediate biophysical and psychosocial crisis for the individual, it is in the post-crisis or recovery period when its effects on sexual expression occur. Having survived the biophysical insult, the individual is now faced with adapting her or his lifestyle to any limitations posed by the pathophysiologic and/or anatomical changes that have occurred. This chapter will explore the effects on sexuality of such events as surgery, hospitalization, chronic kidney failure and renal dialysis, coronary artery disease, mastectomy, spinal cord injury, and learning disabilities.

Sexuality and Hospitalization

Human sexuality is an aspect often ignored by health-care professionals in acute and chronic care settings. The effects of surgical procedures, therapies, and drugs on sexuality receive little attention and are often not even mentioned to the client, partner, or family (Jacobson 1974, 50). In efforts to communicate their needs, clients may sometimes act out sexually. Providers are often ill-equipped to respond appropriately to these behaviors (Withersty 1976, 573).

When a client is confronted with hospitalization and possibly a surgical procedure, health-care professionals sometimes behave as if the person left his or her sexuality at home. The importance of privacy is often ignored. Clients may be transferred or positioned with little regard for feelings about exposure and sexuality. The overt and covert messages the client receives from staff about sexuality may affect his or her perception of the overall care (Alexander 1976, 744). High self-esteem is one ingredient necessary for full expression of sexuality. The client in the hospital may suffer from low self-esteem due to mutilating surgery, debilitating effects of injury or illness, and/or changes in body image (Littlefield 1977, 649). Helping the client to prepare for changes that will affect sexuality, suggesting ways to minimize sexual dysfunction, providing privacy for intimacy between the client and significant other, and offering opportunities for the client to discuss sexuality should be an integral part of care. If hospitalization is prolonged the client needs regular opportunities for sexual expression. He or she should not be made to feel guilty about masturbation or intimacy with a partner.

Preparation for discharge should include discussion of any limitations in sexual activity, any side effects the client may experience from medications, and any residual effects of changes in performance or response that can be expected from the surgery or therapies. When possible or desired, the client's partner should be included in planning. One of the goals in nursing should be to minimize the effects of biophysical assaults and/or hospitalization on all aspects of living, including sexuality. Helping a client achieve a higher level of wellness includes sexual well-being.

Sexuality After Surgery

Certain surgical procedures are especially likely to have an effect on a client's sexuality. Those to be discussed in this section include mastectomy, sexual reassignment, female circumcision, clitoridectomy, ileostomy, colostomy, cystectomy, and pelvic exenteration.

Mastectomy

Loss of one or both breasts alters a woman's body and, thus, alters her self-image. Accustomed not only to the presence of breasts, but also to their role in sexual foreplay, arousal, and intercourse, a woman suffers losses in her image as a woman and also as a sexual being.

Mastectomy is ordinarily done only for carcinoma, so the procedure is an intervention for a serious biophysical assault to a woman's body. She has to cope with loss of her body integrity and the potential for entropy. Postcrisis, she may be unable to achieve a higher level of wellness, but must live with a potentially fatal condition. Facing a life that may be prematurely shortened can also affect a woman's sexuality and sexual expression.

It should be noted that men also experience breast cancer and undergo mastectomy. Although the meaning of breasts to men in our society is different than that to women, men experience a loss of body integrity that may affect their sexuality. However, since the incidence of breast cancer in men is very small, the pronoun "she" will be used in the discussion of mastectomy.

Breast cancer remains a leading cancer-related cause of death. One in every 14 women in the United States will get breast cancer (Michelson 1979, 29). It is the leading cause of death for all women between ages 37 and 55 (Swenson 1980, 7). The lymphatic network of the breasts often acts to facilitate metastasis to other sites (Welch 1980, 8). Thus, early detection is important to prognosis before the axillary lymph nodes are involved. Breast self-examination is the key to early discovery (Garrard 1975, 29), as discussed in Chapter 5. A guide to BSE appears in Figure 5-3.

Assessment and Treatments

The traditional assessment for a breast lump or mass is mammography followed by biopsy, either by surgical removal of the lump or, if it is a cyst, by needle aspiration, and cytology diagnosis. If the mass is malignant, mastectomy has been the treatment of choice. The disease staging of breast cancer is as follows (National Cancer Institute 1979, 136):

Stage I   Breast cancer, no metastasis, tumor less than 5 cm

Stage II   May have lymph node involvement, tumor less than 5 cm, possible fixation on chest wall

Stage III   Nodal involvement, tumor may be attached to chest wall, larger than 5 cm

Stage IV   Extensive metastasis, nodal involvement, tumor any size, extension to chest wall and skin

New approaches to the treatment of breast cancer have evolved over the past few years. Whereas mastectomy was done routinely in the past, current thinking incorporates a combination of treatment modalities. The *Halsted radical mastectomy* is a procedure that involves removal of the breast, skin, pectoralis major and minor muscles, axillary lymph nodes, and fat. An even more radical procedure, an *extended radical,* involves removal of all the tissues in a Halsted plus the internal mammary lymph nodes. A *modified radical* involves removal of the breast, some fat, and most of the axillary nodes. A *simple* or *total mastectomy* involves removal of the breast. Removal of the tumor and 2 to 3 cm of surrounding tissue constitutes a *partial radical.* A local wide excision of the mass may be done. This is called a *tylectomy, lumpectomy, wedge,* or *quadrant excision.* In the least intrusive procedure, called a *subcutaneous mastectomy,* only internal breast tissue is removed (National Cancer Institute 1979, 26–31). Some of the less radical procedures are done followed by radiation treatment if there is nodal involvement (Levene

1977). A biopsy can be done to determine metastasis to nodes. When a subcutaneous mastectomy is done, breast augmentation can be performed at the same time. Chemotherapy is also given as an adjunct to surgery and/or radiation (National Cancer Institute 1979, 31–33) (see Figures 8-1 to 8-4).

There are those who believe cancer cells spread long before a woman can detect a lump and, therefore, chemotherapy is the treatment of choice (Cope 1978). Radiation therapy can be either external or internal through implantation of iridium-192 isotopes in hollow steel needles (Michelson 1979, 30). A comparative study of survivals and treatment modalities has been underway since 1971. It is entitled the National Surgical Adjuvant Breast Project (NSABP) (Alpert 1979, 278). There is considerable disagreement about the efficacy of the different approaches. Thus, the woman must be involved in the decision-making process using the best and most complete information available about the options (Alpert 1979, 285–286). The woman needs to know that breast reconstruction may be possible if the disfigurement is a major concern to her (Townsend 1980, 29; Thomas and Yates 1977).

Effects on Sexuality

The less radical the procedure, the less the impact on the woman's body in terms of mutilating surgery. Nonetheless, her body image will be altered, and that can affect her sexuality. The woman's perceptions of her body after surgery will depend, to some extent, upon the value she places on her breasts (National Cancer Institute 1979, 68–69).

Women's reactions to mastectomy vary, but some common themes are present. Fear of the cancer diagnosis is common, as well as fear of recurrence. Women also express concerns about returning to a normal life: healing of the incision, active use of the arm, and diminution

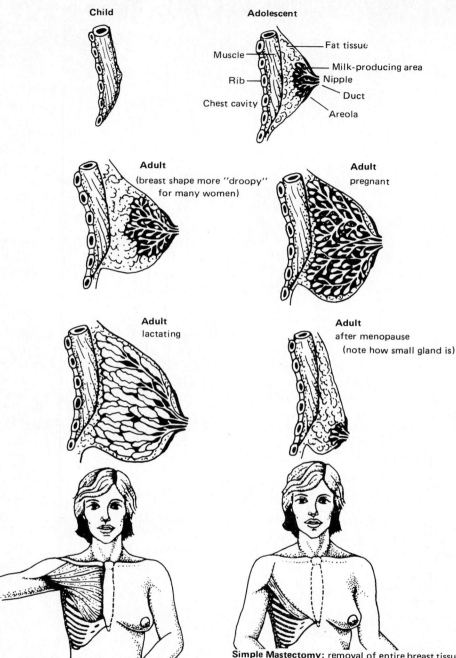

Child

Adolescent

Muscle

Rib

Chest cavity

Fat tissue

Milk-producing area

Nipple

Duct

Areola

Adult
(breast shape more "droopy" for many women)

Adult
pregnant

Adult
lactating

Adult
after menopause
(note how small gland is)

Pectoral Muscles provide support for the breasts and are necessary for many arm movements.

Simple Mastectomy: removal of entire breast tissue, leaving pectoral muscle intact. Some nodes may or may not be removed under the arm. Surgery may be followed by radiation.

FIGURE 8-1
Normal breast configuration across the life span and after mastectomy.

Rebuilding a Breast After Radical Mastectomy

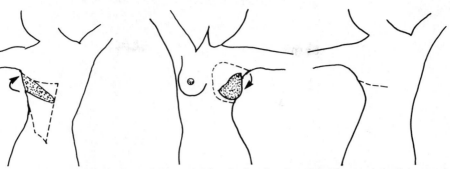

The newest method of reconstructing a breast after radical mastectomy is to move all or part of the broad, thin latissimus dorsi muscle (dotted line) and an "island" of skin (grey tone) from the back to the chest.

A silicone implant is placed under the transposed muscle to replace muscle that was removed from the chest wall during the mastectomy. The skin "island" furnishes skin cover for the reconstructed breast.

A hairline scar remaining on the back can be hidden under a brassiere strap.

FIGURE 8-2
Breast reconstruction.

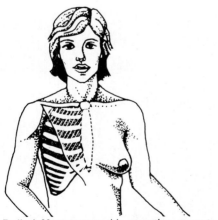

Radical Mastectomy: this operation removes the breast, the entire pectoral muscle and the armpit nodes. Swelling of the arm and restriction of movement must be treated after surgery. The lungs remain vulnerable throughout life.

FIGURE 8-3
Radical mastectomy.

of symptoms in the arm (Miller and Janda 1979).

Effects on sexuality and femininity also vary among women. One woman who underwent a radical mastectomy stated that her fear of cancer was greater than her fear of mutilation or loss of physical attractiveness. She was sure that her long marriage could survive a change in body image and stated, "We could adjust together" (Levinger 1980, 1120). One woman, choosing to be one-breasted after mastectomy (no prosthesis), stated that her sexuality has a new dimension. She now has both a maternal and a youthful, androgynous side (Armel 1981, 23).

Initiating sex after mastectomy needs to be a shared venture. The partner may wait, feeling the woman may be weak or not ready. Instead, she may feel rejected. Communicating needs and desires will give the woman time to feel ready and yet reassure her that she is still loved and desired. Adaptation to the new body is important so that pain or injury to the operative site or affected arm is avoided.

Lymph nodes near the breast, and likely routes of spread in breast cancer

Simple Mastectomy: area removed and stitching

Radical Mastectomy: area removed and stitching

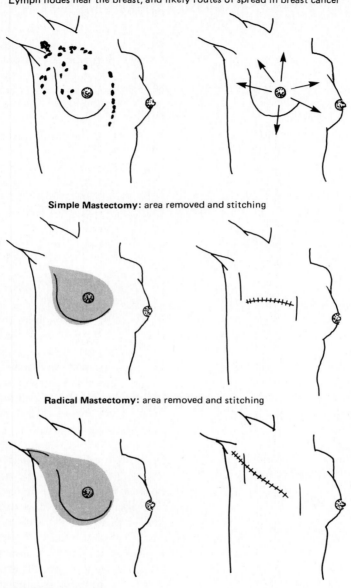

☐ Area removed

FIGURE 8-4
Treatment considerations in breast cancer.

An open sharing of thoughts and feelings about the woman's changed body image and sexual role can create a new closeness. Some women report an improved sex life and a new sexual freedom (National Cancer Institute 1979, 84).

Studies of women's responses to mastectomy indicate that social adjustment is achieved by most women within two years (this includes sexual adaptation). However, a significant number of women do experience changes in sexuality, especially in the three months immediately after surgery (Morris, Greer, and White 1977). In another study, although most women indicated good adjustment, some changes did occur. Some of the married women did not resume intercourse after surgery; nearly one-quarter reported difficulty in achieving orgasm and experienced less sexual satisfaction; frequency of intercourse declined for about one-fifth of the women; and nearly one-fourth did not wish to let their spouses see them naked (Jamison, Wellisch, and Pasnau 1978).

In a study of the responses of male partners of women who have had mastectomies, the men reported adverse effects on sexuality and intimacy from the procedure (Wellisch, Jamison, and Pasnau 1978). Factors that affect the partner's responses include fears of castration and/or mutilation, significance of the woman's physical appearance, and the extent of oral dependency (Schoenberg 1979, 95).

Adjustment: Opportunities for Caring Support

Nurses are the major caregivers for women who have to undergo treatment for breast cancer. As such, they provide care and caring that can facilitate adjustment after the biophysical crisis of the cancer diagnosis and intrusive therapies. If problems arise that appear to be beyond the scope of nursing expertise, referral can be offered.

Preparation for the procedure prior to hospitalization is helpful. The woman needs to know what to bring with her. Preoperatively, she needs information about the kind of dressings and incision to expect, scheduling for follow-up therapy, and physical rehabilitation. Types of prostheses should also be discussed unless breast reconstruction will be done as part of the procedure (Thielen 1980, 58–59; Winkler 1977).

The initial adjustment after the procedure involves the woman's inspection of her body. Women need to be offered a chance to view the incision when dressing changes are done (Kennerly 1977, 1431). They need explanations of any drains in place and how healing is expected to progress.

After mastectomy, the woman is confronted with alterations in her image to herself, to her mate, and to the world (Byrd 1975, 53). All of these can affect her sexuality and her desire for and responses to overt manifestations of sexuality. Recognizing that these changes in image occur for all women may help the woman to feel less alone as she struggles to cope with the many tasks postoperatively. Nurses can offer opportunities for discussion of changes in body image and their effects on sexuality. If the woman wishes, her partner can be included.

Women need to be reassured that they are still loved and desired after mastectomy. Sharing feelings with the partner should be encouraged even before discharge (Thielen 1980, 60 and 63). It is important that the partner be included in the entire experience, in looking at the woman's body, and in resumption of sexual activity. The woman may fear having her partner see her and the partner may not wish to push her or seem insensitive. Open, honest discussion between the woman and her partner should help alleviate such difficulties.

The nurse can help promote communication within the dyad. Exploring fears about and the meaning of mutilating surgery, how the woman and her partner feel about the scar, and the meaning and symbolism of breasts in sexuality can help open up discussion. Using the third person can be a helpful technique: "Some women find that their fears about the appearance of the incision are worse than reality"; "Some men believe that a woman's sexual response will decrease after surgery or that the other breast will no longer be sensitive and responsive during sex." Positive responses to the scar and the healing processes coming from staff can be helpful to the woman's adaptation. Including the partner in learning dressing change and rehabilitation techniques provides concrete ways of being involved and also promotes physical contact. Holding, cuddling, stroking, and other overt signs of caring will help the couple to reestablish closeness prior to attempting intercourse (Schoenberg 1979, 103).

There are a number of resources available for women concerning breast cancer, mastectomy and alternative therapies, and recovery (National Cancer Institute 1979; National Women's Health Network 1980; Kushner 1977; Thielen 1980; Cancer Information Clearinghouse 1979; Napoli 1983). Health-care providers can help women to identify and use resources such as Reach to Recovery (Puhaty 1977, 1437).

Mastectomy should not mean the end of a woman's sexuality. Recognition of the importance of body image to sexuality should be an integral part of nursing women who have breast cancer. Interventions during the crisis and post-crisis periods can help to prevent significant disruptions in sexual expression and promoe the optimal possible levels of wellness for all aspects of life including sexuality.

Sexual Reassignment: Working with Clients

As indicated in Chapter 4 (see Transsexualism), some individuals in our society are struggling with a discrepancy between their biologic sex and their sexual identity. They may see themselves as men trapped in women's bodies, or vice versa.

When an individual makes a decision to undergo surgery for a sex change, he or she is in a situation that has the potential for crisis. The procedures, although relatively safe, still carry the risks of anesthesia and postoperative complications. Although the surgery represents resolution of a long-term identity crisis (Strait 1973, 462), there may be psychological sequelae. It is during the postoperative period that nursing interventions can help to promote resolution and a return to wellness. The nurse can be an important member of the health-care team in caring for these clients.

Procedures for the male-to-female transition include breast augmentation, one-stage reconstruction of the genitals to create a vagina and accomplish female appearance, and hormonal adjustment. The surgery for female-to-male transformation is more complex. Bilateral subcutaneous mastectomy can be done. An abdominal panhysterectomy is performed along with a vaginectomy. During the next phases, the urethra is reconstructed to follow the clitoris, labial tissues are used to lengthen the penis and create the scrotum, and testicular prostheses are implanted (Rowland 1975, 738–739). Repeat admissions for surgery afford staff opportunities to establish rapport over a period of time and offer support to clients undergoing these dramatic procedures.

Emotional outbursts and anger are common responses during the postoperative period. These may be directed at staff members, who need to understand their origins in order to respond appropriately. In a sense, these clients have undergone a mutilating procedure. On the other hand, perceptions may reflect a view of the procedures as restorative, bringing harmony between identity and body image. Clients are struggling with the need to have acceptance as total persons, male or female. Their ways of doing so may sometimes seem bizarre. For example, attempts to appear as an alluring woman may elicit untoward responses from others, who are unaccustomed to seeing persons in the hallway in sheer nightgowns (Strait 1973, 462).

The need to talk about sexuality is often expressed very openly. Nurses may need help with their own feelings about transsexuals and surgery if they are to feel free to discuss sexual issues (Simone 1977, 38). Nurses can also serve as role models for clients as they adapt to their new bodies (Strait 1973, 463). Reassurance that adjustment takes time will help the client to realize he or she is not abnormal. Concerns about meeting new partners, dating, and acceptance by family, friends, and significant others should be discussed. Positive response from others is critical to development of a positive sense of self and sexual adjustment postoperatively. Health-care professionals can foster positive feelings through their behavior and attitude toward clients in the immediate post-crisis period.

Genital Mutilation

Once a common procedure in this country in the form of female circumcision and clitoridectomy (to cure "hypersexuality" and masturbation), genital mutilation has all but disappeared. It is, however, still performed frequently in other parts of the world. While the procedure itself constitutes a biophysical and psychosocial crisis for the individual, it is in the post-crisis period that the effects on sexuality are evident.

It has been estimated that 30 million women suffer from the results of genital mutilation. Some procedures are performed as rituals on children between 3 and 8 years of age. Variations are many, but fall into three main categories: removal of the prepuce and/or tip of the clitoris; excision of the entire clitoris and adjacent labia minora; and *infibulation,* which means suturing of remaining tissue of the labia over the vaginal introitus except for a small opening (Morgan and Steinem 1980, 65). While these practices continue mostly in countries outside North America and Western Europe, some women who have suffered this mutilation live in these parts of the world.

Sudan is a country where female circumcision persists in its most severe form and is still practiced widely. Pharonic circumcision, the most common form, means removal of all of the external genitalia including clitoris, the clitoral prepuce, labia minora, and part or all of the labia majora. The opening is then stitched together so that only a very small orifice is left for the passage of urine and menses. The operation is usually performed by midwives on girls between 5 and 7 years of age. It must be pointed out that women in the Sudan and other countries where these practices persist derive social status and economic security from their roles as wives and mothers. Clitoridectomy and infibulation are seen as a guarantee of virginity that make the girl marriageable (Gruenbaum 1982, 5).

Beyond the immediate risks of hemorrhage, infection, and death, effects of these practices of women include menstrual disorders, dyspareunia, genital and vaginal malformation, incontinence, fistulas, abscesses and cysts, infertility, pregnancy complications, and sexual dysfunction (Morgan and Steinem 1980, 66).

Although male circumcision is widely practiced (despite controversy in recent times about the need for the procedure and its effects), removal of the clitoris is more nearly analogous to penisectomy. Circumcision should in no way disturb sexual pleasure or performance, whereas mutilations of the genitals have serious psychosexual consequences (Morgan and Steinem 1980, 67). The victims of genital mutilation long remember the terror and pain associated with the procedure and may suffer its consequences the rest of their lives (Saadawi 1980).

Interventions

Evidence of genital mutilation can be observed during assessment. Health-care providers need to be cognizant of the risks to women who are its victims and help them to achieve the highest possible level of wellness. Sometimes reconstructive or restorative surgery can be helpful, especially when the introitus is sutured, or when fistulas, cysts, or malformations are present. Explanation of the effects on sexuality can help the woman to achieve at least a degree of normalcy in sexual expression. Assessment for infection and follow-up treatment will remove at least one barrier to sexual pleasure. However, nurses should also be sensitive to the needs of women who feel they must have re-infibulation after delivery of a child in order to honor their cultural beliefs.

In the larger context, nurses as health professionals can support efforts to eradicate these practices. Concerns of women throughout the world are now being heard by groups such as the World Health Organization (Hosken 1980).

Pelvic Procedures: Alterations in Body Image

A number of surgical procedures are performed to treat chronic diseases or carcinoma that result in alterations in anatomy and function of pelvic organs. Usually these extensive procedures are undertaken only after careful consideration of less invasive therapies for a life-threatening condition. The crisis, therefore, is the result of a biophysical assault. It is during the post-crisis recovery period that psychosexual adaptations occur and during this time that clients need help and support in coping with effects on their sexuality.

Ileostomy and Colostomy

Ileostomy and colostomy create significant alterations in anatomy, body functioning, and body image. Functional disturbances experienced by clients include problems in achieving erection, ejaculation, and orgasm. Dyspareunia is reported by some women (Ola-Petter et al. 1977). In one study, the majority of persons undergoing ileostomy reported sexual adjustment, but some attributed marital upsets to the procedure. When rectal excision was performed as part of the treatment, sexual dysfunction occurred for some clients due to pain in the perineal area (Burnham, Lennard-Jones, and Brooke 1977).

Causes of sexual problems may be biophysical and/or psychosocial in origin. In order to help clients in their sexual adjustment, assessment is important. If nerve damage has occurred during excision of the rectum, it is important that the client realize he or she is not a "failure" or a "freak" when impotence or lack of response occurs. The perineal area may also be sensitive or painful (Simmons 1983, 411). A careful explanation of the procedure will help the client understand alterations in anatomy and how the body will function. An understanding of the client's sexual activity before surgery and expectations postoperatively will help the adjustment process. Attention to aspects of general well-being such as sleep, nutrition, and exercise will help maximize sexuality. The client needs the opportunity to discuss feelings about the stoma, changes in body image, sexual desirability and attractiveness, and alterations in sexual activity that occur due to presence of the stoma. Inclusion of the partner in discussion can be helpful in promoting communication between the couple (Lyons 1975).

One author (Simmons 1983) describes

with great sensitivity her experiences after undergoing an ileostomy and offers very practical advice for others. She states that she viewed the period after her surgery as a time to "affirm" her sexuality (1983, 409). Her suggestions include the following: use homecoming as a reacquaintance time with a partner; focus on intimacy and closeness rather than on sexual performance; return to former sleeping habits as long as they feel good, such as sleeping with one's partner; use a plastic sheet to relieve concerns about leakage; spend time away from each other (perhaps at least one full hour a day); and learn to accept one's new body (1983, 409). Simmons emphasizes open communication with one's partner to prevent misconceptions from arising. She suggests that individuals experiment with the best time to empty the pouch before sexual activity, timing of eating and its effects on comfort and flatus production, and the use of a variety of types of pouches for different activities (1983, 410–411). Drainage, leakage, and odor can be dealt with through practice with pouches. Honest communication with one's partner when an accident occurs is recommended (1983, 410–411).

Simmons (1983, 411) suggests that partners experiment with positions for intercourse to find one or more that are comfortable for both persons. She also discusses sexual fantasies that may be generated by the presence of a stoma and the role of fantasy in a healthy sex life.

Cystectomy

Cystectomy is usually performed as treatment for cancer, and sexual dysfunction is an expected result. After the surgery, men are unable to achieve erection and ejaculation. For women, cystectomy is often only part of the procedure, so the uterus may be absent, and in extreme cases, the vagina as well. In addition to adaptation to a stoma, adaptation to alterna-

tive modes of sexual expression may be necessary. Both men and women are still capable of achieving orgasm through manual or oral stimulation, even when vaginal intercourse is not possible. The use of a penile implant can be considered so that vaginal intercourse can be resumed (Montague 1977, 92). Cystectomy need not affect in any way the person's responses to stroking, cuddling, kissing, breast stimulation, or clitoral and penile stimulation.

Discussions of sexuality should be initiated by health professionals to ensure dissemination of correct information about the surgical procedure and its effects on sexuality. The partner should be included, if possible, to help the couple begin to communicate about resumption of the sexual aspects of their relationship.

Pelvic Exenteration

Pelvic exenteration is a radical procedure performed for local carcinomas that are not amenable to other forms of therapy but are unlikely to have metastasized to distant sites. The rectum, distal sigmoid colon, bladder and distal ends of the ureters, internal iliac vessels and branches and all pelvic reproductive organs and lymph nodes are removed. If the client is a woman, her pelvic floor, peritoneum levator muscles, and perineum are also removed (Hamilton and Schlapper 1976, 266). Modifications of the radical procedure can be done depending on the primary site and extent of the carcinoma. Care must be taken preoperatively to assess both the biophysical and psychosocial factors that mediate for or against the procedure.

Deflection of evacuation to the abdominal wall and removal of pelvic reproductive organs alter the body image dramatically. Healing is slow, so body image can be further altered by the presence of drains, dressings, and nasogastric or intestinal tubes. Once the biophysical crisis of the surgery has passed, the client will then focus more intently on living with an altered body. He or she may equate male or female roles with reproduction and/or with vaginal intercourse. Reassurance of completeness as a male or female person, as well as the capacity to respond to other forms of sexual stimulation, can be helpful. Vaginal reconstruction is one alternative that can be offered to women for whom the prospects of success outweigh the risks of this procedure. Most of all, these clients need support from professionals, family, friends, and significant others to endure the risks of complication, adapt to a drastically altered self, and adopt alternatives to the intimacy of vaginal intercourse.

Risks for Adolescents

Adolescents, experiencing a period of maturation preparatory to adult sexuality, are at risk for disruption of that development and expression in the post-crisis, or tertiary, phase of a number of hazardous events. These events, of course, continue through life, but this section focuses on those whose first effects upon sexuality are manifested during this developmental phase. They include scoliosis, seizure disorders, cerebral palsy, and chronic illness.

Scoliosis

Scoliosis is often diagnosed during adolescence, concurrent with the developmental task of discovering one's identity. Scoliosis is defined as "a lateral deviation of the spinal column from the midline" (deToledo 1979, 1588). Not only does the deformity which scoliosis represents affect body image, but the treatments can also interfere with psychosexual social development, including dating. Therapies include use of a brace, an orthoplast jacket, casting, surgery, and/or a special traction system (Anderson 1979, 1595–1597; Micheli, Magin, and Rouvales 1979).

The adolescent is concerned with dependence and independence as well as with body changes and body image. Treatment for scoliosis can offer an improved body. At the same time, the treatment may mean months of increased dependence (Micheli et al. 1979, 1604). Thus, the nurse must be particularly sensitive to the concerns of the adolescent when providing care. Assistance in adaptation to life with a stabilizing device (brace, cast, jacket) is important. Opportunities for peer contact should be offered during hospitalization. The adolescent needs desperately to feel like "one of the gang." She or he should experience minimal disruption of psychosexual development and feel wanted and liked by others. The adolescent who is sexually mature may need privacy for intimacy with friends and needs to feel that masturbation is a normal and healthy method of sexual release. The need for privacy should be respected even if it means excluding parents during certain procedures. Conversely, the need for support should be condoned and fostered. Problems identified by adolescents during treatment include back photography—perhaps because the process of photography raises issues related to body image and privacy—and peer reactions (Schatzinger, Brower, and Nash 1979, 1610).

Seizure Disorders

For the adolescent with a seizure disorder, whether dormant or active, questions about sexuality can arise. Medications to control seizures can lower libido and interfere with response. They can also create changes that alter body image. Information about sexual activity and seizure disorders needs to be shared. It is extremely rare for orgasm to trigger a seizure.

Likewise, a seizure disorder should not interfere with sexual expression. Careful monitoring of drug dosages can alleviate side effects (DeMoya and DeMoya 1980, 104).

Cerebral Palsy

Cerebral palsy is manifested before adolescence and therefore affects sexual development. Young persons with this condition need anticipatory teaching about puberty, menstruation, nocturnal emissions, and social issues concerned with dating (Ziff 1981). Orgasm is possible, as is sexual response to touching, stroking, kissing, massage, and oral-genital contact. If muscle spasms are a problem, alternate positions can be tried. If intercourse is difficult due to severe cerebral palsy, alternative means of sexual activity can be emphasized (Steinbock and Zeiss 1977).

The adolescent with cerebral palsy needs counseling prior to engagement in sexual activity, assurance of normalcy in sexual response, and encouragement in exploring sexual responsiveness through self-stimulation and/or manual stimulation by a partner. Counseling for contraception is also important and must take into account the client's motor abilities as well as method risks and benefits (Ziff 1981, 61–62). With anticipatory guidance, adolescents with cerebral palsy can develop normally with regard to their sexuality.

Chronic Illness

Adolescents with chronic illnesses must struggle with development as sexual beings along with the limitations the hazardous event imposes. The disease may make the adolescent feel "different" or "ugly" and undesirable to peers. It may slow his or her physical development, but not the feelings of adolescence (Frauman and Sypert 1979, 371). Pain may interfere with the pleasures of touching and hugging. The whole spectrum of modes of sharing and intimacy should be discussed. Masturbation, mutual stimulation, caressing, hugging, stroking, touching, and intercourse are among the various alternatives. Adaptation of treatment regimens or medications to accommodate relationships is important to their success. Every effort should be made to foster development of normal sexuality (Frauman and Sypert 1979, 375).

Parents need to be included, but not at the expense of confidentiality. Separate times may be needed for parents to talk about the developing sexuality of their adolescents.

Sexuality and Disability

Any disability can affect sexual development and expression for the affected individual. The disability can be congenital or acquired. If it is congenital, the individual grows up with the condition affecting all developmental tasks. If it is acquired, it probably will precipitate a crisis when the hazardous event occurs. The long-term effects post-crisis will affect one's sexuality. If the insult occurs after establishment of adult sexuality, new patterns of sexual expression may have to be learned.

Taboos imposed by society repress the sexuality that is as much a part of being a disabled person as it is being a person free of disability. Yet the role society defines for the disabled person does not include sexuality (Cohen 1981, A14; Bullard and Knight 1981). One study of attitudes toward sexual behavior of disabled persons revealed that negative attitudes still abound (Haring and Meyerson 1979, 260). Sexual information given to women with disabilities often focuses on reproduction. The implication is that nonreproductive aspects of sexuality are unimportant and inappropriate (Peters 1982, 34). Disabled persons may therefore have to struggle not only with the limitations and stigma of their disabilities in developing as sexual beings, but also with the negative attitudes of society.

Taboos and myths about sexuality pervade our society and in this case the disabled are not excluded. Being able to talk about sexuality, to seek information, ask questions, and to dispel myths can provide a beginning for development as a sexual being. As health-care professionals, we need to be sensitive to the values and cultural beliefs tied to sexuality. "Permission" for exploration can be given, but encouraging masturbation by an individual who believes it is evil can be perceived as intrusive or inappropriate.

Another obstacle faced by disabled persons in expressing their sexuality is finding a partner (Smith and Bullough 1975, 2195–2196). If the disability is essentially lifelong, opportunities for dating and even social contact may be limited or nonexistent. If that hurdle is overcome, and a relationship progresses to the point of mutual desire, then preparation for sex must be accomplished. Sex is usually less than spontaneous for the disabled person. For the person who requires assistance in the activities of daily living, the intrusion of a third person can cause awkwardness. Ideally, the partner can provide any needed assistance and incorporate it as much as possible into foreplay. A successful experience will help to break down barriers, so careful planning and communication at the beginning may be well worth the feeling of contrived sex (see Figure 8-5).

When vaginal intercourse is not possible, other forms of closeness should be encouraged. These include touching, fondling, holding, kissing, mutual masturbation, and oral-genital contact. For disabled persons in particular, sexuality is a concept that must extend far beyond the genitals. Women and

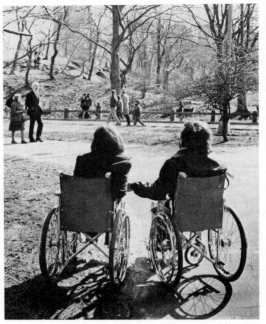

© Geoffrey Gove/Photo Researchers, Inc.

FIGURE 8-5
Sharing intimacy.

men both need opportunities and assistance in being and feeling attractive for social situations (Finch 1977, 19–20). They may need assistance in exploring various forms of intimacy, positions, and other aspects of close relationships. One important reference available to help with details of intimacy is *Toward Intimacy,* by the Task Force on Concerns of Physically Disabled Women (1978).

Sex education is an important component of caring for disabled persons. Whenever possible, preparation for sexuality should be an integral part of the educational program. Special materials may need to be prepared for hearing- and vision-impaired persons so that values and attitudes as well as information can be included (McNab 1978).

Sexuality during Institutionalization

When a disabled person has to be hospitalized for a long period of time or is in a rehabilitation institution, staff members often assume that he or she leaves sexuality behind (Paradowski 1977). The organization of most institutions serves to deter the motivation and independence of clients, and goals are often staff-determined (Struck 1981, 25). Clients are often denied control over their own bodies, including their sexuality. Opportunities for sexual outlet either through masturbation and self-stimulation or intimacy with a partner should be provided. Sometimes weekend passes can be arranged to accommodate relationships. In one innovative program a private room is provided for the sexual aspects of rehabilitation, acknowledging sexual function as a legitimate part of the restoration process. This room can be used for practicing techniques related to sexuality and for intimacy between clients and partners (Griffith and Trieschmann 1977).

Sexuality and Multiple Sclerosis

The effects of multiple sclerosis (MS) on sexuality can be many, depending upon the severity of symptoms and the extent of involvement. Fatigue, depression, sensory numbness, changes in coordination, weakness or paralysis of limbs, and visual disturbances—common symptoms of MS—can interfere with sexual activity and expressions of intimacy. In addition, bowel and bladder problems are both embarrassing and disruptive in social situations. Loss of self-esteem affects ability to respond. Impotence can occur in a man when there are lesions of the sacral cord; women can experience diminished sensation from the same cause (Slater and Yearwood 1980, 276).

Bladder dysfunction can cause incontinence during intercourse, or a catheter may be in place, which can also interfere. Muscle spasms can disrupt sex, necessitating use of alternative positions. Lesions in the central nervous system can alter responsiveness, moods, sensitivity, and human interactions (Catanzaro 1980, 287).

Suggestions to help clients maintain sexual satisfaction include use of alternative methods of stimulation such as a vibrator, exploration of all erotic areas, folding back the catheter and using a condom to cover it, rear entry and other positions, and fostering good communication between partners (McDonnell et al. 1980, 296).

Sexuality and Parkinson's Disease

The symptoms of Parkinson's disease can interfere with or disrupt sexual expression. Tremors, disturbances in voluntary movements, restlessness, weakness, depression, incontinence, drooling, and rigidity can cause embarrassment, make the person uncomfortable in social situations, and make sexual experiences less than successful. Sexual capacity may also decrease (Fischbach 1978). Some of the medications used to treat Parkinson's can also cause disturbances in sexuality such as impotence or diminished sexual response. Alterations in body function affect self-esteem and, in turn, sexual function.

Victims of Parkinson's disease need to be reassured that sexual expression is still possible. Emphasizing nongenital or noncoital forms of intimacy, allowing plenty of time, minimizing effects of medication through dosage monitoring and timing of sexual activity, and promoting communication with the partner are important interventions for health professionals to include in care.

Sex with Arthritis

The limitation of motion and/or pain associated with arthritis can interfere with sexuality. Changes in body image affect comfort and can cause stress in a relationship. Hip and pelvic mobility may be limited. Some medications can impair libido or sexual functioning.

Some suggestions include timing sexual activities to take advantage of medication peaks or minimal pain, using positions that do not cause pain or stress, using aids to comfort such as heat, waterbeds, and pillows, and exploring the many forms of intimacy, including open communication with partners (Halstead 1977). An excellent pamphlet on this subject, *Living and Loving,* has been developed by the Arthritis Foundation (1982).

Sex and Limb Amputation

When a limb must be amputated or is lost through an accident, sexuality is an issue that must be addressed in the post-crisis period. The loss means an alteration in body image and an adjustment to it (Walters 1981). The reason for and extent of the amputation will, of course, affect the client's feelings about the event. So will the client's age, stage in development, support systems, resources, and previous crisis experiences. The client, family, and/or significant others need to know that grieving is normal.

During the grieving stage, interest in or responses to sexual overtures may be delayed or absent. Once the acute phase has passed, the need for closeness and caring will help to renew the desire for intimacy. Preparation for intercourse can include removal of a prosthesis. The partner can be taught to assist and to incorporate touching, stroking, and caressing as part of the process.

Teaching about care and rehabilitation should include not only the client, but also those who make up the support system. In addition to stump care, use of a prosthesis and/or ambulation with crutches, wheelchair, or car, and other aspects of physical care, psychosocial issues such as body image and sexuality should be addressed. Adaptation to a new self takes time. Nurses and other health-care professionals can serve as resources and identify others who can aid in restoration to the highest possible level of wellness.

Spinal Cord Injury

Spinal cord injury is usually the result of an injury resulting from automobile accidents, falls, or shrapnel or bullet wounds (Larrabee 1977, 1321). Because of this, most of the victims are young persons, not yet sexually active or just approaching adult sexual maturity. In fact, 80% of victims of spinal cord injury are between 16 and 24 years old (Garfunkel and Goldfinger, no date, 3). Because of the anatomical structure of lower motor neurons, interruption causes disruption at the level of the lesion. Unless the lesion is at the level of sacral two to four, reflex erection and even ejaculation can still occur. Some success with retraining is also possible (Larrabee 1977, 1326).

Whatever the level of the injury, the victim experiences loss of function and will go through grieving in the crisis phase (Larrabee 1977, 1329). It is in the post-crisis period that the individual will begin to deal with implications for sexuality. Age and developmental stage will affect the process of coping with an altered body image. The adult who has an established identity and independence and has achieved an intimate relationship may cope with a spinal cord injury in a far different way than a 17-year-old who is in the throes of adolescent identity crisis and has not yet achieved intimacy with another. Regression can occur because the person is forced into a dependent position once more and must learn to deal with the drastic alteration in body image (Pepper 1977, 1330).

Once rehabilitation has progressed to the point where the individual has some self-control and a measure of independence, he or she will begin to explore the effect of the injury on sexual functioning and desirability as a sexual partner (Pepper 1977, 1335). Attention may be turned to nursing or medical staff, and sexual overtures may be made to test the responses. Or the individual may repress sexuality completely, sometimes to the detriment of an already existing relationship. It is during this phase that the person needs special help in exploring all the aspects of his or her altered life, including sexuality. The belief that sex is over needs to be dispelled (Chesnutt 1976, 1278). Spinal cord injury does not affect the desire for intimacy, love, or romance, and the enjoyment and sharing of these aspects of life. Most men are capable of erection, and most women are able to respond sexually and bear children. Even if the sensation in the genital area is diminished or absent, other areas of the body are sensitive. If erection or ejaculation is not possible, other modes of sexual expression and intimacy are (Garfunkel and Goldfinger, no date, 13–15).

In studies of sexual activity of spinal cord injured persons, it is evident that even those persons who have impaired sexual function continue to enjoy life as sexual beings (Berkman, Weissman, and Frielich 1978). The extent and level of the lesion determine whether or not the man is capable of erection and ejaculation and the woman of orgasm (Griffith, Tomko, and Tinms 1973, 539; Fitzpatrick 1974). Vibrators, catheter manipulation, hot towels, fellatio, cunnilingus, manual stimulation of the clitoris, and penile protheses are some of the methods used to aid erection and/or ejaculation. Other forms of intimacy including fondling, kissing, and petting also contribute to sexual pleasure (Griffith, Tomko, and Tinms 1973). A review of the literature on women with spinal cord injury reveals that, in addition to childbearing, orgasm may be possible. Little research has been done on the effect on the four phases of sexual response after injury, however (Griffith and Trieschmann 1975).

Nursing Implications

Part of the post-crisis rehabilitation process should address sexuality, because spinal cord injured persons are still sexual human beings. First of all, the spinal cord injured person needs honest and very specific information about the nature of his or her injury and its effects on sexual functioning and fertility, as well as the possible forms of sexual expression and responses available in addition to or instead of vaginal intercourse. When injuries occur at or below the thoracic level, the person will be a paraplegic; if the injury is in the cervical region, he or she will be a quadriplegic. If the cord is severed, paralysis will be complete below the level of the lesion. If the cord is bruised or hemorrhage has occurred, some neurological functioning below the level of the injury is possible; the person may experience weakness and problems with some functions but not total paralysis. Most spinal cord injured men can attain an erection and most women retain full reproductive functioning. Those individuals who experience impaired sensation in the genital area report heightened sensitivity in other parts of the body (Garfunkel and Goldfinger, no date, 13).

Immediately after an injury, it is not possible to predict the degree of function the individual will be able to achieve; return of function can continue for months or even years after an injury. Thus, it is important when working with individuals with a spinal cord injury to emphasize the here and now, to work with functions now present and returning, and to help the person to adapt and adjust as change occurs. Establishment of some control over bladder and bowel functions will help prepare the individual for a return to sexual expression or maturation as a sexual being. This can occur through use of catheters and various retraining programs. As sexual responses and abilities are discussed and explored, inclusion of the partner will help to facilitate communication and mutual exploration of ability and limitations.

Nurses and other health-care professionals working with persons with spinal cord injuries need to recognize that intimacy is the goal, rather than orgasms, erections, and other sexual scoring (Task Force 1978, 5). Intercourse should be considered only one facet of intimacy. Information about sexual response and methods of stimulation can be helpful. "Permission" for exploration and creativity can help to remove barriers to mutual masturbation and oral sex. At the same time, cultural values and beliefs should be respected.

Individuals need to be encouraged to experiment with positions for intimacy; locations other than a standard bed (such as a waterbed or a mattress on the floor); aids such as pillows; showers and baths; range of motion or stretching exercises; massage; and relaxation techniques such as deep-breathing or yoga to promote comfort and relaxation before or as part of intimacy with another (Task Force 1978, 17).

Most of all, individuals with spinal cord injuries need recognition of and attention to sexual issues as part of the provision of total health care. Birth control needs to be considered if a relationship exists that includes the possibility of pregnancy. The method chosen will depend on the preferences of the partners, their physical capabilities (such as the ability to insert foam or a diaphragm), and any limitations due to physical condition (for instance, contraindications for oral contraceptive use due to risk of thrombus) (Task Force 1978, 25–32). In addition to contraceptive counsel-

ing, a pelvic examination, Pap smear, breast examination, testicular exam, discussion of menstrual history, and an opportunity to discuss issues of sexuality should be offered to all persons regardless of their physical abilities.

Sexuality and the Individual with a Learning Disability

The individual with a learning disability that interferes with acquisition of high-level cognitive skills and achievement of developmental tasks is not asexual nor should he or she be labeled as such. Most learning-disabled persons develop physically at a rate comparable to that of persons considered intellectually normal (Mitchell, Doctor, and Butler 1978, 289). The idea that learning-disabled persons have abnormal sex drives is unfounded. Both sexes develop secondary sex characteristics. Women menstruate and men have nocturnal emissions (Caparulo and Kempton 1981, 37). Unless the person is profoundly limited, both physically and intellectually, a desire for closeness, intimacy, and even intercourse can be present. One woman whose adult son has the intellectual abilities of a 6- to 9-year-old speaks of his love of socializing and dancing and love for young women (at a distance). She describes his maturation as a sexual being, his needs to love and be loved, and his desire to express physical feelings and marry (Riddell 1980, 89).

Preparation for sexual development is as important for learning-disabled adolescents as it is for those who are intellectually normal. Young women need to be taught about menstrual self-care and reassured that menstruation is normal. Scarborough's teaching method can be used as a framework to guide levels of instruction (1971). This method is described in a very comprehensive guide for sex education for persons with learning disabilities (Kempton 1975, 79–80). In essence, this method begins with simple concepts and moves to the complex in concert with the individual's abilities. It begins with self-care and implications for social behavior, then moves to biological explanations, psychological and emotional implications, and finally, the social-biological implications of sexuality. In one application of this method, a woman used her own menstrual period to describe and demonstrate self-care (Caparulo and Kempton 1981, 39–40). Most persons are capable of learning concepts of time and place. Thus, the social behavior implications of sexuality— confining sexual activity to socially sanctioned times and places—can be included (Fischer and Krajieck 1974, 78–83). Limitations in judgment and reasoning will influence the choice of contraception for the woman who intends to be or is sexually active. Oral contraceptives and intrauterine devices are the most successful methods, although use of other methods can also be appropriate (Caparulo and Kempton 1981, 41–43). Sometimes sterilization is the optimal choice if informed consent is possible. Breast and pelvic examinations should be performed regularly after careful preparation of the woman. Both men and women need information about and assessment for sexually transmitted diseases.

Gordon and colleagues list key facts for disabled adolescents concerning their sexuality. In addition to information about sexually transmitted diseases, conception, risks of pregnancy, and contraception, they stress normal sexual expression through masturbation and nonexploitive sexual behavior with partners of either sex. The criminal nature of sexual abuse and exploitation is emphasized. The normal experiences of menstruation and nocturnal emission are emphasized, as is use of correct terminology for body parts and functions. The authors stress the multitude of means for expressing closeness and intimacy, deemphasizing genital sex (Gordon, Scales,

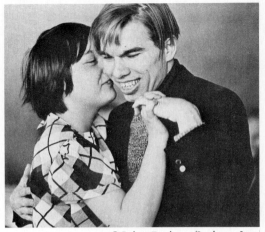

© Robert Foothorap/Jeroboam, Inc.

FIGURE 8-6
Persons with learning disabilities need closeness too.

and Everly 1979, 150–152). Sex education programs for learning-disabled adolescents also focus on appropriate versus inappropriate behaviors, private versus public expressions of sexuality, and social skills and responsibilities (McNab 1978, 304).

Attitudes of caretakers can influence the care and information given to persons with learning disabilities. It is disconcerting that biases among health-care providers still exist concerning sexual expression by these clients (Mitchell, Doctor, and Butler 1978). Information programs for staff might help to dispel myths and assist caretakers to better meet the needs of clients including optimal development as sexual beings (see Figure 8-6).

Living with Chronic Conditions: Issues in Sexuality

A number of chronic conditions have implications for sexuality. While the discussion that follows is in no way meant to be exhaustive, it does attempt to address the problems of a number of common conditions that affect sexuality. Some of these conditions can begin as biophysical and psychosocial crises. During the post-crisis period, effects on sexuality become apparent and should be addressed.

Obesity

Obesity is a major health problem in the United States. It is a condition that affects and is affected by one's self-image (Kahn 1978) and is therefore at least indirectly tied to one's sexuality. Although obesity for some persons can represent disregard for society's standards of attractiveness, or protection against sex, most obese individuals are not apathetic toward sex (Rand 1979, 141). However, in our culture, definitions of sexual attractiveness are quite narrowly defined, especially for women. The obese individual may feel and/or actually be physically unattractive to potential partners. For the adolescent who is struggling with identity and self-esteem, obesity can be devastating. It may isolate the person from the peer group. In adulthood, too, self-esteem is important. Negative self-image can inhibit relationships. The obese individual may not wish to be seen naked by a partner (Jordan and Levitz 1979, 109).

In addition to interfering with social relationships that led to sexual intimacy, obesity can also interfere physically with sexual activity. For the obese person, certain positions may not be possible, shortness of breath on exertion can limit endurance, and physical closeness can be uncomfortable. Obesity can make intercourse difficult if not impossible (Rand 1979, 145). There seems to be no evidence, however, that obese persons have more sexual concerns or problems than nonobese persons (Rand 1979, 150–151). But when the obese individual does express difficulties with sexual activity, health-care professionals need to offer support. The nature of the interventions will be determined by the source of the difficulty.

When obesity is used as a defense against sex, the reasons need to be explored. Professional counseling may be needed to assist the individual in examining his or her attitudes toward sex and the role of body image in sexuality (Jordan and Levitz 1979, 115).

Unsuccessful attempts to disguise body size can contribute to lack of partners. Even without weight loss, counseling about hygiene and clothing can enhance attractiveness, as well as increase confidence and positive self-image (Jordan and Levitz 1979, 115).

When mechanical difficulties occur, discussion of positions, means of intimacy other than vaginal intercourse, and alternate modes of stimulation through masturbation, oral-genital sex, and use of devices such as vibrators can be helpful. Discussion of the problem will help to open up communication between partners and also can lower inhibitions. Closeness, cuddling, and stroking provide reassurance of caring and attractiveness. Encouraging open sharing about problems can stimulate creativity in finding solutions.

The person who loses weight can also face risks. Adapting to a new body image takes time. Rapid weight loss does not allow time for adjustment. Expectations for increased social and sexual activity following weight loss may be unrealistic. When dreams do not materialize, the person's body image and self-esteem may suffer (Jordan and Levitz 1979, 116).

In history-taking with obese persons, age of onset, family attitudes toward obesity, social group and peer acceptance, and the client's own feelings about obesity are all factors to be considered. Health-care professionals need to recognize the potential for risk in obese persons and address them holistically.

Chronic Kidney Disorders

Persons with chronic renal failure face a life of dependency on dialysis unless a successful transplant is accomplished. Fluid, diet, and economic restrictions occur. In addition, lethargy, anemia, and recurrent infection affect clients' sense of well-being. It is not surprising that their sexual expression also is affected (Abram et al. 1975, 221). Impotence is not uncommon among dialysis clients. The majority of persons with chronic renal disease seem to have either decreased sexual activity or reduction in sexual potency (Thurm 1975; Abram et al. 1975). After transplant activity increases and the incidence of impotence decreases (Abram et al. 1975, 225; Salvatierra, Fortmann, and Belzer 1975).

Couples report numerous sexual problems associated with dialysis. These include lack of satisfaction, infrequency of intercourse, and dysfunction including diminished response, lack of orgasm, and impotence (Steele, Finkelstein, and Finkelstein 1976). In one study, decrease in sexual drive was identified as a stressor by individuals on dialysis (Baldree, Murphy, and Powers 1982, 109).

Misinformation is common among persons on dialysis, and these myths extend to aspects of sexuality. Some myths include the belief that sex hormones are removed during dialysis or that one becomes sterile (Hickman 1977, 607).

The high incidence of problems with sexuality related to chronic renal disease warrants the attention of health-care providers. Exploration of sexual issues will help to reveal problems. Clients may be reluctant to bring up difficulties, feeling embarrassed or inadequate. Using the third person can be a useful technique: "Some persons on dialysis find their sexual interest or responsiveness is diminished," or "Decreased interest in intercourse is common." When energy levels are low and impotence present, alternate means of achieving intimacy by less stressful, less energy-sapping means can be encouraged. Desire for soft touching, stroking, and closeness may be present when the energy for intercourse is not. Feelings of anger, depression, sadness, and weakness should be attributed to the disease process and not to relationships. It is important that the many effects of renal failure and dialysis be explored so that couples are not caught up in blame and guilt. It is important, too, to recognize that not all problems are due to dialysis. Careful attention to diet, drug therapy, and management of the psychosocial aspects of renal disease as well as the biophysical aspects can contribute to improved well-being and sexual health (Thurm 1975, 62).

Sexuality and Diabetes

It is now generally recognized that diabetes can be associated with sexual problems. In men, impotence can occur as a result of impairment of the nervi erigentes, the parasympathetic nerves responsible for erection. Diabetic peripheral autonomic neuropathy can affect these pelvic nerves (Ellenberg 1979, 4; Cooper 1972, 35; Kolodny and Kahn 1974; Ellenberg 1971). Problems with fertility also can occur due to impotence or retrograde ejaculation.

It has been estimated that 40% to 60% of all men with diabetes experience some problem with alterations in sexual response due to disruption of peripheral autonomic nerve pathways. (Kolodny and Kahn 1974). These men present with partial or total inability to achieve an erection. Libido is still present, but with deterioration of sexual function over time, feelings of inadequacy may take over and result in loss of libido as well. The onset of sexual problems is usually 6 to 12 months after the onset of diabetes (Block 1982, 19).

Women do not demonstrate an analogous disruption of sexual function as often. There appears to be little correlation between pelvic neuropathy and libido and orgasmic response (Ellenberg 1977; Ellenberg 1979, 7). One study reports lack of orgasm in women with diabetes who were previously orgasmic. However, no correlations with neuropathy or with age, onset, or duration of diabetes were found (Kolodny 1971, 551).

Women experience problems with other aspects of sexuality aside from response. These include fertility, pregnancy, and contraception. The woman who is diabetic may experience some problems with fertility when she desires to become pregnant, although the incidence of infertility seems to be associated with control of diabetes; the woman whose diabetes is well controlled experiences fewer problems getting pregnant. Some methods of contraception may be contraindicated. Oral contraceptives are used with caution in women with insulin-dependent diabetes due to the vascular effects of diabetes and increased risk of thrombus formation with oral contraceptives. Oral contraceptives also seem to alter glucose metabolism; if oral contraceptives are prescribed, insulin dosage may need to be adjusted. Because of the impaired response to infection associated with diabetes, the use of an intrauterine device may also be questioned.

The pregnant woman who is an insulin-dependent diabetic faces many risks, as does her fetus. These risks include increased morbidity and mortality. Morbidity risks include hypertensive disease of pregnancy (toxemia), urinary tract infections, vaginitis, hydramnios (excessive amniotic fluid), a difficult delivery, a higher rate of cesarean births, hemorrhaging, and more birth canal injuries during a vaginal delivery due to the large size of the infant. Risks to the woman's fetus include stillbirth, macrosomia due to the effects of maternal hyperglycemia (stimulation to the fetal pancreas to produce insulin), hypoglycemia after birth (as the pancreas continues to overproduce insulin), respiratory distress syndrome (RDS) due to the need for early delivery to prevent stillbirth, and increased risk of anomalies, probably due to the intrauterine environment. Perinatal morbidity and mortality are higher for infants of diabetic mothers as well (Moore, Bingham, and Keesling 1981, 188–189).

Vaginitis, especially candida albicans, is common in women with diabetes, probably due to the hyperglycemia. A vaginal infection affects sexual response, comfort during sex, and the woman's feelings about her body (Yale Sex Therapy Training Program, no date, 2).

In addition to the organic effects of diabetes on sexuality, important psychosocial consequences also occur for both sexes. Living with a chronic disease affects self-esteem and body image. Organic impairment of sexual function is a threat to femininity or masculinity, creating a vicious cycle of failure. Fear of rejection and feelings of shame can inhibit responses (Schiavi and Hogan 1979, 11).

Interventions are based on a thorough assessment that identifies the origins of sexual dysfunction. It is important to differentiate between organic causes and those that are psychogenic in origin. Nocturnal penile tumescence can be monitored to confirm organic cause. During REM (rapid eye movement) sleep, some erection will occur if there is no neuropathic disruption (Wabrek 1979, 738). A thorough sexual history is also appropriate as part of the assessment process. A man may be able to achieve full erections through masturbation, oral stimulation, or erotic stimuli (Block 1982, 24).

When pelvic neuropathy is present, a penile prosthesis may be one solution (Furlow 1979; Sotile 1979). Several types are now available. Their use, advantages, and disadvantages should be fully explored before any surgery (Block 1982, 24–25).

Sex therapy may be appropriate for some persons and their partners. Nursing care should focus on interpersonal aspects of the relationship, issues of self-esteem and body image, fears, and guilt. Lack of information and misinformation can also contribute to sexual difficulties. When sexual activity has focused on vaginal intercourse, couples may be unaware of other means of sharing intimacy. They should recognize that orgasm can occur for a man even when erection does not (Schiavi and Hogan 1979, 15). Men should also be told that remissions and exacerbations do occur (Block 1982, 25).

Sensitivity of health-care professionals to the sexual needs of persons with diabetes can help avert or alleviate problems. Not all difficulties need the expertise of surgeons or sex therapists. Issues of self-esteem, body image, and sex education and information can be addressed by nurses in the course of providing education for diabetes care. However, special care is needed for the diabetic woman who is pregnant to assure a safe outcome for the women and her fetus (see Hawkins and Higgins, 1981, for complete discussion).

Sexuality and Cardiac Conditions

After diagnosis of coronary disease is made or the acute phase of a myocardial infarction has passed, it is common for persons to experience depression, anxiety, and insecurity. Intermingled among these feelings are concerns about prolonged dependence, adjustments in lifestyle, and implications for sexuality. Both the client and his or her partner may avoid sex, afraid that the exertion will precipitate a crisis (Puksta 1977, 602). In one investigation, sexual activity was found to be the form of exertion most feared by clients with cardiac disease (Schwab, Levenson, and Rossenman 1970).

The effects of sexual activity need to be evaluated in order to advise clients. A number of studies have been done to document the biophysical effects of intercourse (Goldbarg 1970; Hellerstein and Friedman 1970; Masters and Johnson 1966; Ueno 1963; Douglas 1975). The arousal phase is characterized by a slow increase in heart rate and in respiratory rate and mild elevation of the blood pressure. Maximum increases are reached during orgasm and then blood pressure, pulse, and respiratory rates return to normal within seconds (Griffin 1973, 71). Hellerstein and Friedman (1970, 992) found that energy expenditure during sex is modest. It has been compared to the amount of energy required to argue or drive a car. Oxygen consumption is less than that required to walk briskly or to climb a flight of stairs (Hellerstein and Friedman 1970, 987–999). These authors suggest that if a person can perform a Master's "2-step" test, walk vigorously, or exercise at a level that consumes 6 to 8 calories a minute — without experiencing symptoms, adversely affecting blood pressure or pulse, or producing change in a cardiogram — he or she is probably fit to resume sexual intercourse.

If the individual has suffered a myocardial infarction, physical evaluation is done prior to discharge and then as a follow-up in the outpatient clinic or private physician's office. Sexual activity can usually be resumed six to eight weeks after the infarction. A Holter EKG monitor can be worn to monitor effects of intercourse (Scalzi and Dracup 1978, 841 and 843).

In planning education for the cardiac client regarding sex, it is important to evaluate and review lifestyle and symptoms. These factors are relevant: accustomed type and amount of exercise; timing and types of meals; alcohol intake; sleep patterns; sexual activity prior to the infarction; preferred times and positions for sex; any previous problems with sexuality such as impotence, decrease in libido, and associated factors; chest pain before or after intercourse; and sleeplessness or fatigue associated with sexual activity (Puksta 1977, 603).

Counseling should begin as part of education for discharge or following diagnosis of a cardiac problem. Sexual activity should be considered one of the normal activities in a person's life. If possible and desired, the partner should be included (Scalzi and Dracup 1978, 842). Instructions about warning signs should be included: rapid heart and respiratory rates that persist one-half hour or more after intercourse; palpitations which continue for 15 minutes or more; chest pain before, during or after intercourse; sleeplessness following sex; or extreme fatigue the next day (Puksta 1977, 603; Griffith 1973, 72). Clients should be cautioned to avoid intercourse under certain circumstances. After a large meal or drinking alcohol it is best to wait at least three hours. If the temperature is extremely hot or cold, the biophysical demands for temperature maintenance preclude sex. When tension, anxiety, anger, resentment, or other negative feelings are present, or when time is short or the client is extremely fatigued, it is best to wait. Intercourse should occur at a time when leisure and rest are possible, not just prior to strenuous physical activity. Sex with unfamiliar partners is more stressful than with a congenial partner with whom one is comfortable (Puksta 1977, 603; Griffith 1973, 72–73; Scalzi and Dracup 1978, 843).

Positions that are least stressful should be suggested for the person with a cardiac problem. For example, the cardiac partner can sit on a wide chair, assume whatever is the least strenuous position when lying, or lie side by side with his or her partner (Griffith 1973, 73). Nitroglycerin can be taken prophylactically to prevent angina during sexual activity (Cole et al. 1979, 126). Propranolol hydrochloride is sometimes used when nitroglycerin is ineffective (Puksta 1977, 604).

The importance of extended foreplay, of relaxation prior to sexual activity, and of unhurried time with privacy assured should be

stressed (Van Bree 1975, 407–408). Soft music, meditation, a warm shower, and other means of relaxation can help to reduce the stress of sexual activity (Puksta 1977, 604).

The belief that one's sex life is over when one has cardiac disease is untrue and can be detrimental to a relationship, as well as to one's self-esteem. Education about sexuality, a realistic assessment of ability, release from demands to perform, and a sensitive, well-informed partner can help to restore this important part of life.

Sexuality and Respiratory Compromise

For the individual experiencing respiratory compromise — whether from asthma episodes, lung cancer, or chronic obstructive pulmonary disease — interference with sexual activity and expression can occur. The person with asthma that is episodic in nature may be able to adjust the degree of exertion and the kinds of sexual activity engaged in to accommodate any respiratory compromise he or she is experiencing. If the asthma episodes seem to be triggered by sexual activity or are severely limiting or interfering with sexual expression, the advice of health-care professionals should be sought. Perhaps medication can be taken before sexual activity is anticipated. Alterations in modes of expression and open communication with one's partner can allay stress and anxiety and preserve the relationship. Planning ahead does disrupt spontaneity, but it may afford the individual the comfort to engage in strenuous sexual activity without untoward effects. Queries about sexuality may be included appropriately in health assessments and management of the individual with asthma.

Since lung cancer is a life-threatening condition with a poor prognosis, the individual is coping with the possibility of his or her death, and, thus, sexual expression occurs in this context. More information is included later in this chapter in addressing the sexuality of individuals in the terminal stages of their lives.

Individuals living with chronic obstructive pulmonary disease (COPD) experience many disruptions in lifestyle including the impact of disease on sexuality. Dyspnea and fatigue are specific symptoms that interfere with sexual expression. Chronic cough, tenseness, and fear of exacerbation of symptoms may also intrude. The alterations in body image and the guilt and depression that accompany any chronic disease may impede sexual desire and expression. Drugs can impair function: antihypertensives and thiazide diuretics can cause impotence, and corticosteroids can cause muscle weakness, atrophy, and depression. Medications such as spironolactone can cause decreased libido and impotence (Stockdale-Woolley 1983, 16–17). Continuous or intermittent use of oxygen creates a mechanical and perhaps a psychological barrier to intimacy.

Nursing interventions should be based on careful assessment of the limitations the individual is experiencing. Can he or she tolerate the demands of orgasm, equivalent to climbing a flight of stairs? What limitations is the individual experiencing? Does a comfortable room with adequate temperature and humidity help? What timing is best in relation to meals? What positions are most comfortable? Does continuous oxygen increase the individual's tolerance for sexual activity? Suggesting means of intimacy that are less taxing than intercourse can be very helpful in maintaining a close relationship (Stockdale-Woolley 1983, 17 and 20).

Sexuality and Stroke

The individual who has suffered a cerebral vascular accident (CVA) can suffer from a wide range of neurological deficits. The degree of disability during and following reha-bilitation will affect ability to engage in sexual activity. Those who recover sufficiently to return home are most able to resume sexual activity as part of their lives, either alone or with a partner. The needs of the person who must be institutionalized should not be ignored, however.

For the rare individual who experiences a CVA under the age of 45, sexual function is rarely, if ever, disturbed after the crisis (Muckleroy 1977, 115). For the individual left with residual hemiplegia, however, the effects on sexual expression can be considerable. Most of these persons are between 45 and 65 and many have partners in a stable relationship. Some of the problems related to sexuality include fear of damage from another stroke occurring during sex, disability related to paralysis of a limb or limbs, disruptions in communication if speech is affected, changes in personality, and male impotence (Muckleroy 1977, 115–116). One study of sexuality after a cerebral vascular accident indicated that interest does not abate and that sexuality before the stroke is an excellent predictor. If the dominant hemisphere is affected, libido may decrease, but it is altogether likely that no change will occur (Goddess, Wagner, and Silverman 1979, 24).

Counseling concerning sexuality should be an integral part of caring for persons who suffer strokes. During the rehabilitation phase, issues of sexuality should be explored and reassurance given. It is evident that the level of interest in sex remains high when sexual activity was part of the person's life prior to the stroke (Goddess, Wagner, and Silverman 1979, 24). Depression, a common occurrence after a stroke, is more easily lifted when the person is able to resume normal activities. Intimacy may be an important part of the person's life and it need not be deleted because a stroke has occurred.

Education about alternative positions and means of stimulation can be helpful if paralysis is present. Stroking and caressing can be directed to the uninvolved side. However, many persons who have had a stroke want the partner to caress both sides so they can incorporate the affected side into their body image. Touching, feeling, gestures, and other nonverbal communication can be encouraged if aphasia or disturbances in expressive speech persist. Impotence is often present. Assurance of privacy, allowing plenty of time, trying new modes of stimulation, and dispensing with past expectations for "performance" can be helpful. Focusing on intimacies other than vaginal intercourse allows the couple the sharing of softness, closeness, and expressions of love and caring without making unrealistic demands (Muckleroy 1977, 116). Persons who suffer strokes and their partners usually welcome education about sexuality. Part of post-crisis care should include this important aspect of well-being, as plans are directed toward achieving the highest level of wellness possible.

Sexuality and Hypertension

It has been estimated that about 90 million Americans have blood pressures of 140/90 or higher and, of these, more than 90% can be classified as hypertensive (National High Blood Pressure Education Program 1978). Diet and drug regimens are customarily prescribed to decrease risks of sequelae (Hill 1979, 906). The effects on self-esteem and body image of such lifelong restrictions warrant consideration for their impact on sexuality.

A man who has been diagnosed as hypertensive may feel he is somehow less than a complete male. If he adheres to the macho model, he may feel that any defect is an assault on that image of himself. He may be embarrassed by the limits a sodium-restricted diet imposes and wish to hide it from others. He may fear damage to himself if he engages in vigorous sex or, conversely, ignore warnings and medical regimens in an attempt to convince himself that he is fine.

A woman with hypertension may feel that medications and special diets restrict her socially, make her less than desirable as a sex object, or threaten her reproductive capabilities if she is premenopausal. Hypertension does pose a threat to pregnant women and also limits contraceptive choices for women. Use of oral contraceptives is generally contraindicated for the woman who is hypertensive.

It is important to note, however, that hypertension should in no way interfere with normal sexual functioning from a biophysical perspective. Some of the medications used in management of hypertension, however, can produce impotence, inhibition of ejaculation, and occasionally retrograde ejaculation (into the bladder) (Blackford 1981, 270). Clients need to be warned of possible side effects and, if problems occur, told to consult health-care providers for adjustment of the dosage or a change in medication. Some of the drugs that can cause difficulty include: Rauwolfia and derivatives, guanethidine, mecamylamine, trimethaphan, spironolactone, clonidine, propranolol, and metroprolol (Blackford 1981, 270). Sometimes warnings of possible impotence from such medications can become self-fulfilling prophecies. Warnings about sexual effects must therefore be tailored to individual clients and perhaps be included in a more general listing of a variety of untoward effects to be noted and reported (Long et al. 1976, 769). When a client returns for a checkup following prescription of a regimen, assessment can include sexual functioning. If necessary, dosage adjustments can be made at this time.

For the client with severe hypertension and arteriosclerosis, decreasing the dosage of medications may be impossible. Since the penis does not lose sensation, using manual stimulation, patience, and understanding can still make intercourse possible (Blackford 1981, 270).

It is important to help couples find ways to maintain intimacy in spite of use of medications necessary for disease control. Issues of sexuality should be an integral part of education about living with hypertension.

Sexuality, Death, and Dying

In a society in which death is not easily coped with, issues of sexuality for dying persons and their loved ones are rarely confronted. When death is sudden and unexpected, the partner experiences immediate disruption of expressions of intimacy and sexuality with the loved one. But when death is slow and anticipated, as with a terminal condition, the diagnosis should not be considered synonymous with celibacy or death of the sexual being.

Health-care professionals must first confront their own feelings about dying and sexuality in order to help their clients (Wasow 1977, 117). Gideon and Taylor have identified 15 rights of dying persons that pertain to their sexuality (1981, 305). These include knowing oneself as a sexual person and understanding that intercourse and sexuality are two different entities; other rights are related to sexual needs, expression, and communication.

Fear of the death of a close friend or family member can trigger anticipatory grief (Lamerton 1981, 179). During this period, the sharing of intimacy should be encouraged. Both the partner and the person with the terminal condition need to feel it is all right to continue to share closeness, caring, and sexual activity to the extent to which it is desired and comfortable. Sanctioning intimacy gives permission to continue an important aspect of living and dying. It can help a couple resolve feelings, experience a new kind of closeness,

and say good-bye in a way that is peaceful and comforting. When all else seems to be going wrong, continuing sexual activity can help the dying person maintain self-esteem. By contrast, changes and upsets in sex life were among the psychosocial problems experienced by cancer patients in one study (Freidenbergs et al. 1980, 113). Deprivation of physical contact has been identified by dying persons as a source of severe distress (Wellisch 1980, 14).

Maintenance of intimacy can also help the couple share feelings about death and loss. As physical strength wanes, stroking, caressing, touching, and holding one another will extend and preserve the feelings of closeness from former days. If the person chooses to die at home, he or she can continue to share a bed as long as both partners wish. Intimate caretaking activities are sometimes more comfortably performed by the partner, an extension of the caring and concern expressed in sexuality. The individual should be helped to continue maintaining his or her appearance as much as possible. Affirmation of manhood or womanhood is important (Taylor 1983, 54). It should not be assumed, however, that partners wish or are able to be caregivers.

When institutionalization is necessary, privacy should be provided for clients and their partners. Staff need to recognize that the need for intimacy continues for some to the moment of death. Caregivers need to convey the message that terminally ill clients are viewed as having legitimate sexual needs (Wellisch 1980, 15). Hospices offer more personalized, sensitive care and environments for persons to share dying with their loved ones. Even in the critical-care setting, however, the needs of clients for intimacy should not be ignored. Spouses or partners often demonstrate the need to be with their critically ill mates (Breu and Dracup 1978, 53). Flexible visiting hours, a comfortable chair close to the bedside, and relaxation of rules may be in the best interest of both partners. What harm will it do for a partner to hold or caress his or her dying loved one, even lying on the bed together?

It is interesting that the words sex, sexuality, and intimacy do not appear in the indices of the current major works on death and dying. While these topics may not be of supreme interest or importance, it cannot be assumed that all persons divest themselves of sexuality or a need for intimacy when they are diagnosed as terminal or are dying. Perhaps it is time to turn some attention to this aspect of human existence.

Summary of Implications for Nursing Practice

Working with individuals, families, and communities through the post-crisis phase of developmental and situational events involves many important implications for sexuality. Health-care professionals need to be adequately prepared to assist clients and their partners in achieving the optimal desired expression of sexuality as part of restoration to wellness or the highest achievable level of functioning. When death is inevitable, support for maintaining the desired level of intimacy is possible. Only then will we have achieved complete integration of sexuality into all of life, from birth to death.

REFERENCES

Abram, H. S., L. R. Hester, W. F. Sheridan, and G. M. Epstein. 1975. Sexual functioning in patients with chronic renal failure. *The Journal of Nervous and Mental Disease* 160(3):220–226.

Alexander, C. 1976. Nurses ignore importance of sexuality in the OR. *AORN Journal* 23(5):743–746.

Alpert, L. L. 1979. Approaches to breast cancer: A pathologist's perspective. *Women & Health* 4(3):269–286.

Anderson, B. 1979. Carole, a girl treated with bracing. *American Journal of Nursing* 79(9):1592–1597.

Armel, P. 1981. After mastectomy: Choosing to look different. *Ms.,* 10(1):22–23.

Baldree, K. S., S. P. Murphy, and M. J. Powers. 1982. Stress identification and coping patterns in patients on hemodialysis. *Nursing Research* 31(2):107–112.

Berkman, A. H., R. Weissman, and M. H. Frielich. 1978. Sexual adjustment of spinal cord injured veterans living in the community. *Archives of Physical Medicine and Rehabilitation* 59(1):29–33.

Blackford, G. S. 1981. Sexuality and hypertension. *Health Values* 5(6):270.

Block, A. M. 1982. Sexual dysfunction of the male with diabetes mellitus. *The Nurse Practitioner* 7(8):19,24–25.

Breu, C., and K. Dracup. 1978. Helping the spouses of critically ill patients. *American Journal of Nursing* 78(1):51–53.

Bullard, D. G., and S. E. Knight. 1981. *Sexuality and physical disability: Personal perspectives.* St. Louis: C. V. Mosby.

Burnham, W. R., J. E. Lennard-Jones, and B. M. Brooke. 1977. Sexual problems among ileostomists. *Gut* 18(11):673–677.

Byrd, B. F. 1975. Sex after mastectomy. *Medical Aspects of Human Sexuality* 9(4):53–54.

Cancer Information Clearinghouse. 1979. *Breast cancer: Annotated bibliography of public, patient, and professional information and education materials.* Bethesda, Md.: U.S. Department of Health, Education, and Welfare.

Caparulo, F., and W. Kempton. 1981. Sexual health needs of the mentally retarded adolescent female. *Issues in Health Care of Women* 3(1):35–46.

Catanzaro, M. 1980. MS:Nursing care of the person with MS. *American Journal of Nursing* 80(2):286–291.

Chesnutt, J. 1976. He's 34, a quadriplegic, and gets along just fine. *American Journal of Nursing* 76(8):1278.

Cohen, L. 1981. Disabled rebel at sex taboo. *Hartford Courant* 54(319).

Cole, C. M., E. M. Levin, J. O. Whitley, and S. H. Young. 1979. Brief sexual counseling during cardiac rehabilitation. *Heart & Lung* 8(1):124–129.

Cooper, A. J. 1972. Diagnosis and management of "endocrine impotence." *British Medical Journal* 2:34–36.

Cope, O. 1978. *The breast: A health guide for women of all ages.* New York: Houghton Mifflin.

DeMoya, D., and A. DeMoya. 1980. Frank answers to your most delicate patient-counseling questions. *RN* 43(11):104.

deToledo, C. H. 1979. The defect: Classification and detection. *American Journal of Nursing* 79(9):1588–1591.

Douglas, J. E., and T. D. Wilkes. 1975. Reconditioning cardiac patients. *American Family Physician* 11(1):123–129.

Ellenberg, M. 1971. Impotence in diabetes: The neurologic factor. *Annals of Internal Medicine* 75:213–219.

Ellenberg, M. 1977. Sexual aspects of the female diabetic. *The Mount Sinai Journal of Medicine* 44(4):495–500.

Ellenberg, M. 1979. Sex and diabetes: A comparison between men and women. *Diabetes Care* 2(1):4–8.

Finch, E. 1977. Sexuality and the disabled. *The Canadian Nurse* 73(1):19–20.

Fischbach, F. T. 1978. Easing adjustment to Parkinson's disease. *American Journal of Nursing* 78(1):66–69.

Fischer, H. L., and M. J. Krajieck. 1974. Sexual development of the moderately retarded child. *Clinical Pediatrics* 13:78–83.

Fitzpatrick, W. F. 1974. Sexual function in the paraplegic patient. *Archives of Physical Medicine and Rehabilitation* 55(5):221–227.

Frauman, A. C., and N. S. Sypert. 1979. Sexuality in adolescents with chronic illness. *The American Journal of Maternal Child Nursing* 4(6):371–375.

Freidenbergs, I., W. Gordon, M. R. Hibbard, and L. Diller. 1980. Assessment and treatment of psychosocial problems of the cancer patient: A case study. *Cancer Nursing* 3(2):111–119.

Furlow, W. L. 1979. Diagnosis and treatment of male erectile failure. *Diabetes Care* 2(1):18–25.

Garfunkel, M., and G. Goldfinger. no date. *Living with spinal cord injury.* New York: Institute of Rehabilitation Medicine, New York University Medical Center.

Garrard, A. 1975. News about breast cancer—for you *and* your doctor. *Ms.,* 3(9):28–29.

Gideon, M. D., and P. B. Taylor. 1981. A sexual bill of rights for the dying person. *Death Education* 4:303–314.

Goddess, E. D., N. N. Wagner, and D. R. Silverman. 1979. Poststroke sexual activity of CVA patients. *Medical Aspects of Human Sexuality* 13(3):16,23–24,29–30.

Goldbarg, A. N. 1970. Energy cost of sexual activity. *Archives of Internal Medicine* 126:526.

Gordon, S., P. Scales, and K. Everly. 1979. *The sexual adolescent.* 2d ed. North Scituate, Mass.: Duxbury Press.

Griffith, E. R., M. A. Tomko, and R. J. Tinms. 1973. Sexual function in spinal cord-injured patients: A review. *Archives of Physical Medicine and Rehabilitation* 54(12):539–543.

Griffith, E. R., and R. B. Trieschmann. 1975. Sexual functioning in women with spinal cord injury. *Archives of Physical Medicine and Rehabilitation* 56(1):18–21.

Griffith, E. R., and R. B. Trieschmann. 1977. Sexual function restoration in the physically disabled: Use of a private hospital room. *Archives of Physical Medicine and Rehabilitation* 58(8):368–369.

Griffith, G. G. 1973. Sexuality and the cardiac patient. *Heart and Lung* 2(1):70–73.

Gruenbaum, E. 1982. The movement against clitoridectomy and infibulation in Sudan: Public health policy and the women's movement. *Medical Anthropology Newsletter* 13(2):4–12.

Halstead, L. S. 1977. Aiding arthritic patients to adjust sexually. *Medical Aspects of Human Sexuality* 11(4):85–86.

Hamilton, M. S., and N. B. Schlapper. 1976. Pelvic exenteration. *American Journal of Nursing* 76(2):266–272.

Haring, M., and L. Meyerson. 1979. Attitudes of college students toward sexual behavior of disabled persons. *Archives of Physical Medicine and Rehabilitation* 60(6):257–260.

Hawkins, J. W., and L. P. Higgins. 1981. *Maternity and gynecological nursing: Women's health care.* Philadelphia: Lippincott.

Hellerstein, H. K., and E. H. Friedman. 1970. Sexual activity and the postcoronary patient. *Archives of Internal Medicine* 125:987–999.

Hickman, B. W. 1977. All about sex . . . despite dialysis. *American Journal of Nursing* 77(4):606–607.

Hill, M. 1979. Helping the hypertensive patient control sodium intake. *American Journal of Nursing* 79(5):906–909.

Hosken, F. 1980. The politics of female genital mutilation. *Science for the People* 12(6):12–16.

Jacobson, L. 1974. Illness and human sexuality. *Nursing Outlook* 22(1):50–53.

Jamison, K. C., D. K. Wellisch, and R. O. Pasnau. 1978. Psychosocial aspects of mastectomy: I—the woman's perspective. *American Journal of Psychiatry* 135(4):432–436.

Jordan, H. A., and L. S. Levitz. 1979. Sex and obesity. *Medical Aspects of Human Sexuality* 13(10):105,108–109,115–117.

Kahn, A. N. 1978. Group education for the overweight. *American Journal of Nursing* 78(2):254.

Kempton, W. 1975. *Sex education for persons with disabilities that hinder learning: A teacher's guide.* North Scituate, Mass.: Duxbury Press.

Kennerly, S. L. 1977. "What I learned about mastectomy." *American Journal of Nursing* 77(9):1430–1432.

Kolodny, R. C. 1971. Sexual dysfunction in diabetic females. *Diabetes* 20:551.

Kolodny, R. C., and C. Kahn. 1974. Sexual dysfunction in diabetic man. *Diabetes* 23(4):306–309.

Kushner, R. 1977. *Why me? What every woman should know about breast cancer to save her life.* New York: Times Mirror, New American Library.

Lamerton, R. 1981. *Care of the dying.* rev. ed. New York: Penguin.

Larrabee, J. H. 1977. Physical care during early recovery. *American Journal of Nursing* 77(8):1320–1329.

Levene, M. B. 1977. A new role for radiation therapy. *American Journal of Nursing* 77(9):1443–1444.

Levinger, G. E. 1980. Working through recovery after mastectomy. *American Journal of Nursing* 80(6):1119–1120.

Littlefield, V. 1977. The surgical patient's sexuality. *AORN Journal* 26(4):649–658.

Living and Loving: Information about sex. 1982. Atlanta: Arthritis Foundation.

Long, M. L., E. H. Winslow, M. A. Scheuhing, and J. A. Callahan. 1976. Hypertension: What patients need to know. *American Journal of Nursing* 76(5):765–770.

Lyons, A. S. 1975. Sex after ileostomy and colostomy. *Medical Aspects of Human Sexuality* 9(1):107–108.

Masters, W. H., and V. E. Johnson. 1966. *Human sexual response.* Boston: Little, Brown.

McDonnell, M., J. Hentgen, N. Holland, and P. W. Levison. 1980. MS problem oriented nursing care plans. *American Journal of Nursing* 80(2):292–297.

McNab, W. L. 1978. The sexual needs of the handicapped. *The Journal of School Health* 48(5):301–306.

Micheli, L. J., M. A. Magin and R. Rouvales. 1979. Surgical management and nursing care. *American Journal of Nursing* 79(9):1599–1607.

Michelson, M. R. 1979. There *are* alternatives to mastectomy. *Ms.,* 7(7).

Miller, P., and C. A. Janda. 1979. Perceived needs of women undergoing radical mastectomy. *Issues in Health Care of Women* 1(6):27–37.

Mitchell, L., R. M. Doctor, and D. C. Butler. 1978. Attitudes of caretakers toward the sexual behavior of mentally retarded persons. *American Journal of Mental Deficiency* 83(3):289–296.

Montague, D. K. 1977. Sex after cystectomy. *Medical Aspects of Human Sexuality* 11(12):91–92.

Moore, D. S., P. R. Bingham, and O. Keesling. 1981. Nursing care of the pregnant woman with diabetes mellitus. *Journal of Obstetric Gyneologic and Neonatal Nursing* 10(3):188–194.

Morgan, R., and G. Steinem. 1980. The international crime of genital mutilation. *Ms.,* 8(9).

Morris, R., H. S. Greer, and P. White. 1977. Psychological and social adjustment to mastectomy, a two year follow-up study. *Cancer* 40(5):2381–2387.

Muckleroy, R. N. 1977. Sex counseling after stroke. *Medical Aspects of Human Sexuality* 11(12):115–116.

Napoli, M. 1983. Breast cancer: An update. *Network News* (4):2–7.

National Cancer Institute. 1979. *The breast cancer digest.* Bethesda, Md.: U. S. Department of Health, Education, and Welfare.

National High Blood Pressure Education Program. 1978. *New hypertension and prevalence data and recommendations.* Bethesda, Md.: National Institutes of Health. mimeo.

National Women's Health Network. 1980. *Breast cancer*. Washington D.C.: National Women's Health Network.

Ola-Petter, N. Gevner, R. Naass, B. Fretheim, and E. Gjone. 1977. Marital status and sexual adjustment after colostomy. *Scandinavian Journal of Gastroenterology* 12:193–197.

Paradowski, W. 1977. Socialization patterns and sexual problems of the institutionalized chronically ill and physically disabled. *Archives of Physical Medicine and Rehabilitation* 58(2):53–59.

Pepper, G. A. 1977. Psychological care. *American Journal of Nursing* 77(8):1330–1336.

Peters, L. 1982. Women's health care approaches in delivery to physically disabled women. *The Nurse Practitioner* 7(1):34,36–37,48.

Puhaty, H. D. 1977. Confronting one's changed image: Two rehabilitative approaches. *American Journal of Nursing* 77(9):1437

Puksta, N. S. 1977. All about sex . . . after a coronary. *American Journal of Nursing* 77(4):602–605.

Rand, C. S. W. 1979. Obesity and human sexuality. *Medical Aspects of Human Sexuality* 13(1):141–152.

Riddell, R. 1980. Life with my retarded son. *Ms.,* 9(1).

Rowland, W. D. 1975. Surgery for sex reassignment. *AORN Journal* 22(5):735–740.

Saadawi, N. el. 1980. The question no one would answer. *Ms.,* 8(9):68–69.

Salvatierra, O., J. L. Fortmann, and F. O. Belzer. 1975. Sexual function in males before and after renal transplantation. *Urology* 5(1):64–66.

Scalzi, C., and K. Dracup. 1978. Sexual counseling of coronary patients. *Heart and Lung* 7(5):840–845.

Scarborough, W. 1971. Paper presented at the Institute on Retardation and Sexuality, 3–4 December, Philadelphia, Pennsylvania.

Schatzinger, L. H., E. M. Brower, and C. L. Nash. 1979. Spinal fusion: Emotional stress and adjustment. *American Journal of Nursing* 79(9):1608–1612.

Schiavi, R. C., and B. Hogan. 1979. Sexual problems in diabetes mellitus: Psychological aspects. *Diabetes Care* 2(1):9–17.

Schoenberg, B. 1979. Sex after mastectomy: Counseling husband and wife. *Medical Aspects of Human Sexuality* 13(2):88–103.

Schwab, J. J., R. M. Levenson, and R. H. Rossenman. 1970. A summary of a symposium on counseling the cardiac on work and sex. *The Ohio State Medical Journal* 66(10):1003–1007.

Simmons, K. N. 1983. Sexuality and the female ostomate. *American Journal of Nursing* 83(3):409–411.

Simone, C. M. 1977. The transsexual patient. *RN* 40(3):37–44.

Slater, R. J., and A. C. Yearwood. 1980. MS facts, faith, and hope. *American Journal of Nursing* 80(2):276–281.

Smith, J., and B. Bullough. 1975. Sexuality and the severely disabled person. *American Journal of Nursing* 75(12):2194–2197.

Sotile, W. M. 1979. The penile prosthesis and diabetic impotence: Some caveats. *Diabetes Care* 2(1):26–30.

Steele, T. E., S. H. Finkelstein, and F. O. Finkelstein. 1976. Hemodialysis patients and spouses. *The Journal of Nervous and Mental Disease* 162(4):225–237.

Steinbock, E. A., and A. M. Zeiss. 1977. Sexual counseling for cerebral palsied adults: Case report and further suggestions. *Archives of Sexual Behavior* 6(1):77–3.

Stockdale-Woolley, R. 1983. Sexual dysfunction and COPD: Problems and management. *The Nurse Practitioner* 8(2):16–17,20.

Strait, J. 1973. The transsexual patient after surgery. *American Journal of Nursing* 73(3):462–463.

Struck, M. 1981. "Disabled doesn't mean unable." *Science for the People* 13(5):24–28.

Swenson, N. 1980. Breast cancer: The problem. In *Breast cancer,* 7–15. Washington, D.C.: National Women's Health Network.

Task Force on Concerns of Physically Disabled Women. 1978. *Toward intimacy.* 2d ed. New York: Human Sciences Press.

Taylor, P. B. 1983. Understanding sexuality in the dying patient. *Nursing 83* 13(4):54–55.

Thielen, P. G. 1980. Nursing concerns for patients undergoing mastectomy. *Issues in Health Care of Women* 2(3–4):55–56.

Thomas, S. G., and M. M. Yates. 1977. Breast reconstruction after mastectomy. *American Journal of Nursing* 77(9):1438–1442.

Thurm, J. 1975. Sexual potency of patients on chronic hemodialysis. *Urology* 5(1):60–63.

Townsend, C. M. 1980. *Breast lumps.* Summit, N.J.: CIBA.

Ueno, M. 1963. The so-called coition death. *Japanese Journal of Legal Medicine* 17:333–340.

Van Bree, N. S. 1975. Sexuality, nursing practice, and the person with cardiac disease. *Nursing Forum* 14(4):397–411.

Wabrek, A. J. 1979. Sexual dysfunction associated with diabetes mellitus. *The Journal of Family Practice* 8(4):735–740.

Walters, J. 1981. Coping with a leg amputation. *American Journal of Nursing* 81(7):1349–1352.

Wasow, M. 1977. Human sexuality and terminal illness. *Health and Social Work* 2(2):105–121.

Welch, D. A. 1980. Spinal metastases from carcinoma of the breast. *The Nurse Practitioner* 5(4):8,10.

Wellisch, D. K. 1980. Sex and the cancer patient. *Cancer News* Spring/Summer, 14–15.

Wellisch, D. K., K. C. Jamison, and R. O. Pasnau. 1978. Psychological aspects of mastectomy: II —the man's perspective. American *Journal of Psychiatry* 135(5):543–546.

Winkler, W. A. 1977. Choosing the prosthesis and clothing. *American Journal of Nursing* 77(9):1433–1436.

Withersty, D. J. 1976. Sexual attitudes of hospital personnel: A model for continuing education. *American Journal of Psychiatry* 133(5):573–575.

Women's Issues Task Force of the National Council of Jewish Women. 1980. *Women helping women.* New York: National Council of Jewish Women.

Yale Sex Therapy Training Program. no date. *Sexuality resource book.* New Haven, Conn.: Yale University.

Ziff, S. F. 1981. The sexual concerns of the adolescent woman with cerebral palsy. *Issues in Health Care of Women* 3(1):55–63.

Methods of Contraception: Implications for Nursing Practice

Method

Condoms (Figure A-1)
Rubbers, skins, prophylactics, safes, sheaths

Types:
- Thin, latex rubber (0.0025 in)
- "Skin" condoms made from animal membranes. Thinner and more porous, more expensive
- Various colors, textures, either blunt or reservoir-tip ends, dry or prelubricated types, all about same size (7½ inch)

How Method Works

Condom fits snugly over penis and acts as a mechanical barrier; traps ejaculate in closed end, preventing semen from escaping into vagina/uterus.

How Method Used

Rolled on erect penis before contact with labia/introitus. Sperm contained in preejaculatory fluid trapped. Open end has rubber ring which helps keep condom in place.

Method Advantages

1. Readily available and easily carried.
2. Can be used as a "back-up" to other methods: missed birth control pills, early pill and IUD use, or as adjunct to other methods—spermicides, mid-cycle natural family planning.

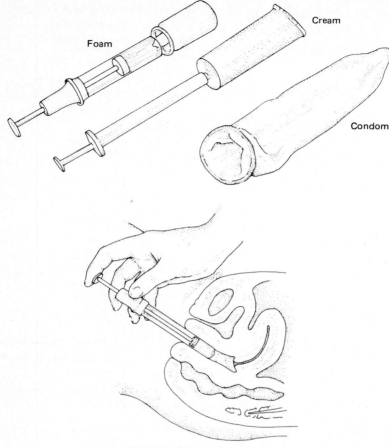

Insertion of foam or cream

FIGURE A-1
Condoms and spermicides.

3. Completely reversible method.

4. Decreased risk of STD.

5. No medical prescription or exam needed.

6. Can be incorporated by either partner into foreplay.

7. Women can carry to ensure partner use.

8. Often effective for males with erectile dysfunction (premature ejaculation).

9. In rare cases women have developed anti-bodies to response to sperm antigens, causing infertility. Use of condom decreases antibody build-up.

10. No hormonal or systemic effects.

Method Effectiveness

(Rates number of pregnancies during first year of use/100 nonsterile women partners) (Hatcher 1980–1981)

	Theoretical	*Actual*
Condom alone	3/100	10/100
Condom and spermicide	less than 1/100	5/100

Possible Side Effects/Constraints

1. Allergy or sensitivity to rubber/animal "skin," prelubrication substance. Rare.
2. Can tear — pregnancy possible.
3. Some say decreased sexual sensitivity with use.
4. May decrease sexual spontaneity.

Method Cost/Acquisition

1. Can purchase without prescription in family planning clinics, drug stores, supermarkets, vending machines. Vending machine condoms frequently of poor quality and not dated for shelf life.
2. Individually wrapped.
3. Prelubricated, textured, colored, and "skins" more expensive.
4. Box of 3 latex — $1.00 – $1.50. Often cheaper by the dozen.

Nurses' Health Teaching

1. Sex-dependent method.
2. Will deteriorate unless stored away from heat including body heat (if kept in billfold).
3. Use adjunct, spermicide especially with thinner "skin" condoms.
4. Do not use with petroleum jelly as lubricant. Water-soluble K-Y jelly, contraceptive foam, cream or gel are safe.

5. Avoid using condoms more than once, even when ejaculation occurs more than once during an encounter.
6. Do not use condoms over two years old.
7. Flaccid penis will increase chance of semen escaping from condom and inadvertently leaving condom in vagina. Immediately withdraw penis after ejaculation, holding onto condom rim.
8. Prelubricated condoms slip off more easily.
9. Suggested readings for clients — (A) See Health Teaching Oral Contraceptives, (B) *Consumer Reports,* 1979 October, pp. 583 – 89.

Method

Spermicidal agents (Figure A-1)
Spermicidal vaginal foam, suppositories, cream, jellies (gels), tablets, and polyurethane sponges (2 in, one size fits all).

How Method Works

Agents mechanically block cervical os by coating with chemicals that immobilize and kill sperm. Can be used individually or in combination with condom.

Suppository: Melts and effervesces with body heat to coat cervix.

Foam: Some effervesce and coat cervix; others do not effervesce.

Cream or jelly: Coats cervix. Used primarily with a diaphragm.

Sponge: Permeated with spermicide. Releases spermicide continuously and absorbs semen so fewer sperm are free in cervical canal.

How Method Used

Foam:
- Shake multidose canister well — 15–20 times
- Fill reusable applicator to appropriate levels. Different brands require varying amounts — check label.
- Some foams come in preloaded applicators.
- Spread labia, insert deep (like tampon) into vagina.

Suppository: With fingers insert deep in vagina.

Cream and gel: Often come in preloaded applicator (see above).

Sponge: Moisten with water and insert like diaphragm. To remove, pull gently on attached loop.

Method Advantages

1. No medical prescription or exam needed.
2. Adjunct to "natural" vaginal lubrication.
3. Readily available and easily carried (small size).
4. Increases effectiveness of condom and diaphragm use (except sponge).
5. Some decreased risk to STD.
6. Warmth from effervescent effect can be erotic.
7. Completely reversible method of contraception.
8. Insertion can be incorporated by either partner into foreplay.
9. Can be additionally used as (1) a "backup" to other methods: missed birth control pills, early pill and IUD use, if condom tears, (2) as adjunct to other methods: condoms, mid-cycle natural family planning, diaphragm, and (3) interim use, postpartum, during lactation.
10. No hormonal or systemic effects.

Method Effectiveness

(Rates number of pregnancies during first year of use/100 nonsterile women users)

	Theoretical	Actual
Foam*	3/100	22/100
Suppository*	3/100	20–25/100

Sponge (new) 1983 clinical trials suggest effectiveness rates approximately same as diaphragm.[†]

Possible Side Effects/Constraints

1. Occasional male/female mucous membrane or skin sensitivity or allergy to particular brand. Itching/rash may occur. Switch brands or discontinue.
2. Unpleasant taste. May have anesthetic effect on tongue/oral mucous membrane if used prior to cunnilingus.
3. Some evidence of increased risk of congenital defects and spontaneous abortion (if method fails and pregnancy results).
4. May decrease sexual spontaneity.

Method Cost/Acquisition

1. Multidose container (foam) medium size — $3.

---

* Hatcher, R. A., G. K. Stewart, F. Stewart, F. Guest, D. Schwartz, and S. A. Jones. 1980. *Contraceptive technology 1980–1981.* 10th ed. New York: Irvington.
† Sponge gets OK. 1983. *Science News* 123(17):261.

2. Preloaded foam (box of 6) — $3.

3. Jellies/creams (tube for 10/12 uses) — $3 – $4; (20 uses) — $5 – $8.

4. Sponges: approximately $1 per sponge.

5. Can purchase without prescription in family planning clinics, drug stores, supermarkets, some physicians' offices (sponges).

Nurses' Health Teaching

1. Sex-dependent method.

2. Woman needs to feel comfortable touching genitals.

3. Woman should lie down after insertion; if she gets up, liquified spermicide will leak out and decrease effectiveness.

4. No douching for eight hours.

5. Messy; postcoital leakage. Use tampon or pad.

6. Not able to measure contents of foam container or see remaining contents. May run out. Keep extra on hand.

7. Subsequent intercourse requires an additional suppository, application of foam, cream, or gel.

8. Jellies are water soluble and become watery at body temperature (increases mess). Creams are in water-insoluble base and may be drying. Do not spread as easily (conflicting data on this).

9. Creams and jellies recommended for diaphragm use only.

10. Can store foam about 1½ years. Keep away from heat.

11. Be sure container says CONTRACEPTIVE foam when purchasing.

12. Wash reusable applicators with soap/water after use.

13. Emphasize these are *vaginal* rather than rectal suppositories.

14. Following insertion of suppository wait 20 minutes for melting/effervescent action to be complete (directions may say 10 minutes).

15. Suppositories (tablets should be inserted 20 minutes to one hour before intercourse, foam no more than 15 minutes before intercourse).

16. Sponges can be used during multiple acts of intercourse without adding extra spermicide. Each sponge effective for 24 hours.

17. Suggested readings for clients — see Health Teaching Oral Contraceptives.

Method

Diaphragm (Figures A-2, A-3, A-4, A-5) Dome-shaped, individually-sized, latex rubber cup with a generally flexible (flat, coil, or arcing spring) rim. Available size range, 50 – 110 mm.

How Method Works

Acts in two ways: as a mechanical barrier and to hold spermicidal cream or jelly in place against the cervix. Held in place by suction of rim against vaginal walls. Diaphragm completely covers cervix; posterior rim is below and behind cervix against cul-de-sac and anterior rim snugly behind pubic bone.

How Method Used

Insertion:

1. 1 – 1½ tsp. of spermicide applied to rim and inside dome.

2. Diaphragm held in one hand, squeezing

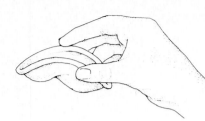
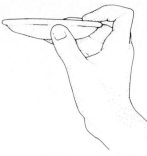

Arcing diaphragm   Coil spring or flat diaphragm

FIGURE A-2
Types of diaphragms.

rim together in center. Other hand spreads labia and inserts.

3. While woman standing with one leg on chair, squatting or lying supine with knees flexed, diaphragm is inserted downward and deep into vagina, anterior rim tucked into place last. Can use plastic or metal inserter.

4. Check proper placement. Cervix should be felt underneath dome; feels like tip of nose.

Removal:

5. To break suction, place index finger between diaphragm and pubic bone.

6. Hook finger behind (underneath) anterior rim, bear down (as if defecating) and remove; a squatting position helps.

Method Advantages

1. Insertion can be incorporated by either partner during foreplay.

2. Completely reversible method.

3. Can be used as temporary barrier during menstruation.

4. The contraceptive jelly and creams offer some protection against STD.

5. No hormonal or systemic effects.

6. Small, easily carried but if forgotten not easily replaced.

Method Effectiveness

(Rates number of pregnancies during first year of use/100 nonsterile women users) (Hatcher 1980–1981)

	Theoretical	*Actual*
Diaphragm with spermicide	3/100	17/100

Possible Side Effects/Constraints

1. Occasional sensitivity or allergy to spermicide or latex rubber.

2. Bladder pressure, foul smelling discharge and uterine cramping may occur if left in too long.

3. Women with uterine prolapse or other abnormalities, chronic constipation, recurrent urinary tract infections or an inadequate pubic arch may be unable to wear diaphragm comfortably or at all. Improper

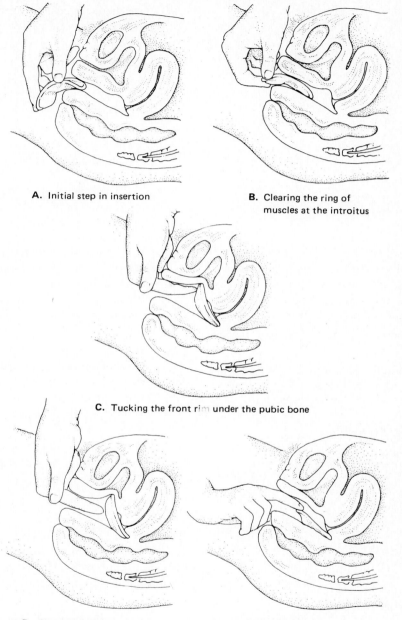

A. Initial step in insertion

B. Clearing the ring of
muscles at the introitus

C. Tucking the front rim under the pubic bone

D. Checking placement

E. Breaking the seal and
pulling the diaphragm up and out

FIGURE A-3
Insertion and removal of the diaphragm.

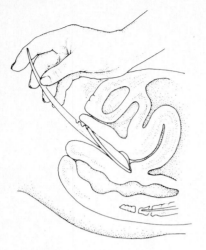

FIGURE A-4
Insertion of a diaphragm with an introducer.

fit can increase recurrent bladder infections.

4. Requires high motivation, readiness, and planning. May decrease sexual spontaneity.

Method Cost/Acquisition

1. Fit, prescription, and teaching done by professional: nurse, practitioner, midwife, physician. Services offered by clinics and private practices.
2. Costs include diaphragm, professional fees, and spermicide (ongoing). Diaphragm about $7–$10.

Nurses' Health Teaching

1. Sex-dependent method.
2. Woman/couple needs to be highly motivated and comfortable touching genitals.
3. No douching while diaphragm in place.

4. Leave diaphragm in 6–8 hours after intercourse but avoid leaving in more than 24 hours.
5. Subsequent intercourse requires additional insertion of 1 tsp of spermicide into upper vagina with applicator. Don't remove diaphragm.
6. Diaphragm care:
   • Wash with mild soap, rinse, dry, and store in container (cool, dry, dark place) after use.
   • Check for defects; hold up to light, fill dome with water.
   • Don't use petroleum jelly. Dusting with talcum or scented powders may deteriorate rubber. Even with care, rubbber deteriorates and diaphragm will need periodic replacement (3–4 years). Latex rubber normally darkens with time and use.
7. Follow-up:
   • At yearly pelvic and Pap smear exams, diaphragm can be checked for size.
   • May need refitting after childbirth, some pelvic surgery, abortion, or weight loss/gain more than 10–15 pounds.
8. Diaphragm can be dislodged with the female superior position and during multiple acts of intercourse.
9. Pain, pressure, or slipping of diaphragm are signs of improper fit.
10. The diaphragm and spermicide can be inserted anytime; however, unless intercourse follows in less than two hours, insert 1 additional tsp of spermicide. No need for removal.
11. Special care is needed during vaginal infection (see STD).
12. History and physical exam (with pelvic) prerequisites to fitting.
13. Written informed consent important.

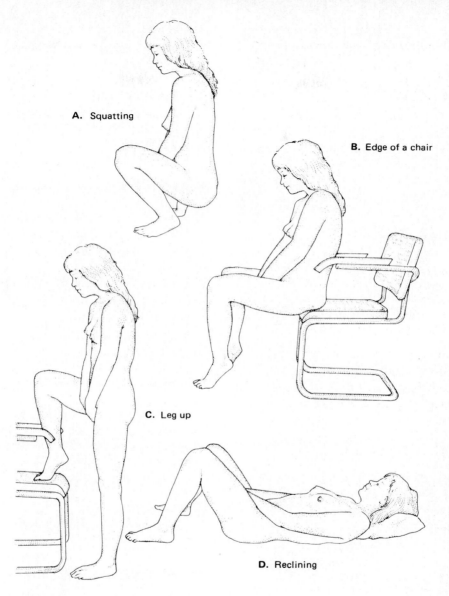

A. Squatting

B. Edge of a chair

C. Leg up

D. Reclining

FIGURE A-5
Positions for insertion and removal of the diaphragm.

14. Suggested readings for clients — see Health Teaching Oral Contraceptives.

Method

Cervical Cap (Figures A-6, A-7)
Can be custom fit or comes in three common shapes and several sizes. Made from firm plastic and soft rubber. Fits over cervix as a thimble over a finger.

How Method Works

Acts in two ways: as a mechanical barrier and to hold spermicidal cream or jelly in place against cervix. Forms suction and air-tight seal with rim snugly around cervix at cervical-vaginal junction.

How Method Used

Insertion:
1. Fill cap ⅓ – ½ full of spermicide.
2. In squatting or partially reclining position separate labia with one hand.
3. Grasp cap between thumb and index finger, squeezing sides together.
4. Slide deep into vagina.
5. Use index finger to press cap around cervix until dome covers cervix.

Removal:
6. Lift rim away from cervix by breaking suction with finger.
7. Grasp dome, pull down and out.

Method Advantages

1. Some women who find diaphragm difficult (urinary infections, cystocele, rectocele) can wear cap.
2. Some find fit erotic.
3. No hormonal or systemic effects.

Method Effectiveness

Accurate method effectiveness figures not available at present.

Possible Side Effects/Constraints

1. Some women unable to wear (cervical erosion, cysts, lacerations, cervicitis, or abnormally shaped cervix).
2. Avoid if client has pelvic inflammatory disease/STD — until infection cleared.
3. Requires high motivation, readiness, and planning.
4. May decrease sexual spontaneity.

Method Cost/Acquisition

1. Not manufactured in this country. Obtained through some feminist health-care centers, clinics, private practice. Fit, prescription, and teaching done by professional: nurse practitioner, physician, midwife.
2. Costs include device and provider fees plus spermicide. Approximately $6 – $12/cap.

Nurses' Health Teaching

1. Not F.D.A. approved. Dispensed through research projects. Need written informed consent.
2. Sex-dependent method.
3. May produce odor if left in too long. Soak in 1 cup water with 1 tbsp cider vinegar or lemon juice for 20 minutes.
4. May be difficult to insert/remove.

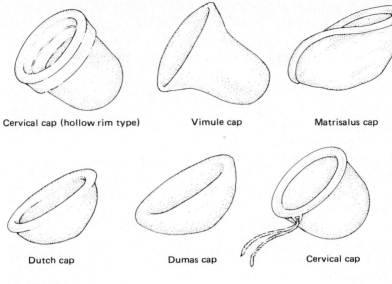

Cervical cap (hollow rim type)   Vimule cap   Matrisalus cap

Dutch cap   Dumas cap   Cervical cap

FIGURE A-6
Types of cervical caps.

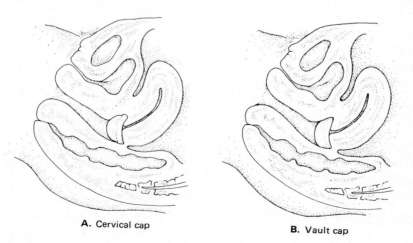

A. Cervical cap   **B.** Vault cap

FIGURE A-7
Placement of the cervical cap.

5. Need to be comfortable touching genitals.

6. May need to be removed frequently when menstruating or cap will fill, breaking suction.

7. May dislodge with deep penile thrusting during intercourse. Use condom for back-up first 8–10 times.

8. Conflicting advice about length of time for wearing: 24 hours to 3–4 days. Wash and reinsert if desired.

9. If vaginal discharge increases may need to remove more frequently.

10. Use with spermicidal creams or jelly.

11. Needs refitting after an abortion, birth, physical growth, or weight gain or loss.

12. Should not remove for 6–8 hours after intercourse. No douching during this time.

13. Suggested readings for clients—see Health Teaching Oral Contraceptives.

Method

Periodic abstinence, "natural" family planning or fertility awareness
Based on calculation of female fertile (unsafe) and infertile (safe) days in menstrual cycle. These are caused by hormonal fluctuations that produce detectable biophysical signs and symptoms (result of hypothalamic-pituitary-ovarian feedback cycles). These methods may be used to achieve or avoid pregnancy.

Cervical mucus method (ovulation method or Billings method)

Calendar rhythm method

Basal body temperature (BBT) method (Figure A-8)

Sympto-thermal method (combines BBT and cervical mucus method, or all three)

Combination methods are thought to be most effective.

How Method Works

Calendar: Using menstrual cycle, individual records length of shortest and longest cycles over eight month–one year period. Calculates future based on past fertile/infertile days. Abstains from unprotected intercourse on fertile days to avoid pregnancy (and intercourse to achieve pregnancy).

BBT: BBT will decrease 0.2–0.3°, 24–36 hours prior to ovulation and increase 0.7–0.8° 24–48 hours after ovulation and remains plateaued until day before menses. Use abstinence 24–48 hours before ovulation and 72 hours after ovulation if pregnancy is undesired (and intercourse if desired).

Cervical mucus (Billings): Based on assessment of changes in cervical mucus during cycle; fertile and infertile day calculated. (See Table A-1.)

Sympto-thermal: Combines methods. Increases validity and reliability.

How Method Used

Calendar: Reviews calendar records. Determines earliest fertile days—subtract 18 days from shortest cycle. Determines latest fertile days by subtracting 11 days from longest cycle. Example: Longest cycle = 34 days, shortest cycle = 26 days; earliest fertile day = 8th day of cycle, latest fertile day = 23rd day of cycle. (Day 1 is 1st day of menses.) Avoid unprotected intercourse on fertile days if wish to avoid pregnancy.

BBT: Take temperature daily with BBT

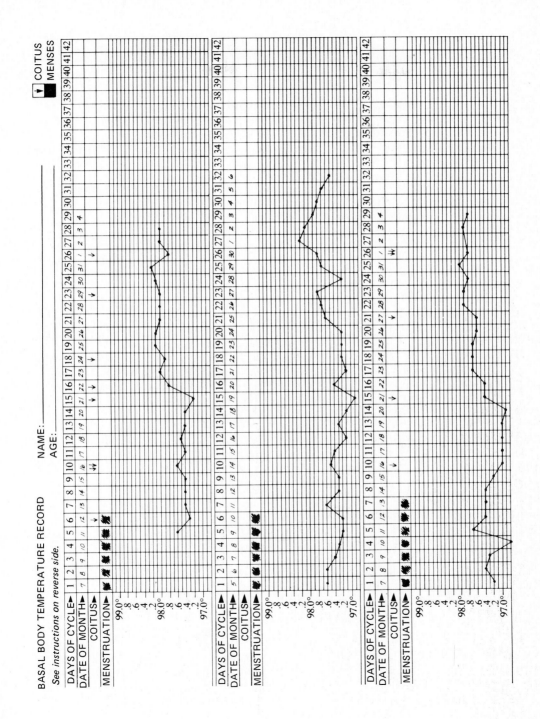

FIGURE A-8
Basal body temperature chart.

TABLE A-1   *Changes in Cervical Mucus During Menstrual Cycle*

Stage of Cycle	Amount	Viscosity	Color	Spinnbarkeit	Ferning
Post-menstruation	Moderate	Thick	Cloudy, yellow, or white	<1″	No
Nearing ovulation	Increasing	Somewhat thick to thin	Mixed cloudy and clear	1–1½″	Moderate
Ovulation	Maximum	Very thin and slippery	Clear	6–8″	Well developed
Post-ovulation (about 3 days)	Decreasing	Thin	Mixed cloudy and clear	4–6″	Minimal or no
Nearing menstruation	Minimal	Thick	Cloudy	<1–1½″	No

SOURCE: From Hatcher et al. 1980. *Contraceptive technology 1980–1981.* 10th ed. New York: Irvington. Reprinted by permission.

thermometer. Record for approximately 3–4 successive months.

Cervical mucus: Based on assessment of vaginal/cervical secretions.

Sympto-thermal: Correlate all subjective and objective signs and symptoms to determine fertile/infertile days.

Method Advantages

1. All methods acceptable to most religious groups.
2. Physically safe—no drugs, devices. Non-hormonal.
3. Joint contraceptive responsibility (preferable).
4. Increase awareness of female anatomy, physiology. Mittelschmerz (dark red/brown spotting at ovulation lasting few minutes—24 hours; may have pain). Occurs in about ⅕ women.
5. Does not require medical intervention.
6. Assists couples who wish to achieve as well as avoid pregnancy.
7. Little cost (except BBT kit).

Method Effectiveness

(Rates number of pregnancies during first year of use/100 nonsterile women users) (Hatcher 1980–1981)

	Theoretical	*Actual*
Calendar only	13/100	21/100
BBT only	7/100	20/100
Cervical mucus only	2/100	25/100

No data on combined use

Possible Side Effects/Constraints

1. Animal studies suggest increased fetal abnormality if conception occurred in post-ovulatory period ("old egg theory").

2. May decrease sexual spontaneity.

3. Requires high motivation, readiness, and planning.

Method Cost/Acquisition

1. BBT thermometer or kit (contains records).

2. Cervical mucus — may use vaginal speculum — cost about $4. Can be obtained from most women's health centers or write: Women to Women Publications, 6520 Selma Avenue, Box 551, Los Angeles, California 90028.

3. Family planning counselor/physician, midwife, or nurse practitioner *may* be able to assist and interpret findings; not all are skilled.

4. Women/couples may increase knowledge from Couple to Couple League (training by lay couples).

Nurses' Health Teaching

1. All: Long periods of abstinence may require high motivation levels.

2. Unpredictable ovulation. Can be influenced by stress, illness, infection, fatigue, irregular sleep patterns, physical activity, electric blankets. These will influence all signs and symptoms.

3. Calendar method *alone* most commonly used and most often ineffective. Women with irregular cycles (especially young adolescents and pre- and postmenopausal women) should avoid.

4. Often confusing to determine cervical mucus. Can be altered by ejaculate, lubricants and spermicides, and infection. Douching contraindicated, disturbs normal secretions.

5. Mucus method requires comfort with touching genitals and vaginal secretions.

6. BBT: Temperature must be taken in the morning before getting out of bed, smoking, eating, or drinking.

7. Can increase woman's/couple's awareness of reestablishment of ovulation (positive fact for breastfeeding women or after discontinuing birth control pill).

8. Not all women have easily identifiable temperature fluctuations in presence of ovulation.

9. Abortion should be acceptable if pregnancy *totally* undesired.

10. Methods more successful in women who have regular menstrual cycles and more permanent relationships.

11. Characteristics:
    - Sperm survival after intercourse, up to five days (norm about 72 hours)
    - Ovum survival about 24 hours
    - Ovulation occurs ($\pm$ two days) 14 days *prior* to the menses

12. Most miscalculations and "accidents" occur prior to ovulation.

13. Suggested readings for clients — see Health Teaching Oral Contraceptives.

Method

Intrauterine devices (IUDs or IUCDs) (Figure A-9)
Inert plastic or nonreactive metal devices available in varying sizes and shapes, medicated (CU-7, CU-T, Progestasert-T) and non-medicated (Saf-T-Coil, Lippes loop).

How Method Works

Exact mechanism of action is unknown. Suggested action:

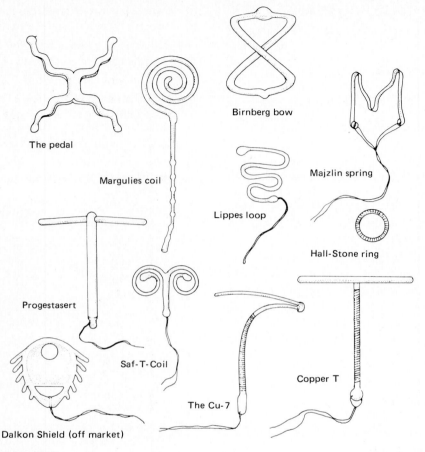

FIGURE A-9
IUDs (Intrauterine devices).

1. Endometrial inflammatory response which destroys sperm and inhibits implantation.
2. Immunologic antifertility mechanism (increases immunoglobin G and M levels).
3. Increased prostaglandin effect.
4. Adjunct effect of copper decreases sperm mobility and implantation.
5. Mechanical dislodging of blastocyst and increased mobility of ovum in tubes.

How Method Used

1. Practitioner measures size and position and sounds uterus. Slowly inserts IUD into uterus via insertion barrel by push or withdrawal technique.
2. Insert is removed and tails cut to leave approximately two inches outside external cervical os.

3. Clients should feel for tails following exam.

Method Advantages

1. Female only responsibility (may be seen as advantage or disadvantage).
2. Sex-independent method.
3. Requires less motivation than most other methods.
4. No further cost after insertion except for follow-up exams or reinsertion.
5. Does not interfere with sexual spontaneity.

Method Effectiveness

(Rates number of pregnancies during first year of use/100 nonsterile women users) (Hatcher 1980–1981)

	Theoretical	*Actual*
IUD	1–3/100	5/100

Effectiveness rates vary among different IUD types.

Possible Side Effects/Constraints

1. Increased occurrence of:
   - abdominal and low back pain
   - menorrhagia
   - between period spotting/bleeding
   - dysmenorrhea
   - dyspareunia
   - pelvic inflammatory disease
   - ectopic pregnancies
   - uterine and cervical perforation
   - leukorrhea
2. Undetected expulsion (partial or complete) pregnancy. May occur without client awareness.

3. IUD tails (strings) may cause irritation to penis or vagina.
4. Allergy or sensitivity to copper. Look for rash.
5. Pregnancy may occur with IUD in place.
6. Individuals who are uncomfortable touching genitals see checking IUD tails as a constraint.
7. Contraindications:
   Absolute
   - pelvic infection (acute or chronic)
   - pelvic inflammatory disease (acute or chronic)
   - septic abortion
   - postpartal endometritis
   - pregnancy
   - cervical or uterine malignancy
   - abnormal Pap smears
   - uterine abnormalities
   - history of ectopic pregnancy
   Relative
   - hypermenorrhea
   - dysmenorrhea
   - acute cervicitis
   - valvular heart disease
   - endometriosis
   - anemia
   - uterus less than 6 cm
   - marked antiflexion or retroflexion
   - abnormal uterine bleeding
   - no previous pregnancies

Method Cost/Acquisition

1. Insertion and teaching done by professional: nurse practitioner, midwife, physician. Services offered by clinics and private practices.
2. Costs include device plus professional fees — $30–$100. Clinics often have sliding scales for payments.

Nurses' Health Teaching

1. History and physical exam (with pelvic) prerequisite to insertion and laboratory tests (Pap smear, GC culture, other).

2. Insertion procedure:
   - Done during menses (increased ease of insertion with slight dilation of os and assume no pregnancy).
   - May experience mild to severe cramping. Temporary vasovagal response may be elicited with pressure on cervix; pallor, tachycardia, feel faint and diaphorese.
   - Local anesthesia may be used.
   - Due to possibility of adverse temporary insertion reactions need support person who can take client home after release.

3. Need written informed consent.

4. Check IUD strings frequently in first months and after every menstrual period.

5. Cu-7 and T-Cu need replacement every 2–3 years, Progestasert every year.

6. Will often increase menstrual flow and cramping (especially in first months).

7. Need adjunct contraception for first 1–2 months (condom, foam, etc.).

8. Never self-remove IUD.

9. See provider if danger signals occur (Hatcher 1980–1981):
   P eriod late or no period
   A bdominal pain
   I ncreased temperature, chills, fever
   N asty discharge, foul discharge
   S potting, bleeding, heavy periods, clots

10. When taking antibiotics, aspirin, or other anti-inflammatory drugs use adjunct methods. These drugs will decrease IUD inflammatory effect.

11. Can use tampons but check carefully on removal as strings (and IUD) may attach to fabric.

12. If anemic avoid or may need exogenous iron and diet high in iron. Preinsertion and follow-up hemoglobin and hematocrits.

13. No protection against STD. IUD tails can increase pathway for microorganism invasion of uterus (especially during menses).

14. IUD should not be removed midcycle if intercourse has occurred within 4–5 days.

15. If pregnancy occurs, IUD should be removed by provider. If pregnancy is suspected, call provider immediately.

16. Need yearly follow-up exams with laboratory testing.

17. IUD should be removed after menopause (see Menopause section for further discussion).

18. Suggested readings for clients—see Health Teaching Oral Contraceptives.

Method

Oral contraceptives (birth control pills, BCP, "the pill")

1. Combined pill with synthetic forms of estrogen and progesterone; available in a wide variety of formulas and dosages.

2. Progestin-only pill (minipill).

How Method Works

Primary

1. Synthetic estrogen's effect on hypothalamus inhibits production and release of FSH and LH from anterior pituitary. In absence of FSH and LH, which stimulate maturation and release of ovarian follicles, ovula-

tion is suppressed (some exceptions with 50 μg of estrogen or less). Exogenous estrogen also accelerates ovum tubal transport: has an antiprogestational effect of altering endometrial secretory developing and decreasing pH. Both of the latter interfere with implantation and fertilized ovum survival.

2. Progestins alter cervical mucus, promoting an increased viscosity which acts as a sperm barrier and partially inhibits capacitation. They also decrease ovum tubal transport, alter endometrial proliferation so that implantation is inhibited, and inhibit preovulatory LH surge.

How Method Used

21-day combination pill:

1. Start 5th day after menses onset.
2. Take one pill/day for 21 days until packet finished.
3. Take no pill for seven days. Menses will occur at this time.
4. Begin new packet of pills on same day of week you ended — one week later.

28-day combination pill:

1. Start 5th day after menses onset.
2. Take one pill/day for 28 days until packet finished. The last seven pills of 28-day pill regimen are inert substances, often of a different color. These may contain iron or vitamins.
3. Begin new packet the day following completion of old packet.

Progestin-only pill:

1. Start first day of menstrual cycle.
2. Take one pill/day until packet completed.
3. Next day start new packet.

Method Advantages

1. Sex-independent method — highly effective.
2. May decrease dysmenorrhea, menstrual flow, and length of periods.
3. May decrease iron deficiency anemia.
4. Helps regulate cycles — predictable bleeding occurs.
5. Mini-pills: Often effectively used if estrogen side effects have been problematic with combined pills (headaches, weight gain).
6. Easily carried.
7. Female only responsibility (may be seen as advantage or disadvantage).
8. Does not interfere with sexual spontaneity.
9. BCP users have lower incidence of ovarian cysts.
10. May be more acceptable to clients who are uncomfortable handling genitals.

Method Effectiveness

(Rates number of pregnancies during first year of use/100 nonsterile women users)

	Theoretical	Actual
Combined pill	0.34/100	4–10/100
Progestin only	1–1.5/100	5–10/100

(Pills containing <35 μg slightly lower theoretical effectiveness.)

Possible Side Effects/Constraints

1. Combination pill affects almost every organ system. About 40% of pill users have

some side effects ranging from relatively minor to very serious. A sample:

- thrombophlebitis, thromboembolus
- hypertension
- gallbladder disease
- myocardial infarction
- nausea
- migraine headaches
- chloasma and may increase skin cancer incidence
- monilia vaginitis
- breast tenderness and cystic changes
- hirsutism
- depression
- fatigue
- weight gain
- increased varicosities

Etiology of side effects classified as estrogen/progestin in excess or deficiency.

2. Contraindications to estrogen containing birth control pills (Hatcher 1980–1981)
   Absolute contraindications:
   - thromboembolic disorder (or history thereof)
   - cerebrovascular accident (or history thereof)
   - coronary artery disease (or history thereof)
   - impaired liver function
   - hepatic adenoma (or history thereof)
   - malignancy of breast or reproductive system (or history thereof)
   - pregnancy

   Strong relative contraindications:
   - termination of term pregnancy within past 10–14 days
   - severe vascular or migraine headaches
   - hypertension with resting diastolic blood pressure of 110 or greater
   - diabetes, prediabetes, or a strong family history of diabetes
   - gallbladder disease, including cholecystectomy
   - previous cholestasis during pregnancy
   - elective surgery planned in next four weeks
   - long-leg casts or major injury to lower leg
   - over 35–40 years old
   - fibrocystic breast disease and breast fibroadenomas

   Other relative contraindications (may contraindicate initiation of pills):
   - failure to have established regular menstrual cycles
   - cardiac or renal disease (or history thereof)
   - history of heavy smoking
   - conditions likely to make patient unreliable at following pill instructions, such as mental retardation, major psychiatric problems, history of alcoholism, history of repeatedly taking pills incorrectly, or being a young teenager
   - lactation (oral contraceptives may be initiated as weaning begins and may be an aid in decreasing the flow of milk)
   - patient with profile suggestive of anovulation and infertility problems: late onset of menses and very irregular, painless menses

3. Mini-pills side effects: irregular menses, shortened length and amount of flow, spotting, and amenorrhea.

4. Birth control pills can also alter effects of anticoagulants and insulin and the results of some lab tests (sed rates, tests for protein-bound iodine (PBI) or thyroxine, blood corticotrophins, and even Pap smear) and diagnostic endometrial and cervical biopsies.

Method Cost/Acquisition

1. Acquired from professional. Services offered by clinics and private practice.

2. Costs include pill supply plus professional fee. Month's supply $7–$10.

Nurses' Health Teaching

1. Complete history and physical exam and laboratory tests (urine, Pap, and GC) prerequisite to prescription.

2. Caution about danger signs. Call provider immediately.

   A bdominal pain (severe)

   C hest pain (severe) or SOB

   H eadaches (severe)

   E ye problems: blurred vision, flashing light, or blindness

   S evere leg pain (calf or thigh)

Plus:

   dizziness/faintness
   jaundice
   severe depression
   speech disturbance
   muscle weakness/numbness
   breast lump

3. Do not borrow or lend pills as various types and dosages differ.

4. Combination pills are not used as or to be confused with progestin-only or "morning after pills" (DES).

5. Missed pills: Combination
   - One. Take as soon as remembered and today's (or next) pill at regular time. Pregnancy unlikely.
   - Two. Take both as soon as remembered and two next day. Finish packet and use adjunct birth control until completed.
   - Three or more. Stop taking pills. Use adjunct birth control. Start new packet in one week even if bleeding. Continue using adjunct contraception for two more weeks.

Missed pills: Progestin only
   - One. Take as soon as remembered and today's (or next) pill at regular time. Use adjunct birth control.
   - Two. Take two pills as soon as remembered. Next day take two pills, continue packet and adjunct birth control until next period.
   - If no period 45 days after last, see provider immediately for pregnancy test.

6. Missed periods:
   - One or more missed pills and no period, possible pregnancy, see provider.
   - No pills missed and no period, pregnancy unlikely.
   - Two periods missed and no missed pills, possible pregnancy (not as likely with mini-pill). See provider.

7. No protection of STD.

8. Tell provider caring for you that you are on BCP. This is especially important if you are ill, have an infection (STD), or before surgery. Certain drugs (both OTC and prescription) can decrease BCP effectiveness: some tranquilizers, some sedatives, some antidepressants, some drugs taken for arthritis, TB, and epilepsy. Use a back-up method while taking medication.

9. Take pills on regular schedule at about same time of day (especially important with mini-pill) to maintain blood levels of hormone(s).

10. Use adjunct contraception for first month of combined pill use; to increase effectiveness of mini-pills, use first 3–6 months and mid-cycle thereafter.

11. Informed written consent a must after a thorough discussion of all aspects of method.

12. Pill use may increase/decrease headache and migraines, ache, libido, depression, other effects — depends on type.

Traditional Tubal Ligation   **Laparoscopy**

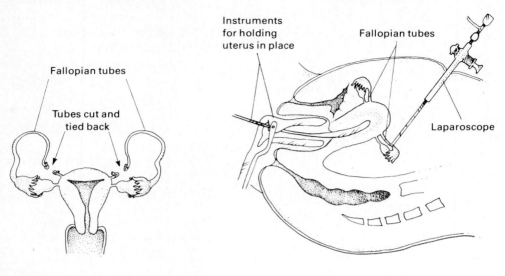

FIGURE A-10
Tubal ligation.

SOURCE: From *Sexual Choices,* 2nd ed., by G. D. Nass, R. W. Libby, and M. P. Fisher. Copyright © 1984, 1981 by Wadsworth, Inc. Reprinted by permission of the publisher, Wadsworth Health Sciences, Monterey, California.

13. Need for follow-up visits (may be 3–6 months); thereafter, annually.

14. Suggested readings for clients
    • *Changing Bodies, Changing Lives,* by Bell. Especially written for teenagers.
    • *My Body, My Health,* by Stewart et al.

15. BCP may cause significant vitamin B_6 deficiency which can, in turn, cause depression. Supplementary B_6 (20 mg/day) may alleviate depression.

16. BCP high in progestin or progestin-only may cause increased skin oiliness.

17. BCP may cause increased sensitivity to sunlight — more easily sunburned. Avoid overexposure.

18. Contact lens wearers may need prescriptions changed or may be unable to wear them while on BCP (increases fluid retention, which causes alteration in shape of eyeball).

19. Caution about hazard of smoking and BCP use*
    <1 pk/day ↑ risk of 3.4 × more incidence of MI
    >1 pk/day ↑ risk of 7 × more incidence of MI
    >1 pk/day and >35 y/o ↑ risk of 39 × more incidence of MI

Method

Female Sterilization (Figure A-10)
Tubal ligation: vaginal, abdominal, laparosco-

---

* Weinberg, J. S. 1982. *Sexuality: Human needs and nursing practice.* Philadelphia: Saunders.

pic. Hysterectomy, not primarily done as contraceptive method.

Male Sterilization (Figure A-11)
Vasectomy

How Method Works

Female: Prevents fertilization by surgical interruption of fallopian tube continuity (or removal of uterus).

Male: Prevents fertilization by surgical interruption of vas deferens continuity. Considered to be primarily a permanent method of contraception. Reversal microsurgery effectiveness rates vary.

How Method Used

Female: Method, approach, and anesthesia vary according to client health status and choice, practitioner's skill, and recommendation.

1. Client prepped.
2. Anesthesia administered.
3. Incision made.
4. Tubes isolated and ligated, plugged, cauterized, or clips applied.

In most cases one must be 21-years-old and wait 30 days after consent form signed. Consent form effective for 180 days.*

Male: 1. Client prepped.
      2. Anesthetic administered.

---

* Madoras, L. and J. Patterson. 1981. *Woman care.* New York: Avon.

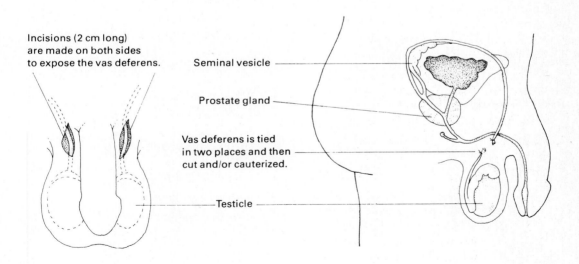

Incisions (2 cm long) are made on both sides to expose the vas deferens.

Seminal vesicle

Prostate gland

Vas deferens is tied in two places and then cut and/or cauterized.

Testicle

FIGURE A-11
Vasectomy.

SOURCE: From *Sexual Choices*, 2nd ed., by G. D. Nass, R. W. Libby, and M. P. Fisher. Copyright © 1984, 1981 by Wadsworth, Inc. Reprinted by permission of the publisher, Wadsworth Health Sciences, Monterey, California.

3. Vas deferens located.

4. Incision made, vas deferens exposed and ligated or cauterized.

Method Advantages

1. Considered permanent. Most effective method.

2. May increase libido, spontaneity, and sexual responsiveness with decreased fear of pregnancy (see side effects).

3. No further cost for contraception.

Method Effectiveness

(Rates number of pregnancies during first year of use/100 nonsterile women users and partners) (Hatcher 1980–1981)

	Theoretical	*Actual*
Female — tubal ligation	0.04/100	0.04/100
Male — vasectomy	0.15/100	0.15 +/100

Possible Side Effects/Constraints

Both:
At risk for common adverse effects of surgery and anesthesia: increased risk of thrombophlebitis and embolism; decreased respiratory, cardiac, GU, and GI patency and regulation; decreased fluid/electrolyte balance; hemorrhage and shock.

Male (side effects):

1. Incisional hematoma (rare).

2. Edema, infection, discharge, and bleeding possible at incisional site. Scrotal and testicular edema.

3. Possible decreased libido and erectile difficulties and depression due to psychogenic response to loss of reproductive ability and genital surgery.

4. Sperm antibody development (½ – ⅔ men — no known medical problem yet documented).

5. Spontaneous reanastomosis vas (rare) with possible pregnancy.

Female (side effects):

1. With laparoscopic technique — shoulder/chest pain (associated with CO_2 instillation during surgery).

2. Incisional discomfort, edema, infection, discharge, bleeding.

3. Possible decreased libido and sexual response and depression due to psychogenic response to loss of reproductive integrity and sexual self-concept.

4. Spontaneous reanastomosis of fallopian tubes with possible pregnancy.

Male (possible constraints):

1. Hydrocele or varicocele.

2. Fixed, undescended testicle.

Female (possible constraints):

1. Large fibroids (myomas).

2. Some ovarian cysts.

3. History of endometriosis or PID.

Method Cost/Acquisition

1. Procedure done by physician in hospital, clinic, office.

2. Costs include agency charge plus professional fees. Vasectomy—about $300. Tubal ligation—$900–$1200.

Nurses' Health Teaching

Both:

- Operative permit written.
- Informed consent required.
- History and physical exam with appropriate lab tests prerequisite.

Male:

1. Not immediately sterile. 10–15 ejaculations needed to decrease stored, mature sperm in prostate/seminal vesicles. Two consecutively negative, fresh sperm counts verify sterility. Will need to use other contraceptive method for interim.

2. Postsurgical: moderate activity, ice bags to decrease edema, use of athletic supporter, sitz baths, and mild analgesic to decrease discomfort. Resume sexual activity when comfortable. Caution: call provider if temperature rises above 100°F, acute pain, bleeding.

Female (depends on method used):

1. Laparoscopic tubal ligation (common), postsurgical: moderate activity, shower or bath—most sutures dissolveable, mild analgesic for discomfort. Resume sexual activity when comfortable. Caution: see above #2.

2. Postpartum tubal ligation often done 1–3 days after delivery with sub-umbilical incision.

Methods of Abortion: Implications for Nursing Practice

Method

Early induced
Menstrual extraction or induction, mini-abortion, endometrial aspiration. Dilation of cervix not needed.

When: Most often before 6 weeks after LMP (varies with practitioner—may be done up to 8 weeks).

Where: Clinics, private office, rarely in hospital.

Cost: Varies with agency and professional fees.

Note: Informed, written consent needed.

How Method Used

- Anesthesia: regional or none.
- Speculum inserted, vagina and cervix prepped.
- Products of conception removed via small flexible catheter inserted into uterus and rotated cavity.
- Gentle, negative pressure from suction machine or large syringe.

Method Advantages

- No cervical dilation.
- Little blood loss: 1–2 oz for 6-week gestation.
- Short procedure (varies with gestational age): usually 5–10 minutes.

Possible Side Effects/Constraints

- Low risk, few complications.
- Potential side effects: cervical trauma, retained tissue, perforation, products of

conception missed—continue pregnancy, infection, bleeding.

• If procedure is done before pregnancy confirmed, it may be unnecessary.

Note: If acute pelvic infection or STD exists, abortion may be delayed for treatment.

Method

Dilation and evacuation
Suction abortion or aspiration, vacuum abortion or aspiration, vacuum or suction curettage (variety of methods)

When: 6–16 weeks after LMP most common (in some places may be done up to 24 weeks after LMP).

Where: Clinics, hospitals (often on outpatient basis), private office by professional.

Cost: Varies with agency and professional fees. $250–$1,000. Insurance coverage varies.

• 80% of all induced abortions in the United States.

• Method will depend on gestational age and amount of dilatation needed.

Note: Informed, written consent needed.

How Method Used

• Anesthesia: Regional or general.

• Speculum inserted, vagina/cervix prepped, tenaculum applied to stabilize cervix.

• Cervix dilated with dilators or laminaria (more gradual/less discomfort) done prior to procedure.

• Products of conception removed via curette or cannula attached to suction.

• 13–16 plus weeks: crushing instruments may be needed prior to vacuum curettage/aspiration (larger volume of fetal/placental tissue).

• Following suction/vacuum aspiration, instrumental curettage may be used and/or IV oxytocin drip to increase contractions post-procedure and decrease blood loss.

Method Advantages

• Minimal time (depends on procedure and gestational age): 15–45 minutes. May be released 1–4 hours after abortion, depends on anesthesia, complications.

• Minimal blood loss, approximately 12–16 oz for 12-week pregnancy.

• Laminaria decreases procedure time (done prior), cervical trauma, and risk of uterine perforation.

Possible Side Effects/Constraints

• Hemorrhage, uterine perforation, infection. The shorter the gestational age, generally fewer risks.

• An incompetent cervical os may result in future pregnancies if damage to cervical muscle fibers.

Note: If acute pelvic infection of STD exists, abortion may be delayed for treatment.

Method

Dilation and curettage (D & C)
When: Most common during first trimester. Occasionally done up to 20 weeks after LMP.

Where: Hospital, some clinics, often on outpatient basis by physician.
Cost: Varies with agency and professional fees. Hospital stay varies.

Note: Informed, written consent needed.

How Method Used

- Anesthesia: Regional or general.
- Speculum inserted, cervix/vagina prepped, tenaculum applied to cervix.
- Cervix dilated. Laminaria may be used prior to procedure.
- Products of conception removed by scraping uterine endometrium with sharp metal curettes.

Method Advantages

- Procedure familiar to most physicians (used for a variety of gynecological treatments and to diagnose).

Possible Side Effects/Constraints

- Uterine perforation (increases with longer gestation), bleeding, retained tissue, infection.
- General anesthesia often given (associated risks).
- Longer recovery than suction methods and frequently more discomfort and bleeding.

Note: If an acute pelvic infection or STD exists, abortion may be delayed for treatment.

Method

Hypertonic saline, prostaglandins, and urea
When: Second trimester abortions 15–24 weeks after LMP (varies with practitioner).
Where: Hospital. Many hospitals do not provide this resource. Hospital stay may be several days.
Cost: Varies with agency and professional fees. $400 to $1,500. Insurance coverage varies.

Note: Informed, written consent needed.

How Method Used

Amnioinfusion method
- Abdomen prepped and area of amniocentesis tap is locally anesthetized.
- Amniotic fluid removed; amount varies with material to be infused.
- Substance infused after a small test dose: Saline (20% sodium chloride)—50–250 cc
Prostaglandin F_2a—40–60 mg
Urea (30%-C)—200 cc in 5% D/W
- IV oxytocin often used as adjunct to stimulate contractions and reduce time.
- Laminaria also used as an adjunct to dilate cervix (reduce time and cervical trauma).
- With laminaria and oxytocin use labor process may last 5–48 hours, up to 72 hours without these.
- May be interim period (30 minutes–several hours) before onset of labor.

Other:
- Prostaglandins (F_2a or E_2) may also be used via intravaginal, oral, intravenous, and intramuscular routes as abortifacient. IV, oral, and IM routes have many side effects.

- Increasingly, a combination of agents is used to dilate the cervix, stimulate contractions, as feticides.

Method Advantages

Prostaglandins:
Lower complication rates than saline. Labor usually shorter than with saline.

Urea:
Feticidal effects, low cost, fewer complications.

Saline:
Feticidal effects, inexpensive.

Possible Side Effects/Constraints

Prostaglandins: Expensive, increased risk of cervical trauma, fetus may be born alive, increased occurrence of GI side effects, headache, and increased temperature, infection. *Contraindicated* for women with hypertension, respiratory problems, glaucoma, heart disease, and epilepsy.

Urea: Dehydration, alteration in coagulation factors, high failure rate when used as sole abortion, infection.

Saline: High rate of complications: hemorrhage, hypernatremia, water intoxication, disseminated intravascular clotting, myometrial necrosis, infection, others. *Contraindicated* in women who have kidney or severe heart disease.

Note: If an acute pelvic infection or STD exists, abortion may be delayed for treatment. Some women feel a need to see the fetus after delivery, whether dead or alive. This may make it easier to deal emotionally with the situation.

Suggested Health Teaching (Appropriate for all methods)

1. Return for follow-up exam (10 days – 3 weeks). A pelvic exam is usually done at this time and some providers request repeat pregnancy tests (especially after first trimester abortion).

2. Avoid intercourse for one – two weeks or until bleeding stops, douching for one – two weeks, strenuous activity/exercise for several days or until ready.

3. Use mild analgesic for discomfort; sanitary pads for flow — some providers recommend tampons after first few days.

4. Menstrual periods should resume in 4 – 6 weeks. If no period within 8 weeks, notify provider.

5. Caution, danger signs:
   - Temperature above 100°F or chills, malaise, aching
   - Abdominal pain/tenderness and severe cramping
   - Heavy flow/clots (soaking two pads/ hour or more)
   - Foul-smelling and/or green vaginal discharge

   Women should be given a 24-hour emergency number to call in case of emergency.

6. Will experience mild-moderate cramping, minimal – moderate flow (about same as menstrual period 4 to 5 pads per day) for first week or two. May spot 3 – 4 weeks post-abortion.

7. Contraception is needed to avoid pregnancy. Ovulation may occur before menses resume. Oral contraceptives are often started at once if gestation less than 12 weeks, in one week if gestation more than 12 weeks. Diaphragms and cervical cap may need refitting. Condoms and

spermicides are an excellent method. Insertion time for IUD varies; may be immediately (early abortions) or at follow-up exam.

8. Many women will experience the grieving process in variable ways. This response is normal, most often temporary, and of relatively short duration (sleep disturbances, loss of or increased appetite, lethargy, depression, difficulty concentrating, crying, etc.). The emotional impact is unique to each individual. However, if symptoms increase, are severe or prolonged, professional help may be necessary. A number of women say their overwhelming response after an abortion is relief.

9. Women who have additional complicating health problems *may* need to have abortion performed in a hospital setting, for example, bleeding disorders, drug or anesthesia allergies, chronic debilitating diseases, anemia, etc.

10. Women who are Rh negative and eligible for Rhogam (based on laboratory testing) need this administered within 72 hours post-abortion. Informed, written consent needed. Costs $35–$55. May be less if gestational age under 12 weeks (smaller dose).

11. Bathing, showering are appropriate.

12. Wearing a snug bra for several days may decrease discomfort and stimulation if breast milk develops after abortion. Do not attempt expressing milk: may stimulate milk flow.

13. Some physicians prescribe ergotrate every 4 hours post-abortion to maintain uterine contraction (methergine is sometimes used also). This may increase cramping. Women with hypertension should not be given these drugs.

Common STD: Implications for Nursing Practice

Insult to Body

Herpes simplex type II, virus
Herpes type I, virus

Effect of Insult, Infection

Herpes simplex type II (genital herpes, herpes progenitalis, HSV II, herpes vaginitis)

Influencing Factors

1. Primarily sexually transmitted by type II (85%) or by type I (less common) and by oral-genital-anal intercourse. Autoinocculation may occur to other areas of the body.

2. Epidemic — approximately 500,000 new cases per year and affecting 5 to 20 million Americans. More common and severe in women. No known cure or vaccine yet available.

3. Can remain dormant for long periods of time. During latency, virus thought to migrate along sensory nerves into sacral ganglia (type II) and trigeminal ganglia (type I). Recurrence with more than 50% of infected individuals. Outbreaks may be frequent or infrequent.

4. May have subclinical disease: shedding virus and yet asymptomatic.

Body Reactions

- Two to ten days (average, six) after contact — multiple, small, painful blisters develop. May be preceded by tingling and itching in genital area or "flu-like" symptoms.
- Blisters occur on vulva, cervix, penis, anus, scrotum, buttocks, inner thighs.
- Blisters will rupture, leaving superficial ulcers/erosions leading to
  a. increased itching.
  b. increased pain with ulcers (especially on voiding).
- increased edema.
- increased lesion discharge. May have increased fever, inguinal adenopathy, malaise.

Nursing Interventions

A. Screening

1. Immunofluorescence — scraping from lesion
2. Tzanck smear — scraping from lesion
3. Viral culture — scraping from lesion
4. Papanicolaou smear
5. Serum viral titre
6. Visual exam of lesions

B. Medication

Treatment is symptomatic. Acyclovir ointment (Zovirax®) is not a cure but will shorten episodes. New in 1982. Now available in intravenous form also. Other: Oral analgesics, topical neosporin, xylocaine, zinc oxide, Bacitracin/Betadine scrub, vitamin E oil, and 2-deoxy-D-glucose cream. Lysine has been said to prevent recurrent HSV II, but clinical studies are inconclusive.

C. Health teaching

1. Warm sitz baths, cool wet tea bags, and L-lysine taken orally have proven to be effective for some.
2. Women need Pap smears every 6 to 12 months for rest of life. Strong link to cervical cancer. Definitive diagnosis made with culposcopy and biopsy.
3. Abstinence or condom use with active lesions and for ten days (some recommend six weeks) after ulcer healing.
4. Keep genital area dry. Petroleum jelly applied to lesions before urinating may decrease discomfort, however.
5. Initial infection more severe and lasts up to three weeks. Peaks at 10 to 14 days. Recurrence is milder, less painful, of shorter duration, and heals more rapidly.
6. Secondary bacterial infection of genital lesions should be treated appropriately.
7. Air drying (hair dryer) may avoid irritation of a towel.
8. Precipitating factors can trigger recurrences: physical or emotional stress, fever, illness, ovulation, menstruation, exposure to heat and sunlight, fatigue, and intercourse. Varies with the individual.
9. Support groups: HELP (Herpetics Engaged in Living Productively — now called Herpes Resource Center) is a national group with more than 40 local chapters. Sponsors hotline (415-321-5134) and newsletter (The Helper), P. O. Box 100, Palo Alto, California 94302.
10. Complications increase vulnerability to crisis:
    a. Severe dysuria and urethral lesions

may cause dehydration and/or urinary retention. Individuals may avoid fluids because of painful voiding, which will concentrate urine and increase problem. Encourage fluids, voiding in sitz bath, or under running water.

b. Viral encephalitis — rare.

c. Pregnancy and newborn:

- Herpes increases spontaneous abortions (5× increase with primary infection, 3× increase with recurrence) and premature births.
- Incidence of congenital anomalies (rare) include severe mental retardation, patent ductus, and CNS sequelae.
- High mortality with neonatal infection.
- Cesarean birth recommended if the woman has active lesions at or close to term.
- Viral cultures are recommended to monitor status in third trimester if infection known or history warrants. Routine testing is often not done.
- Herpes infection may be more severe for pregnant women.

11. Vaginal and cervical lesions are often painless. A woman may be unaware of infection; the only symptoms may be intermittent vaginal discharge.

12. Resources: *The Herpes Handbook* by Gunn and Stenzel-Poore; *Herpes* by Santa Cruz Women's Health Center.

Insult to Body

Candida albicans, a fungus

Effect of Insult, Infection

Monilia (yeast infection, Candida)

Influencing Factors

1. Common vaginal infection. Occurs when vaginal pH/environment is altered. Often *not* acquired sexually, but can be sexually transmitted. Can be spread to other parts of body by finger.

2. Proliferation may increase with antibiotics and steroid use, diabetes, poor nutrition (high carbohydrate intake), compromised general health, oral-genital contact, pregnancy, birth control pills, poor genital hygiene, menopause.

3. Candida exists as part of normal flora of mouth, intestines, and vagina.

Body Reactions

- Female: increased vaginal discharge, white, "curd-like" cheesy patches (on vaginal wall, cervix), thick, thin, or watery. Vulvar irritation, also thighs, buttocks.
- Male: increased itching, penile rash.
- Male and female: white patchy exudate, oropharyngeal area (thrush).

Nursing Interventions

A. Screening

Microscopic exam of discharge with KOH/wet mount, urethral, seminal, vaginal cultures.

B. Medications

Nystatin (mycostatin) suppositories bid × 7 to 14 days OR miconiazole (Monistat) vaginal cream qd × 7 days OR Nystatin oral suspension (for oropharyngeal infection).

C. Health teaching

1. Partners need to be screened and treated (if needed) to avoid "ping-pong" effect.

2. Infection may be persistent and take as long as six to eight weeks (or longer) to be resolved.

3. A fungus infection (for example, athlete's foot) on other parts of body may be spread to vaginal area.

4. Neonatal thrush can develop if woman has infection at time of a vaginal birth.

5. If infection persists or frequently recurs, a blood sugar test may be needed to rule out diabetes.

6. Nutritional assessment is needed to monitor for carbohydrate and sugar intake (including alcohol, beer, and wine). Yeast grows well in a glucose-rich vaginal environment.

7. Symptoms may increase during menstruation; pH more conducive at this time (blood pH more alkaline) to growth of monilia.

8. Sitz baths may help to alleviate symptoms. Hot water and soap can aggravate an inflamed perineal area. Warm or tepid water is more appropriate.

9. Yogurt (plain), used with water in a douche and inserted into vagina, or eaten, may help to restore/maintain vaginal flora and acidity of vagina. Vinegar douches may also be helpful (1 to 2 tbsp white vinegar to 1 qt of warm water).

10. Complications — rare.

11. Use of antibiotics, steroids, birth control pills may need to be discontinued during treatment if infection persists.

Insult to Body

Protozoan — Trichomonad

Effect of Insult, Infection

Trichomonas vaginalis (trich)

Influencing Factors

1. May be asymptomatic (more common in men).

2. Often associated with venereal warts.

3. Can survive several hours on moist objects: toilet seat, towels, swimming pools, although more commonly sexually transmitted.

4. May be difficult to examine with speculum if vagina and labia are very irritated.

Body Reactions

- 4 to 28 days incubation period.
- Male: Increased penile discharge, dysuria.
- Female: Increased vaginal discharge: watery, frothy, greenish-gray color. Increased foul odor, itching/burning, pain, reddened "strawberry" appearance of cervix and vaginal walls. May have increased dysuria, dyspareunia, postcoital bleeding.

Nursing Interventions

A. Screening

Microscopic examination of wet mount (NaCl) of penile and vaginal discharge. May do GC culture to rule out gonorrhea.

B. Medications

Oral metronidazole (Flagyl) 2 g stat or 250 mg tid × seven days.

C. Health teaching

1. Both partners will need to be screened and treated (if needed), or "ping-pong" re-infection may persist (60% of cases recur if both partners are not treated). Commonly carried under uncircumcised foreskin and in semen.
2. Abstinence or condom use during treatment.
3. Flagyl not used in treating pregnant or lactating women. Use Betadine gel topically.
4. Take all medication prescribed. But never take Flagyl on an empty stomach — take right after each meal.
5. When beer or alcohol is used during Flagyl therapy there is a high incidence of nausea, headache, vomiting and abdominal cramps, diarrhea, dry mouth.
6. Flagyl may temporarily cause WBC depression. Do a WBC before/after Flagyl prescription.
7. Flagyl stains the urine a dark color.
8. Complications are rare but can cause epididymitis and prostatitis.
9. Class II Pap smear may result from Trich infection. Some evidence of possible link of Flagyl use and cervical cancer.

10. Need to be rechecked a week after treatment.

Insult to Body

Human Papilloma virus

Effect of Insult, Infection

Condylomata accuminata (venereal/genital warts)

Influencing Factors

1. May be self-inoculated but frequently sexually transmitted through anal, vaginal, or oral sex.
2. Similar to common skin warts.
3. Pregnancy can stimulate growth.
4. Often concurrent with other vaginal infections.

Body Reactions

- Incidence occurs one to three months after exposure.
- Single/multiple raised papillary or sessile growths (1 mm — several cm).
- Warts occur on vulva, introitus (most common in women), cervix, vagina, penis (most common glans), scrotum, urethra, anus, and anal canal. May occur in clusters. Appearance differs from moist (vagina) to dry (shaft of penis) parts of body. Dry skin appearance: hard, yellow-grey, usually small. Moist skin appearance: soft, white, pink, or red; warts

often have "cauliflower-like" appearance.

• Intense itching and foul discharge.

• Often painless but discomfort increased with growth in size and often felt with intercourse, tampon use, or defecation.

Nursing Interventions

A. Screening

Clinical appearance and history of contact. VDRL — appearance mimics condyloma lata (secondary syphilis). GC culture: the two may coexist. Lab testing — rarely necessary (electron microscopy, histology).

B. Medication

Podophyllin 10% to 25% (in tincture of benzoin) applied directly to lesions with swab 1× per week until disappearance of warts.

C. Health teaching

1. Partner needs to be examined and treated (if needed) to avoid "ping-pong" re-infection.

2. Condom use necessary during symptoms.

3. May need to stop use of oral contraceptives if lesions persist. Warts tend to be estrogen-dependent.

4. Podophyllin is caustic. Following application it needs to be washed off with soap and water in four to six hours. Chemical burns may result if this is not followed.

5. Podophyllin not used on vaginal or cervical lesions.

6. Podophyllin cannot be used during pregnancy; may cause spontaneous abortion or premature birth; possible teratogenesis.

7. Complications are rare. Possible malignant changes can occur, but rare.

8. If warts are unresponsive to treatment or are massive, medical intervention may be necessary: electrocautery, curettage or cryotherapy, and/or laser treatments.

9. Treat any coexisting infections.

10. May produce abnormal Pap smear but not related to cancer. Pap will return to normal after successful treatment.

Insult to Body

Bacteria. Most common: *Chlamydia trachomatis* and *Hemophilus bacterium* (later classified as *Corynebacterium vaginale;* now called *Gardnerella vaginalis*). *Ureaplasma urealyticum,* others.

Effect of Insult, Infection

Bacterial vaginitis, cervicitis, urethritis or *Gardnerella vaginalis* and Chlamydia — common. If microorganism unknown: Nonspecific vaginitis or urethritis (NSU) or nongonococcal urethritis (NGU).

Influencing Factors

1. Infections can be sexually transmitted or arise spontaneously.

2. Chlamydia:
   • Perhaps the most common STD with over 3,000,000 reported cases per year.
   • Class II and III Pap smears associated with Chlamydia.

- The genital strains of Chlamydia have been implicated in a number of nonsexually transmitted and sexually transmitted diseases: trachoma, inclusion conjunctivitis of the newborn, neonatal pneumonitis, nonspecific plus nongonococcal and postgonococcal urethritis, nongonococcal pelvic inflammatory disease, salpingitis, and cervicitis.

3. NGU and NSU — primarily asymptomatic in women and some men; 30% of NGU and NSU occurs after treatment for a gonococcal infection. Recurrences common.

4. With a bacterial vaginitis, 10% to 40% may be asymptomatic.

Body Reactions

- Vaginitis: Increased discharge: thick or thin, grey-white, often frothy, "fishy" odor (from cervical hypertrophy and discharge). Increased vulvar irritation and itching. May have dysuria.

- Urethritis: Symptoms often do not occur in less than ten days after exposure. Increased urethral discharge: purulent to mucoid, increased dysuria.

Nursing Interventions

A. Screening

- Vaginitis: Microscopic exam of exudate with Gram stain/KOH wet mount. Immediate "fishy" odor and appearance of "clue cells." Culture of exudate (Chlamydia). GC culture to rule out gonorrhea.

- Urethritis: Based on negative GC cultures/smears.

B. Medication

- Vaginitis: Ampicillin (oral) 500 mg qid × 7 to 10 days (Gardnerella) OR metronidazole (Flagyl) 250 mg tid × 7 days (Gardnerella) OR tetracycline (oral) 500 mg qid × 7 to 14 days (Chlamydia — NGU).

- Urethritis: Tetracycline 500 mg qid × 7 days OR erythromycin 500 mg qid × 7 days.

C. Health teaching

1. Partners need to be screened and treated (if needed) to avoid "ping-pong" effect.

2. Sulfa creams and suppositories are sometimes prescribed but are of questionable value. They often relieve itching but may not kill organisms.

3. Tetracycline and Flagyl should not be used during pregnancy. Erythromycin can be used to treat Chlamydia in pregnant women or those sensitive to tetracycline.

4. Hemophilus vaginalis often related to soap allergies, poor natural lubrication, and vagina insertion after anal intercourse.

5. Complications from NSU/NGU can also increase vulnerability to crisis: epididymitis, prostatitis, proctitis, and sterility.

Insult to Body

Phthirus pubis, a parasite.

Effect of Insult, Infection

Pediculosis pubis (crabs, crab lice, pubic lice)

Influencing Factors

Can be contracted through exposure to bedding, clothes, sleeping bags, toilet seats used by infected individual. More commonly, sexually transmitted.

Body Reactions

- Intense itching and skin irritation. Nits/lice cling to pubic hair (especially) and may spread if individual is very hairy (chest hair, underarms, and, rarely, scalp). Increased skin discoloration from puncture wounds.
- Symptoms usually appear one to three weeks after exposure.

Nursing Interventions

A. Screening

Microscopic findings of nits/lice/larvae on mineral oil wet mount.

B. Medication

1% gamma benzene hexachloride (Gamene, Kwell). A prescription shampoo, cream, or lotion.

C. Health teaching

1. Secondary infection may occur and will need specific antimicrobial treatment.
2. Complications are rare but can increase vulnerability to crisis: impetigo furunculosis/pustulas, eczema.
3. Pubic lice can survive 24 hours off the body, eggs, about six days. Launder bedding and clothes with high temperature water or dry clean and spray mattresses and pillows.

4. Do not use Kwell or Gamene during pregnancy; Eurax cream prescription is appropriate.
5. Follow medication package directions closely. These are pesticides and have harmful side effects.

Insult to Body

Gram-negative intracellular diplococcus *Neisseria gonorrhea*.

Effect of Insult, Infection

Gonorrhea (GC, clap, dose, PPNG)

Influencing Factors

1. Transmitted sexually (vaginal, anal, oral-genital contact) or congenitally.
2. Sensitive organism. Dies in seconds outside body's mucous membranes.
3. Frequently asymptomatic—females: 50% to 80%; males: 40% to 50%.
4. Rarely see "classic textbook case." Symptoms may go unnoticed until gonorrhea ascends (or descends) reproductive tract.
5. PPNG (penicillinase-producing *Neisseria gonorrhea*) strains, although rare, are painful and complications can be severe. This strain produces an enzyme that destroys penicillin. Treat with spectinomycin.
6. Of those exposed to gonorrhea for first time, 75% become infected.

Body Reactions

- Males: 3 to 30 days after contact (usually three to five days): increased frequency, increased penile discharge (more common in morning, often purulent).

- Females: 3 to 30 days (may be indefinite) after contact: increased vaginal discharge (may be purulent, of endocervical origin). Increased vulvar irritation and burning.
- Males and females: sore throat (if oropharyngeal), increased dysuria.
- If untreated: increased lower abdominal or back pain, increased fever, increased dyspareunia/postcoital bleeding, and testicular pain.

Nursing Interventions

A. Screening

- Male: Gram stain microscopic exam of exudate (GC smear), cultures.
- Female: GC culture on Thayer Martin medium + CO_2. Gram stain not reliable for women. Cultures take 48 hours to complete.
- Cultures: Should include endocervix, nasopharynx, rectum, urethra.
- VDRL: Syphilis may coexist.
- Young children can develop gonorrhea. Sexual abuse and incest are often the causes.

B. Medication

Initial/uncomplicated gonorrhea: Aqueous procaine penicillin G — 4.8 million units (two sites) IM OR tetracycline 0.5 gm qid × five days (oral) OR amoxicillin 3 g (oral). Spectinomycin 2 g IM male, 4 g IM female. All above given in conjunction with probenecid 1 g (oral) 30 minutes prior to initial dose. This will decrease rate of excretion of antibiotic by kidneys, increase serum levels, and increase absorption.

C. Health teaching

1. Individuals are contagious until a negative smear/culture. Follow-up cultures done five to seven days after end of therapy. Symptoms may disappear, however, two or three days after beginning treatment.

2. No easy method of detection in females. Must have a vaginal exam and culture.

3. A reportable communicable disease. Notifying partners is essential for their screening and treatment.

4. Avoid anal, genital, and oral intercourse until negative culture, or use condoms if abstinence impossible.

5. Focus on prevention of recurrence and sexual health care.

6. Complications can increase vulnerability to crisis:
   a. Systemic involvement rare but possible if untreated; arthritis, meningitis, endocarditis.
   b. Pharyngitis and tonsilitis incidence is increasing.
   c. Gonococcal ophthalmia neonatorum can infect an infant at delivery. Within approximately 48 hours after birth infant may exhibit red, edematous eyes with pussy drainage which can destroy vision within several days. A simple, inexpensive treatment, silver nitrate or penicillin by drops, will prevent. Unfortunately, some states no longer require this treatment.
   d. Gonococcal conjunctivitis may result when infection is spread by fingers to the eye.
   e. Without treatment, reproductive tract complications can occur: epididymitis, proctitis, skenitis, bartholinitis, salpingitis, oophoritis, peri-

tonitis. Complications can cause sterility and increase the incidence of ectopic pregnancies.

7. Avoid drinking alcohol, coffee, and tea while infection persists as these are irritating to the urethra.

8. Tetracycline therapy:
   - Do not give during pregnancy: will produce discolored teeth in these infants and decrease fetal bone growth.
   - Take tetracycline on an empty stomach; especially avoid milk, milk products, and antacids for one hour before and two hours after ingestion.
   - Tetracycline can cause skin rash if there is prolonged exposure to sun during medication course.

Insult to Body

Virus

Effect of Insult, Infection

Hepatitis B infection (and possibly A)

Influencing Factors

1. Can be sexually transmitted, but not always. May be transmitted by oral-rectal contact as well as blood serum of carrier (contaminated needles). Urine, feces, semen, saliva, and vaginal discharge have been known to harbor viruses.

2. Common among homosexuals and those with other STD.

3. Some individuals are asymptomatic carriers.

4. Communicable during incubation periods

and several days following onset of symptoms.

Body Reactions

Insidious onset, often 60 to 180 days after contact. Vague symptoms: increasing abdominal discomfort, anorexia, nausea, increased fever, increased jaundice, joint pain.

Nursing Interventions

A. Screening

Radioimmunoassay detection of Hepatitis B surface antigen (HB_SAg) in blood.

B. Health teaching

1. Treat symptomatically; may include bedrest.

2. Complications include liver damage. Death is rare.

3. Active or recent hepatitis infection is absolute contraindication for "minipill" use.

4. Avoid vaginal intercourse after anal insertion or use condom when anal insertion occurs before vaginal. Finger or penile insertion into anus should be followed with soap and water scrub to avoid contamination with virus from GI environment.

Insult to Body

A spirochete, *Treponema pallidum*

Effect of Insult, Infection

Syphilis (syph, bad blood, sores, lues, pox)

Influencing Factors

1. Increased incidence in past several years.
2. Premarital VRDL required in 45 states. Prebirth and postbirth VRDL required in 42 states.
3. Curable in primary/secondary stages only.
4. Not contagious during incubation period.
5. Sexually or congenitally transmitted.
6. Positive serology four to seven weeks after contacting disease.
7. Chancres may be misdiagnosed or unnoticed (cervix/anus).

Body Reactions

- Primary syphilis: 10 to 90 days after exposure, appearance of painless eroded watery lesion (chancre) or multiple lesions.
- Sites: Vagina, male/female external genitalia, cervix, anus, rectum, mouth, fingers, nipples. Unilateral/bilateral lymph node enlargement may occur.
- Secondary syphilis: Highly variable skin/mucous membrane lesions and rash usually bilateral, symmetrical, macular, papular, or papulosquamous cherry-red or greyish-blue in blacks. Alopecia, mild URI symptoms, and anorexia that may last several days, can occur. Highly contagious in secondary stage
- Sites: Most common on palms and soles of feet. Generalized lymph nodes involved.
- Tertiary of late syphilis: Rarely seen today.
- If untreated: Chancres will heal spontaneously without treatment in one to five weeks but infection becomes systemic. Three to six days after chancre heals,

secondary stage may occur. Chancres can recur up to two years if no treatment in secondary stage. Untreated individual enters latent period after two years and is no longer contagious. Two to forty years later, systemic late stage may begin. At this stage only 25% of untreated syphilis can be arrested, not cured.

Nursing Interventions

A. Screening

VDRL or RPR reagent tests. Specific and definitive—FTA/ABS or MHA-TP— effective four weeks after contact. Expensive and difficult test.

B. Medication

Benzathine penicillin G, 2.4 million units IM (one-half dose in each buttock at a single visit). For treatment of syphilis of unknown length of longer than one year's duration: 2.4 million units a week × three weeks OR IM aqueous procaine penicillin G—4.8 million units (600,000 u/day × eight days). Requires multiple visits OR tetracycline HCl 500 mg qid × 15 days if allergic to penicillin or oral erythromycin, which is used for pregnant women who are allergic to penicillin.

C. Health teaching

1. Inaccurate results from VDRL can occur. Because VDRL is not disease-specific, a false-positive can often result. Results may be due to other disease: mononucleosis, measles, hepatitis, chronic collagen disease, other Spirochete disease.
2. Syphilis is a reportable communicable disease. Casefinding is important to decrease spread. Notifying partners is es-

sential for their screening and treatment.

3. Following successful treatment — VDRL does not become negative for 6 to 12 months after primary stage and 12 to 18 months after secondary stage.

4. Condyloma lata, a second syphilitic lesion resembling venereal warts, may become extensive during pregnancy.

5. Untreated syphilis acquired during pregnancy will produce a congenitally syphilitic infant, a stillborn, or, rarely, a second trimester abortion. The affected newborn needs to be treated with penicillin as soon as a positive diagnosis is made.

Insult to Body

Immune deficient syndrome. Etiology unknown; may be viral-caused.

Effect of Insult, Infection

Acquired immunodeficiency syndrome (AIDS). Highly associated with a rare malignant neoplasm called Kaposi's sarcoma (KS), pneumocystis carinii pneumonia (PCP), and other opportunistic infections.

Influencing Factors

- Manifested by immunosuppressed (often previously healthy) individuals.
- Possible risk factors (thought to be both biologic and lifestyle).
  1. Transmitted by direct sexual contact. Often seen in homosexual and bisexual men, although syndrome not limited to this population. Women, children, and heterosexuals have been AIDS victims. New evidence links disease to those only having prolonged household contact with individuals who have AIDS.
  2. Those at high risk:
     - Abusers of intravenous drugs, amyl/butyl nitrites
     - Multiple sex partners and those with incidents of STD
     - Hemophiliacs and those who received transfusions or other blood products
     - Immigrants from Caribbean island countries
  3. May be genetic predisposition; a congenital immune defect.
- No known cure for AIDS.
- Almost 80% of reported AIDS cases in the United States have been concentrated in six metropolitan areas on East and West coasts.

Body Reactions

- Continual deterioration of immune system; constant fatigue and malaise.
- May progress to more severe form of KS, PCP, or other opportunistic diseases.
- Kaposi's sarcoma: purple, vascular, nodular lesions on skin and mucus membranes (often lower extremities) which do not itch or cause pain. Increase in lymphadenopathy including visceral involvement.
- Pneumocystis carinii pneumonia: initial symptoms of upper respiratory infection. May progress in months to severe illness and death; increase in dyspnea, increase in temperature, tachypnea, cyanosis, night sweats, weight loss.

Nursing Interventions

A. Screening

Immunologic studies; histology or culture.

B. Medications

- Some success with high doses of purified interferon.
- PCP: trimethoprim (Bactrim) and sulfamethoxazole (Septa), oral or intravenous.

C. Teaching

1. Diagnosis of AIDS *does not necessarily* mean one will progress to KS, PCP, or other opportunistic disease.
2. Regular medical follow-up essential.
3. Medication (Bactrim and Septa)
   Oral — take one hour before meals, or two hours after with a large amount of water. Drink large amounts of fluids daily. Contact health-care provider if any adverse effects: skin rashes, sore throat, fever, oral lesions, light sensitivity.

Avoid sun exposure and preparations containing PABA.

4. Avoid unknown sexual contact and those with known infection.
5. Use condom and avoid oral and anal sex.
6. National Gay Task Force Crisis hotline:
   Monday through Friday, noon to 6 P.M.
   1-800-221-7044
   (Allen and Mellin 1982, 1720; Centers for Disease Control 1983, 101–103; AIDS Update 1983).

Enteric Infections

There appear to be a number of enteric or intestinal diseases becoming more commonly transmitted sexually today. These were previously not considered STD but appear to be more prevalent in homosexual than heterosexual individuals. Diagnosis can be made from stool cultures and the diseases are treated according to the protocols for the specific infection. Among these diseases are bacteria-caused shigellosis, and protozoan-caused amebiasis, salmonellosis, and giardiasis.

Film Resource List

Abortion. Spontaneous and elective abortion. NASCO. Filmstrip/cassette.

Abortion — Woman's Right. The right of women for control of their bodies. Great Atlantic. Cassette.

About Conception and Contraception. A factual teaching film — animated drawings, no narration. Planned Parenthood.

About Sex. Rap session with mixed group of teens; open discussion of issues related to sexuality. Planned Parenthood.

Adolescent Sexual Conflict — Are We Still Going to the Movies? Conflicts over sexuality in an adolescent relationship. Planned Parenthood.

Anatomy of the Female Pelvis and Reproductive Organs. Describes anatomy of external and internal reproductive system. NASCO. Filmstrip/Cassette.

Are You Ready for Sex? Clarification of values and responsible decision-making. Planned Parenthood.

Battered Women. Lives of women, the work of shelters. Great Atlantic. Cassette.

Choosing a Method of Birth Control. Methods of FP — for patients. National Audiovisual Center. 16 mm.

Cindy and Jack. A film about a young man with gonorrhea. Planned Parenthood.

Contraception. Discusses seven methods. NASCO. Filmstrip/cassette.

Engagement Ring. Spanish-English subtitles. Romance versus reality in relationships. Planned Parenthood.

Family Planning. Animated cartoon for elementary and junior high students. Planned Parenthood.

A Family Talks about Sex. One family's discussion over the years. Planned Parenthood.

Female Sterilization. Discusses facts and myths. National Audiovisual Center. 16 mm.

For Men: Sterilization as a Method of Contraception. About vasectomy—pros and cons. National Audiovisual Center. 16 mm.

Four Young Women. Decision-making about abortion. Planned Parenthood.

A Full Life for Sara: Growing up Different. Growing up. Living in an able-bodied world. Living with a handicap. Ibis. Slides/cassettes.

Gay Male Liberation. Oppression of men who are gay. Great Atlantic. Cassette.

Greta's Girls. A film about a day in the life of two lesbians. Women Make Movies.

Happy Family Planning. Animated cartoon on methods. Planned Parenthood.

Herpes Simplex II. Facts about herpes. Milner-Fenwick. 16 mm.

Hope is not a Method. Basic anatomy and physiology and methods of contraception. Planned Parenthood.

Human and Animal Beginnings. Basic information on reproduction for young children. Planned Parenthood.

Human Growth III. Adolescent sexual development. Planned Parenthood.

Human Reproduction: Male and Female Anatomy and Conception. Development of reproductive systems; includes adult sexuality. Career Aids. Filmstrip/cassette.

Human Sexuality. A variety of topics, including pregnancy and sexuality, helping parents teach children. AJN Co.

It Couldn't Happen to Me. Topics of premarital sex, birth control, pregnancy. Junior high through adult. Planned Parenthood.

It Happens to Us. Unwanted pregnancy—termination. Planned Parenthood.

Jennifer: A Revealing Story about Genital Herpes.

Information about herpes 2. National Audiovisual Center. 16 mm.

The Lavender Menace. Lesbian feminists discuss their politics, the women's movement and other issues. Great Atlantic. Cassette.

Linda's Film—Menstruation. Menstruation and the myths. Junior and Senior high. Planned Parenthood.

Living with a Mastectomy. Return to normal life after mastectomy. Includes exercises, self-examination. Career Aids. Filmstrip/cassette.

Mack and Susan. Drama of a parked car. Planned Parenthood.

Margaret Sanger. Life of the leader of the American birth control movement. Planned Parenthood.

Menstruation. Exposes myths and old wives tales; discussion of menses. Phoenix.

The Neurologically Disabled Patient. Preparation for Home Care. Discusses aspects of sexuality. AJN Co.

The Nurse in Child Abuse Prevention. Antecedents and manifestations of child abuse; role of the nurse in detection, treatment, and prevention. AJN Co.

Old Enough to Know. Attitudes about sex—parents' concerns. Planned Parenthood.

One in Eleven. Breast Cancer. Pyramid.

Oral Contraception: Current Thinking on Metabolic Effects and Clinical Concerns. Update on O.C. ACOG.

Parents' Voices. Role playing after sex (teens). Planned Parenthood.

Pelvic Inflammatory Disease. All about PID. Milner-Fenwick. 16 mm.

Psychosocial Sexual Development: Infant-Preadolescent. Defines sexuality and describes sexual health. Presents biological determinants and developmental sexuality. AJN Co.

Psychosocial Sexual Development: Adolescent-Aged. Development of sexuality; emphasis on behavioral aspects. AJN Co.

Rape Culture. A film on the phenomenon of rape. Cambridge Documentary.

Reproduction. Genetics, male and female anatomy, ovulation, intercourse, conception, fetal development. Career Aids. Slides and booklet.

Reproduction: The Origin, Development, and Genetics of Life. Reproductive system including genetics. Career Aids. Filmstrip/cassette.

The Reproductive System. Anatomy and physiology. Career Aids. Filmstrip/cassette.

Sexism and Juvenile Justice. Problems in the legal system that victimize juvenile women. Great Atlantic. Cassette.

Sexual Desires vs. Sexual Restraints. Conflicts and contradictions of society and values. Ibis. Slides/cassettes.

Sexual Health Care in the Nursing Process. Defines sexual health care in the context of nursing process. AJN Co.

Sexually Transmitted Diseases. All about STD and how transmitted. Milner-Fenwick. 16 mm.

Street Harrassment. A movie on the verbal harrassment of women on the street. Women Make Movies.

Susana. Autobiographical portrait of a young Argentine woman who is a lesbian. Women Make Movies.

Teenage Pregnancy and Prevention. The Problem. The Choices. The Solutions. Magnitude of the problem; choices for abortion, parenting, foster care, marriage; need for sex education. Ibis. Slides/cassettes.

Teen Sexuality — What's Right for You. Issues in sexuality for teens. Junior high. Planned Parenthood.

Teens Having Babies: Getting Prenatal Care. A model program for pregnant teens. Polymorph.

Then One Year. Changes in puberty. Planned Parenthood.

Too Soon Blues. Conflicts about sex and pregnancy scare. Planned Parenthood.

Trial for Rape. Record of an actual rape trial in Italy (English subtitles). Women Make Movies.

VD A New Focus. Information of VD; dispels myths. Planned Parenthood.

VD Prevention. Methods of prevention. Junior and Senior high. Planned Parenthood.

VD Quiz. Quiz format to teach about VD. Planned Parenthood.

Violence in the Family. Battered Wives. Adolescent Abuse. Problems of battering; sexual abuse in the family. Ibis. Slides/cassettes.

We Will Not Be Beaten. Story about battered women. Transition House. 16 mm.

What about McBride? Issues in homosexuality for teens. Planned Parenthood.

What Every Woman Should Know About Breast Cancer. Case histories of some well-known women; SBE; physiology of the breast. Ibis. Slides/cassette.

When Teens Become Parents. Aspects of parenting as a teen. Polymorph.

When Teens Get Pregnant. Prenatal interviews with pregnant teens in Boston. Polymorph.

Why Women Stay. Documentary of women living with violence in the home. Women Make Movies.

Woman-Loving Women. Explores misconceptions about lesbians. A sensitive presentation on lesbian culture. Lavender Horizons.

Film Companies and Distributors

ACOG Film and Video Service. Box 299, Wheaton, Illinois 60187.

American Cancer Society. Check local chapter for films available.

AJN Co. American Journal of Nursing Company. 555 West 57th Street, New York, New York 10019.

ASPO. American Society for Psychoprophylaxis in Obstetrics. 1411 K Street, NW, Suite 200, Washington, D.C. 20005.

Bullfrog Films, Inc. P. O. Box 114, Milford Square, Pennsylvania 18935.

Cambridge Documentary. P. O. Box 385, Cambridge, Massachusetts 02139.

Career Aids, Inc. 8950 Lurline Avenue, Department N, Chatsworth, California 91311.

Department of Audio-Visual Communications. Fairview General Hospital, Room AU1, 18101 Lorain Avenue, Cleveland, Ohio 44111.

EDC Distribution Center. Department 130, 55 Chapel Street, Newton, Massachusetts 02160.

Feminist Women's Health Center. 1112 South Crenshaw Boulevard, Los Angeles, California 90019.

The Great Atlantic Radio Conspiracy. 2743 Maryland Avenue, Baltimore, Maryland 21218.

Ibis Media. Department HD, P. O. Box 308, Pleasantville, New York 10570.

March of Dimes Birth Defects Foundation. Public Health Education, 1275 Mamaroneck Avenue, White Plains, New York 10605.

Milner-Fenwick, Inc. 2125 Greenspring Drive, Timonium, Maryland 21093.

NASCO Health Care Educational Materials. 901 Janesville Avenue, Fort Atkinson, Wisconsin 53538.

National Audiovisual Center. Washington, D.C. 20409.

Phoenix Films, Inc. 470 Park Avenue South, New York, New York 10016.

Planned Parenthood. Check local chapter for films available.

Polymorph Films. 118 South Street, Boston, Massachusetts 02111.

Pyramid Film & Video. Box 1048. Santa Monica, California 90406-1048.

Transition House Films. 25 West Street, Fifth Floor, Boston, Massachusetts 02111.

Women Make Movies. 257 West 19th Street, New York, New York 10011.

Index